Health, Technology and Society

Series Editors
Andrew Webster
Department of Sociology
University of York
York, UK

Sally Wyatt
Faculty of Arts and Social Sciences
Maastricht University
Maastricht, The Netherlands

Medicine, health care, and the wider social meaning and management of health are undergoing major changes. In part this reflects developments in science and technology, which enable new forms of diagnosis, treatment and delivery of health care. It also reflects changes in the locus of care and the social management of health. Locating technical developments in wider socio-economic and political processes, each book in the series discusses and critiques recent developments in health technologies in specific areas, drawing on a range of analyses provided by the social sciences. Some have a more theoretical focus, some a more applied focus but all draw on recent research by the authors. The series also looks toward the medium term in anticipating the likely configurations of health in advanced industrial society and does so comparatively, through exploring the globalization and internationalization of health.

More information about this series at
http://www.palgrave.com/gp/series/14875

Caragh Brosnan • Pia Vuolanto
Jenny-Ann Brodin Danell
Editors

Complementary and Alternative Medicine

Knowledge Production and Social Transformation

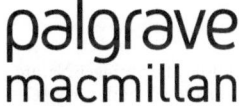

Editors
Caragh Brosnan
School of Humanities and Social Science
University of Newcastle
Newcastle, NSW, Australia

Pia Vuolanto
School of Social Sciences and Humanities
University of Tampere
Tampere, Finland

Jenny-Ann Brodin Danell
Department of Sociology
Umeå University
Umeå, Sweden

Health, Technology and Society
ISBN 978-3-030-08889-7   ISBN 978-3-319-73939-7   (eBook)
https://doi.org/10.1007/978-3-319-73939-7

Cover illustration: iStock / Getty Images Plus

Printed on acid-free paper

This Palgrave Macmillan imprint is published by Springer Nature
The registered company is Springer International Publishing AG
The registered company address is: Gewerbestrasse 11, 6330 Cham, Switzerland

Series Editors' Preface

Medicine, healthcare, and the wider social meaning and management of health are undergoing major changes. In part, this reflects developments in science and technology, which enable new forms of diagnosis, treatment, and the delivery of healthcare. It also reflects changes in the locus of care and burden of responsibility for health. Today, genetics, informatics, imaging, and integrative technologies, such as nanotechnology, are redefining our understanding of the body, health, and disease; at the same time, health is no longer simply the domain of conventional medicine, nor the clinic. The 'birth of the clinic' heralded the process through which health and illness became increasingly subject to the surveillance of medicine. Although such surveillance is more complex, sophisticated, and precise as seen in the search for 'predictive medicine', it is also more provisional, uncertain, and risk laden.

At the same time, the social management of health itself is losing its anchorage in collective social relations and shared knowledge and practice, whether at the level of the local community or through state-funded socialised medicine. This individualisation of health is both culturally driven and state sponsored, as the promotion of 'self-care' demonstrates. The very technologies that redefine health are also the means through which this individualisation can occur—through 'e-health', diagnostic tests, and the commodification of restorative tissue, such as stem cells, cloned embryos, and so on.

This series explores these processes within and beyond the conventional domain of 'the clinic' and asks whether they amount to a qualitative shift in the social ordering and value of medicine and health. Locating technical developments in wider socio-economic and political processes, each book discusses and critiques recent developments within health technologies in specific areas, drawing on a range of analyses provided by the social sciences.

The series has already published 20 books that have explored many of these issues, drawing on novel, critical, and deeply informed research undertaken by their authors. In doing so, the books have shown how the boundaries between the three core dimensions that underpin the whole series—health, technology, and society—are changing in fundamental ways.

This new book, with its focus on complementary and alternative medicine (CAM), contributes to furthering understanding of the series' themes in multiple ways. Instead of focusing, as is often the case in this area, on the struggles that CAM practitioners have faced as they seek professional recognition by the traditional biomedical community, contributors to this volume analyse CAM as a set of practices shaped by, and implicated in, epistemic and social transformations. By drawing on approaches from science and technology studies, including actor network theory and theories of boundary work, social worlds, co-production and epistemic cultures, this book calls attention to CAM's contingency, situatedness, materiality, and co-production within various spheres of governance and knowledge production. Contributors examine a variety of complementary and alternative medicines in different countries, ranging from traditional and indigenous medicines to herbal supplements, therapeutic touch, and homeopathy. The theoretical and empirical richness offers fruitful ways of comprehending what CAM is and how and why it is evolving.

York, UK   Andrew Webster
Maastricht, The Netherlands   Sally Wyatt

Contents

Notes on Contributors

Joana Almeida is a medical sociologist with research interests in health and illness and the professions. She is a Lecturer in Applied Social Studies at the University of Bedfordshire, UK. Previously she was a teaching fellow in Sociology in the School of Law, Royal Holloway, University of London. Joana holds a PhD in Medical Sociology from Royal Holloway, a Masters in Communication, Culture and Information Technologies from the University of Lisbon, and a BSc in Sociology from the University of Coimbra, Portugal. She was a Mildred Blaxter postdoctoral research fellow funded by the Foundation for the Sociology of Health and Illness, UK, in 2013–2014.

Charlotte Baarts is Associate Professor and Head of Studies at the Department of Sociology, University of Copenhagen. Her research interests cover particularly learning, knowledge, and expertise. Her work is situated within the field of sociology of health and illness, sociology of work, and educational sociology. She is investigating learning with particular interest in students' and researchers' reading practices.

Nelson Barros is a social scientist with research interests in sociology of health, illness and care. He is an Associate Professor at the Faculty of Medical Sciences, University of Campinas, São Paulo, Brazil. He holds a PhD in Collective Health from the same university. Nelson has been the coordinator of the Brazilian Laboratory for Alternative, Complementary and Integrative Health Practices (LAPACIS) since 2006. He held visiting scholar posts at the University of Leeds in 2006–2008 and the University of London in 2017.

Heather Boon BSc.Phm., Ph.D. is Professor and Dean at the Leslie Dan Faculty of Pharmacy, University of Toronto, Canada. Her research focuses on the safety, efficacy, and regulation of natural health products and traditional medicine. She served as the president of the International Society of Complementary Medicine Research from 2013–2015 and is the 2015 winner of the Dr Rogers Prize for Excellence in Complementary and Alternative Medicine.

Caragh Brosnan is Associate Professor of Sociology in the School of Humanities and Social Science at the University of Newcastle, Australia. Her work explores the construction of legitimate knowledge in scientific and health professional practice and education. She recently led the Australian Research Council-funded project, 'Complementary and Alternative Medicine Degrees: New configurations of knowledge, professional autonomy, and the university'. Previous publications include the edited volumes *Handbook of the Sociology of Medical Education* (with Bryan S. Turner, Routledge, 2009) and *Bourdieusian Prospects* (with Lisa Adkins and Steven Threadgold, Routledge, 2017).

Geoffroy Carpier is a PhD research scholar in socio-anthropology at Laboratoire des Dynamiques Sociales (DySoLab, EA 7476), Université de Rouen Normandie—Normandie Université. Before joining DySoLab, he studied law, history, anthropology, and sociology at Université Paris I Panthéon-Sorbonne, Université Paris V Descartes, Cardozo, and the New School for Social Research. In 2016–2017, he was an invited research scholar at NYU—department of anthropology and a guest researcher at the Office of Cancer CAM (OCCAM) (NCI-DCTD). He is finalising a PhD thesis, under the supervision of Patrice Cohen, on processes of legitimisation of cancer CAM in the United States. His research received a three-year funding support from the French National Cancer Institute (INCa).

Patrice Cohen is Professor of Anthropology at Université de Rouen Normandie—Normandie Université, and a researcher at Laboratoire des Dynamiques Sociales (DySoLab, EA 7476). For about 30 years now, he has been working on various themes in the anthropology of food, health, and illness including the relationships between nutrition and health. His work focuses on different geographical and cultural areas such as Reunion Island, a French overseas territory in the Indian Ocean (anthropology of food and research on young people affected by the HIV/AIDS epidemic), Southern India (medical pluralism and research on mother-to-child HIV transmission), and France (CAM, food, and cancer). Since the mid-2000s, he is developing a multi-centre approach to the study of unconventional forms of health and healing for patients with cancer, within a 'therapeutic pluralism in motion' (*pluralisme thérapeutique en mouvement*): illness trajectories of patients and the social construction of medical institutions when patients' use of CAM is concerned. In that regard, his work has led to international comparisons between France, Belgium, and Switzerland. More recently, he has been questioning nutrition and eating trajectories of patients with cancer in France, the making of legitimisations of CAM in the United States (with Geoffroy Carpier) and the social construction of therapeutic fasting and diet in France.

Jenny-Ann Brodin Danell is Associate Professor in Sociology at the Department of Sociology, Umeå University, Sweden. Her work focuses on how CAM is established as a scientific field and on how CAM knowledge is produced, received, and negotiated by different actors. This is achieved with help from both bibliometric and qualitative methods.

Cathy Fournier is a PhD student at Dalhousie University and a research fellow at the Wilson Centre in Toronto. Her interests include the integration of indigenous knowledges and practices into biomedical education and healthcare settings. She has worked as a 'complementary and alternative medicine' health practitioner for 27 years in a variety of integrative medicine settings in Canada.

Nadine Ijaz is a critical qualitative health services researcher with substantive interests in the statutory regulation of traditional and complementary medicine practitioners, health professional education, health policy, gender-based violence, and food justice. She is also a medical herbalist with over a decade of clinical and teaching experience. Nadine is a postdoctoral fellow at the Leslie Dan Faculty of Pharmacy, University of Toronto, and a sessional instructor at McMaster University.

Jaroslav Klepal is a researcher in the Institute of Sociology of the Czech Academy of Sciences where he works on a project 'Medicine Multiple: Ethnography of the interfaces between biomedical and alternative therapeutic practices'. He received his PhD in Anthropology from Charles University in Prague. His dissertation focuses ethnographically on multiple enactments of post-traumatic stress disorder among war veterans in Bosnia and Herzegovina. His primary research interest is medical anthropology.

Ana M. Ning is a medical anthropologist and Associate Professor in the Department of Sociology and Criminology at King's University College at Western University. Her research expertise and interests are in the areas of addiction and mental health, biomedicine, and complementary and alternative medicine (CAM) with wider application in public policy and clinical settings. While her published research has focused on health-related issues, her interests and perspectives are also relevant to diverse anthropological and sociological concerns including social theory, crime, social control, as well as culture, gender, and ethnicity.

Robin Oakley is an anthropologist at Dalhousie University in the Critical Health Area of Social Anthropology. She is interested in the relationship between economy, culture, and health and has conducted research in the former South African Namaqualand reserves and in India on forms of health, wellness, and ancient science that survived selective healthcare biomedical erasures.

Inge Kryger Pedersen is Associate Professor at the Department of Sociology, University of Copenhagen. Her research concentrates on health-related issues concerning forms of knowledge and practice within medical technologies. She draws on the sociology of knowledge, body, and culture when she investigates knowledge-creating and norm-setting institutions such as health sciences and medical technology, and how actors optimise their bodies and different forms of everyday and professional practices.

Danuta Penkala-Gawęcka received her PhD and post-doctoral degrees in ethnology and cultural anthropology and works as Associate Professor at the Department of Ethnology and Cultural Anthropology, Adam Mickiewicz University in Poznań, Poland. She specialises in medical anthropology; her interests focus on medical pluralism and health-seeking strategies in Central Asia. She has published books on transformations of traditional medicine in Afghanistan and on complementary medicine in Kazakhstan, and edited volumes on medical anthropology in Poland. Her articles have appeared in *Anthropology & Medicine* and *Central Asian Survey*, among other journals.

Pâmela Siegel is a Brazilian psychologist and specialist in Analytical Psychology. Her main field of interest is the interface between psychology, religion and health. She earned her post-doctorate degree in the field of Collective Health, at the State University of Campinas (Unicamp), Brazil, where she focused on yoga and the use of acupuncture, medicinal herbs and Reiki by cancer patients. She is currently a member of the Laboratory for Alternative, Complementary and Integrative Health Practices (LAPACIS), at Unicamp.

Tereza Stöckelová is a researcher in the Institute of Sociology of the Czech Academy of Sciences and Associate Professor in the Department of General Anthropology at Charles University. Her work is situated in between sociology, social anthropology, and science and technology studies, and draws upon actor network theory and related material semiotic methodologies. She has investigated academic practices in the context of current policy changes, science and society relations, and most recently, the interfaces between biomedical and alternative therapeutic practices.

Pia Vuolanto is a researcher at the Research Centre for Knowledge, Science, Technology, and Innovation Studies at the University of Tampere, Finland. She specialises in science and technology studies. Her work centres on controversies over legitimate knowledge and CAM knowledge production. Her PhD thesis in sociology (2013) examined two controversies over CAM therapies: fasting and therapeutic touch. Her articles have been published in *Minerva, Science and Technology Studies* and *Scandinavian Journal of Public Health*.

Fabian Winiger completed a MSc in Medical Anthropology at Oxford University and is a doctoral candidate at the University of Hong Kong. His research, funded by a four-year grant by the Hong Kong Research Grants Council and a Sin Wai-Kin Fellowship at the Institute of Humanities and Sciences, follows the transnational circulation of East Asian techniques of body-cultivation, in particular 'qigong'-practice and its attendant neo-socialist, cultural-nationalist, and alternative medical discourses. Winiger is a visiting assistant in research at the Yale Institute of Cultural Sociology.

List of Figures

1

Introduction: Reconceptualising Complementary and Alternative Medicine as Knowledge Production and Social Transformation

Caragh Brosnan, Pia Vuolanto,
and Jenny-Ann Brodin Danell

Introduction

CAM is a controversial topic. In the media, in the doctor's office, in comedy routines, and around dinner party tables, CAM frequently provokes debate, mirth, and even anger. Discussions are often polarised (Gale and McHale 2015): CAM is dismissed as 'quackery' by some, while others ardently defend it based on their own experiences of use. CAM has

C. Brosnan (✉)
School of Humanities and Social Science, University of Newcastle,
Newcastle, NSW, Australia

P. Vuolanto
School of Social Sciences and Humanities,
University of Tampere, Tampere, Finland

J.-A. B. Danell
Department of Sociology, Umeå University, Umeå, Sweden

© The Author(s) 2018
C. Brosnan et al. (eds.), *Complementary and Alternative Medicine*, Health,
Technology and Society, https://doi.org/10.1007/978-3-319-73939-7_1

1

become a staple research area in the sociology of health and illness, as sociologists have sought to understand CAM's status and the appeal to patients that underpins its widespread uptake. It is not clear whether CAM use has actually risen, but it has certainly garnered widespread attention in clinical, public health policy, and academic circles since the turn of the century (Chatwin and Tovey 2006; Gale 2014). Its new prominence is understood as reflecting wider changes in healthcare and society, including shifts in the locus of healthcare, increased scepticism towards scientific expertise and the mobilisation of lay health consumer groups, the commodification of techniques and technologies of well-being (such as yoga, vitamin supplements, and massage), and a new focus on personal responsibility for health, along with the globalisation of plural healing modalities.

Much sociological work has positioned CAM in relation to these wider transformations. The popularity of CAM has also, typically, been interpreted as a threat to medical dominance, and numerous studies have examined the relationship between CAM and the medical profession. However, what remains relatively unexamined until now is how CAM *itself* is shaped by social processes. In existing research, the actual content of CAM is often taken for granted, and the focus is on how CAM is perceived by, experienced by, or mediates relationships between, people. Rather than problematising the polarised views of CAM, sociological studies have often taken these as starting points: CAM has been treated as a provocative entity, something that can be used to increase or undermine the power of patients and practitioners. Rather than being understood in their own right, CAM and CAM use are read as signifiers of other, broader societal shifts.

The purpose of this volume is to take sociological studies of CAM in a new direction. Our goal is to show that CAM not only reflects, but is *shaped by*, and *implicated in*, social transformations. We aim to shift the focus away from CAM as a stable entity that elicits perceptions and experiences, and towards an examination of the forms that CAM takes in different settings, how global social transformations elicit varieties of CAM, and how CAM knowledge and practices are co-produced in the context of social change. To achieve this, the volume draws strongly on Science and Technology Studies (STS)—an area that has influenced sociological and anthropological thinking in relation to other domains of health practice (Martin 2012; Webster 2002) but which is only beginning to inform studies of CAM. STS approaches are particularly attuned to studying knowledge-making practices and to unpicking controversies. The chapters in this volume demonstrate that the combination of a sociological focus on social transformations with an STS-informed perspective can offer new understandings of the material, social, and cultural dimensions of CAM.

This introductory chapter begins to lay out these approaches to CAM. It starts by discussing the set of concerns that have dominated existing sociological studies of CAM and highlights some of the gaps that have emerged as a consequence. It then explores what it means to reconceptualise CAM as knowledge production and social transformation, introducing a range of perspectives from STS that could help us to understand CAM in new ways. Finally, the structure of the book and the chapters that comprise the three parts of the volume are outlined.

Current Sociological Understandings of CAM

CAM has been a key topic area within the sociology of health and illness for at least the past 15 years. Gale (2014) has provided a comprehensive overview of this body of work. Here, we outline some of the main trends and gaps in this area, most notably, what we see as an emphasis on the role of medical dominance at the cost of other theoretical perspectives. Additionally, empirical sociological research on CAM has most often centred on patients, practitioners, and their interrelationship, while CAM's constitution and knowledge-making practices in different contexts have been less well-studied.

Patterns of and reasons for CAM use have been a major theme. Common explanations for why people turn to CAM include dissatisfaction with biomedical interventions and the conventional doctor-patient relationship, coupled with a search for greater fulfilment offered by the longer consultations and individualised focus on holistic well-being within CAM therapies (Chatwin and Tovey 2006; Lee-Treweek and Heller 2005; Siahpush 2000). These interactional factors are often situated in the context of postmodern emphases on plurality and reflexive identity construction through consumption practices (Fries 2013; Gale 2014; Rayner and Easthope 2001).

Another key research area is CAM practitioners, with studies largely centring on professionalisation strategies (Gale 2014; Lee-Treweek and Heller 2005), such as CAM groups' attempts to gain practising rights, statutory regulation, accredited education, and public healthcare funding, typically in the face of opposition from the medical profession. Most studies have taken a neo-Weberian perspective to understanding the professionalisation process, highlighting the struggles between different occupational groups as they try to achieve social closure and protect their own scope of practice (Gale 2014; Kelner et al. 2006; Saks 1995). Studies of conventional practitioners' attitudes to, and integration of, CAM have also revealed the ongoing influence of medical dominance on which practices are legitimated within healthcare arenas (Gale 2014). Much of the emphasis in practitioner studies has therefore been on understanding inter-professional relationships and power dynamics, through the lens of CAM.

Work on professionalisation has also considered the status of CAM knowledge, sometimes including knowledge production, again largely in relation to the dominance of biomedical knowledge. In an early essay on 'deviant science'—knowledge claims or systems that contravene prevailing scientific norms—Dolby (1979) argues that because deviant medical systems must compete with orthodox medicine that models itself on science, they are more likely to succeed by establishing their scientific base. In the same volume, Webster (1979) discusses acupuncture's relationship to science as it is practised and taken up by allopathic professions and by traditional acupuncturists in the West, concluding that the higher status of the former groups had allowed them greater control over which knowledge claims were accepted or rejected. Later work by Cant and Sharma (1996) argues that the grand narrative of scientific progress has declined and asks to what extent CAM knowledge challenges the legitimacy of scientific paradigms and blurs categories of lay and expert knowledge. They attempt to problematise the CAM-biomedicine dichotomy—chiming with more recent work on CAM's hybridity (Gale 2014; Keshet 2010) (something that this volume aims to further develop)—yet still they argue that CAM and its knowledge base must be understood in relation to biomedicine (p. 7).

An overriding concern in the sociology of CAM has therefore been CAM's status relative to biomedicine. As Gale (2014: 806) points out, the very name 'complementary and alternative medicine'—CAM[1]— invokes the 'absent presence' of biomedicine. There is, of course, a long history of very active processes of exclusion and subordination of CAM by the medical profession, and sociologists have played a key role in documenting their effects (Gale 2014; Willis 1983). Many efforts to define CAM do so in reference to its marginalisation within mainstream medical practice, medical education and healthcare systems (Saks 1995; Gale and McHale 2015; Wieland et al. 2011). Sociologists have studied these representations and debates over terminology, and the underlying power relations that shape them (Gale 2014; Saks 1996). At the same time, sociology has often relied on these frameworks to direct its inquiries: 'Sociological accounts of contemporary society tend to use the terms "complementary", "alternative", "heterodox" or "holistic", to contrast with "conventional", "orthodox" or "biomedicine"' (Gale 2014: 806). However, drawing on these binaries can produce inaccuracies, blind spots, and simplistic representations of both CAM and biomedicine (Gale 2014: 806–7; Ning 2013). Although sociology's focus to date on CAM representations, users, practitioners, and professional power struggles has produced rich insights and been used to challenge CAM's marginalisation (e.g. see Myers et al. 2012), there are a number of reasons why we believe the field would be strengthened by new approaches.

Firstly, the strong reliance on medical dominance and neo-Weberian perspectives means that CAM is often interpreted through pre-existing categories and defined by its marginalisation from mainstream healthcare. This can produce a black-boxing effect where the content of CAM is rarely treated as an object of analysis. Attention to the actual constitution of CAM, including in a material sense, is, we argue, necessary for sociology to contribute to answering what Gale (2014) calls 'the big question': understanding how and whether CAM therapies work. Social scientists and CAM scholars have identified the limited scientific evidence base for CAM's efficacy and effectiveness as the most pressing problem CAM faces (Chatwin and Tovey 2006; Gale 2014; Fischer et al. 2014). The push for systematic evidence has intensified in recent years and has accompanied the rise of research programmes—sponsored by public funding, CAM product manufacturers, or pharmaceutical companies—that study CAM's biological mechanisms and clinical effects. Within CAM communities, however, there is a wide variety of views on whether CAM therapies require a scientific underpinning and how to go about developing one (Barry 2006; Brosnan 2016; Lee-Treweek and Heller 2005). Major disciplines with an established place in higher education systems around the world—particularly, chiropractic, osteopathy, naturopathy, and Chinese medicine—have been pursuing scientific validation for some time; other therapies remain on the margins, and across CAM the validity and applicability of the hierarchy of evidence within evidence-based medicine (EBM) is strongly contested (Barry 2006; Flatt 2012; Jackson and Scambler 2007). Rather than sidestepping these debates, there are calls for sociology to tackle questions such as, 'how [in a CAM context] can we value diversity of knowledge and different perspectives, while also working towards high quality and safe practice?' (Gale and McHale 2015: 8; see also Gale 2014; Keshet 2010). Gale (2014) identifies an emerging, yet nascent, interest within sociology in these issues and notes the influence of STS, anthropology, and other fields on a turn towards studying processes of scientific knowledge production in relation to CAM. This volume seeks to develop this body of work further and suggestions of how to do so are discussed in the next section.

Another related issue arises from the tendency in existing research to ascribe characteristics such as 'holism', 'vitalism', and 'experientialism' to the CAM field (Cant and Sharma 1996; Ning 2013; Zhan 2014). This can lead to the ontology of CAM practices being taken for granted and depicted as homogenous and unchanging. In fact, CAM practices and technologies are increasingly hybridised in a similar but perhaps even more significant way to other emerging health technologies which often draw from different scientific domains (Webster 2006). Rather than being 'timeless' traditions, various CAM therapies and techniques merge ancient philosophy with cutting-edge bioscience, vitalistic with biomechanical ontologies, or Eastern with Western customs. Some CAM modalities date back thousands of years, and others are newly invented (Lee-Treweek and Heller 2005). Hybridisation is facilitated by processes of globalisation which have seen knowledge and practices flow from their original settings to new locations. There is therefore a need to problematise dominant views of CAM and the prevailing juxtaposition between

CAM and biomedicine and to explore the new forms that CAM takes as it shifts and resurfaces in different cultural contexts.

Finally, by framing CAM use and practice as reflective of wider trends, sociological studies have tended to overlook the potential for CAM to influence social change. The relationship between CAM and society has largely been conceptualised as one-way: CAM is an entity that is given more or less prominence according to other social transformations. Yet this relationship can be two-way. For instance, it has been noted already that CAM's ubiquity has prompted conventional medicine to pay greater attention to interactional factors in the clinical encounter which often distinguish CAM (e.g. patient-centredness) (Chatwin and Tovey 2006). This shows that CAM itself can be an agent of change, embedded in and constitutive of social transformations. A central aim of this volume is therefore to open up the black box of CAM and to trace its effects in multiple domains.

Reconceptualising CAM as Knowledge Production and Social Transformation: Engaging with STS

CAM is only beginning to emerge as an empirical research area in STS. Where it has been conceptualised in STS literature, this has sometimes been as 'an escape from medicine' or a trend that turns away from highly technological medical practice (Webster 2007: 147). This is seen as part of the development where new medical technologies have, during the past century, changed the ways in which people define the meaning of medicine (Brown and Webster 2004). In this context, CAM modalities are framed as 'alternative' health technologies. Central to CAM from the point of view of STS have been its challenges to medicine, pointing to the failure of medicine to find solutions and to address the side effects of drugs (Webster 2007: 147, 158). CAM has also been conceptualised as a health social movement that 'mounts challenges to medical knowledge' (Hess 2004: 695). One way to frame CAM in STS has thus been to focus on its tendency to resist the technologisation of medicine and to challenge the dominant modes of scientific and medical knowledge production

(Goldner 2004; Hess et al. 2008: 479). However, as discussed earlier, CAM communities have increasingly come to embrace the push for 'scientific evidence'.

The fact that CAM has rarely been a topic of STS inquiry probably reflects the historical construction of CAM as 'non-science' and its relatively recent move into the sites of scientific knowledge production that have been the predominant focus of STS. This development in itself raises interesting questions both for STS and CAM scholars about what counts as 'science' and how scientific research methods and practices long deemed unscientific interact. STS has had, at its heart, an interest in the methods and 'machineries' of scientific knowledge production (Knorr Cetina 1999: 2) and how these are shaped by or co-constructed through social factors. From the sociology of scientific knowledge (Bloor 1976; Barnes 1974), to the tradition of laboratory ethnographies (Latour and Woolgar 1979; Knorr Cetina 1999), to work going beyond formal scientific settings to explore how science is taken up and challenged in everyday life (Epstein 1996; Callon 1999), scientific knowledge has been treated as something that is made collectively through social processes and deployed variously across different social terrains (Sismondo 2008). STS therefore offers a wide range of approaches that can help us to understand CAM as a set of knowledge-making practices, to follow CAM actors to their places of knowledge production, and to understand their perceptions of knowledge and science. STS is also primed to study the controversies that attend CAM use and practice (discussed further in a later section). Such controversies are often paradigmatic of wider debates over what counts as scientific knowledge and which forms of expertise are most reliable. The remainder of this section outlines three broad ways to conceptualise CAM—each of which addresses some of the gaps in existing sociological work outlined earlier—by introducing a range of theoretical approaches from within STS.

Boundary Work and Social Worlds Frameworks in the Study of CAM

The first STS approach captures CAM as a contested space where legitimate science and knowledge are negotiated and given meanings.

Controversies over CAM concern individual and public health, freedom of choice in healthcare, and value systems and worldviews related to health and illness, which make the debates most heated and active in the media, social media, and the political domain. Many different organisations such as hospitals, healthcare centres, universities, and professional associations are involved in such debates.

STS offers good tools to study the complex and controversial conflicts around CAM. The demarcation question 'What belongs to science?' has been at the core of STS research since the early philosophers of science (Popper 1990/1934; Kuhn 1970), continuing through to studies of controversies and conflicts in science (Bloor 1976; Nowotny 1975; Nelkin 1979; Collins 1981). Studies have concentrated on scrutinising the actors and complex interactions and negotiations of controversies, the social structures influencing conflict situations, the incompatible goals and interests of actors, the arguments of different parties in conflict, and the closure processes of controversies (Brante and Elzinga 1990; Martin and Richards 1995; Taylor 1996; Gieryn 1999). Delving into the reflexivity of the social scientist studying scientific controversies has been a significant contribution of STS. For example, focussing on debates over fluoridation and Vitamin C and cancer—which resonate and overlap with some CAM debates—Martin and Richards (1995: 514) emphasise that analysing the nuances of controversy dynamics requires a multi-perspective account in order to avoid providing 'de facto support' either for orthodox medicine or its opponents.

Central to CAM controversies is the contested knowledge base underpinning CAM practice and education. In recent years, there have been active campaigns against CAM by individuals and groups loosely identified as 'sceptics', often with key spokespeople holding high-ranking positions in academic science or medicine. Similar movements are evident in the UK (Givati and Hatton 2015; Caldwell 2017), Australia (Brosnan 2015), Canada (Villanueva-Russell 2009; Derkatch 2016), the Czech Republic (Stöckelová and Klepal, this volume), and Sweden (Forstorp 2005). These sceptics typically use a mix of social media, news media, and political lobbying to call for CAM to be de-funded, de-registered, and removed from public education systems, arguing that it is 'non-science', 'pseudoscience' or 'anti-science'.

STS-oriented studies on CAM have shown that CAM experts and other allies have countered this by pointing to the growing evidence base supporting CAM use and to the significant levels of basic science within CAM education programmes (Brosnan 2015). CAM activists have been lobbying for CAM modalities and practices to be integrated into, or applied within, conventional medicine (Goldner 2004). These developments might be thought of as social movements that 'address disease, disability or illness experience by challenging science on etiology, diagnosis, treatment and prevention' (Brown et al. 2004: 52).

STS research on social movements highlights the political nature of attempts to professionalise and regulate CAM, similar to experiences of inequality based on race, ethnicity, gender, class, and/or sexuality, regarding freedom of choice of patients and professional rights (Hess et al. 2008; Brown et al. 2004). However, there is a need to see CAM as not just one movement but several movements with different societal goals. Some of these movements aim at integrating CAM into biomedicine (Goldner 2000); others might more directly resist biomedical knowledge, like anti-vaccinationism (Blume 2006). Lumping these together as one movement would not do justice to the variety of movements involved and threatens to stabilise the juxtaposition between CAM and biomedicine instead of opening it up to scrutiny.

The boundary work approach (Gieryn 1999; Amsterdamska 2005) has been deployed to study the debates and juxtapositions between CAM and biomedicine (Danell and Danell 2009; Derkatch 2008, 2012; Goldner 2000; Mizrachi and Shuval 2005; Mizrachi et al. 2005; Shuval et al. 2012; Polich et al. 2010) or what Derkatch (2016) terms 'biomedical boundary work', meaning how medical practitioners and researchers separate CAM from medicine. While more studies on biomedical boundary work are required to understand it in different contexts, there is a need to also make visible the other actors involved in the debates besides medicine, for example, nursing and midwifery (Adams and Tovey 2008; Vuolanto 2015), sceptics (Forstorp 2005; Brosnan 2015), researchers in different disciplines, and varied CAM communities including practitioners of different therapies (see Vuolanto, this volume).

With regard to CAM, it is important to unveil different parties' understandings of the role of knowledge and science in society, in order to understand better the reasons why people are committed to boundary work that reproduces and continues the societal debates and juxtapositions around CAM. There is also potential in this approach to study not only conflict situations that tend to dichotomise the issue but to extend even further to the boundary work that takes place in writing research articles or in meetings between patients and healthcare professionals— 'routine boundary work' (Mellor 2003) that CAM practitioners, activists, and researchers are committed to in their everyday lives and workplaces. This could open up new research questions about subtle hierarchies between different ways of knowing that are hidden in everyday actions.

The social worlds framework within STS (Clarke and Star 2008) offers some useful starting points for exploring the 'multiplicities of perspective' (Clarke and Montini 1993: 45) around CAM issues (see both Vuolanto and Winiger, this volume). Studies to explore the complex whole of the CAM debates are needed to understand how different social worlds centre on different expectations around healthcare and thus emphasise different goals and aims for CAM. In situations where there is no consensus around a mutual concern, the concept 'boundary object' (Star and Griesemer 1989; Star 2010) could be used to trace the factors that unite the social worlds (see Ijaz and Boon, this volume).

The social worlds perspective could also be applied to understand the legitimation processes (Gerson 1983) through which the boundaries between science and different knowledge systems such as CAM are established and enforced. One possible future direction of social worlds research is to use it to tackle the multiplicity within the CAM social world or rather to make known the intersections but also incompatibilities between the different social worlds within CAM, for example, homeopathy, anthroposophy, or Chinese medicine. Owens (2015) has made inroads here through her comparison of acupuncture and Christian Science's differential success in mobilising boundary objects to advance their mainstream integration. Further work would help to understand the different traditions of knowledge production and the different perceptions about knowledge and science behind the category of CAM.

CAM and Actor-Network Theory: Exploring Materiality and Relationality

A less explored STS approach to CAM is actor-network theory (ANT). This approach is known for the provocative inclusion of non-human agency in sociological analysis and its critique of established concepts and dichotomies, such as society–nature, body–mind, human–non-human, micro–macro, or truth–falsehood. According to ANT there are no hidden agendas, external powers, or invisible structures (Latour 2005). Instead, reality is analysed in terms of actors, interlinked in heterogeneous networks within a 'flat' ontology. Actors appear, as John Law (1992) puts it, in any shape or material. What constitutes them is their relation to other entities (Law 1999) and the capacity to cause difference or change (Latour 2005). Some networks, such as relations between CAM and conventional medicine in Western societies, are relatively stable and taken for granted. Others are weak, fluid, contested, and short-lived. The focus in ANT analysis is usually on the processes—on how networks assemble and on what is mobilised and enrolled to stabilise or weaken them (e.g. Callon 1986). A key notion is generalised symmetry and openness towards what or whom to include in the analysis (Latour 2005).

Anne L. Scott (1998) has conducted a pioneering analysis of CAM from an ANT perspective. She challenges the taken-for-granted biomedical perspective, and argues that it is not fruitful to ask how CAM can work within conventional medicine, or a modernistic ontology. Rather, we should turn the questions around. What is needed is an ontology 'in which the natural body can be both subject, the ground of perception, and object, a thing-in-itself' (p. 26). Scott also shows how some CAM therapies, such as homeopathy, can serve as good examples of how heterogeneous networks operate and that we might not need the sharp divisions between the natural–social and body–mind. In her study, homeopathic substances emerge as actors, with their own capacities, within complex networks of metaphors, dreams, myths, plants, practitioners, and many other objects.

Another good example of using an inclusive ANT approach is the work of Andrews, Evans, and McAlister (2013). Coming from human geography, the authors have a special focus on space and place, but, as they point out, instead of thinking of these as discrete or fixed locations, "'relational thinking" conjures an image of spaces and places as produced through their connections with other spaces and places' (p. 100). Using mixed methods, they explore holistic medical settings in Canada. By focussing on relations between all sorts of objects, such as bodies, gestures, emotions, therapists, physical settings, and different kind of devices, they unpack what happens in specific therapeutic moments. As a consequence, they also expand the understanding of taken-for-granted concepts, such as holism and healthcare.

In addition to relationality, ANT is centrally concerned with materiality (Sismondo 2004). The role of bodies and physical experiences in CAM has been explored by a number of authors. These studies show how ANT can be a fruitful approach to investigate the material dimensions of individual and lived experiences of CAM, by expanding the analysis to non-human objects. For example, Johannessen (2007) has studied experiences of body and self, among Danish CAM users and practitioners. She shows how individual bodies, emotions, and practices are interlinked with devices, technology, and healthcare systems. A similar approach to the body in CAM—as existing in constant translations and negotiations in shifting networks—is proposed by Meurk et al. (2012) and Danell (forthcoming). In both of these examples, bodily experiences and physical sensations are linked to how CAM users form knowledge.

Questions on knowledge production and scientific boundaries are also clear themes among ANT studies on CAM. For example, Yael Keshet (2009) asks how we can know if CAM treatments are beneficial or not. By following debates and scientific controversies, she identifies a number of rhetorical strategies to establish evidence, as well as the untenable boundaries and ambiguity of conventional medicine. This work is a good example of how ANT can be combined with boundary work. Another example is a study by Brossard (2009), which follows the debate on homeopathy and reveals the non-linear processes of scientific communication. It also highlights the variety of actors (such as scientists, academic journals, mass media, intellectuals, and the general public), and the complex relations between them, involved in the processes of stabilising truths and facts on CAM (see also Danell, this volume).

The ANT approach clearly moves away from taken-for-granted concepts and distinctions that have underpinned many prior sociological CAM studies—not only in relation to medical dominance but also CAM itself. By rejecting analyses that rely on predefined notions of power, it allows the ontology of CAM to emerge through studying what actually happens in practice. Through close empirical analysis, ANT has been shown to be fruitful for unpacking everyday practices, interactions, and material aspects of CAM, but there is certainly much more to explore.

CAM as Epistemic Object

A third conceptual move is to understand CAM as constituted through, and implicated in, technologies, modes, and communities of knowledge production. To a large extent, it is CAM's resistance to biomedical ways of knowing and its historical exclusion from biomedical sites of knowledge-making and knowledge transmission (e.g. hospitals and universities) that has defined it as CAM. Such epistemological boundaries have begun to erode with the rise of integrative medicine and the professionalisation of many CAM types, including their move into tertiary education settings. These developments have seen CAM increasingly evaluated against the evidence hierarchy of EBM, and in research centres around the world, CAM therapies and technologies are now the subject of clinical and basic scientific research, with all the infrastructure, personnel, and funding that this implies. That is, CAM is undergoing a transformation from healing practice to 'epistemic object' (Knorr Cetina 2005)—a shift for which the social science of CAM must account.

Critical reflections on the characteristics of scientific objects may offer new perspectives on CAM that help to move beyond current impasses in CAM knowledge production. Attempts to bring bioscientific methods to bear on CAM therapies have not been straightforward. There is a large literature within CAM and social science on the problems of trying to study what are typically 'holistic', relational, multi-faceted, and individualised therapeutic interventions through randomised control trials (RCTs) or laboratory research (e.g. Barry 2006; Flatt 2012; Lee-Treweek and Heller 2005; Kim 2007; Verhoef et al. 2005). Some see these problems of epistemology and ontology as explanations for why CAM still lacks a strong 'evidence base'. One of the challenges faced includes controlling for the placebo effect: if interaction with the practitioner is part of the therapy, as claimed in many CAM modalities (Chatwin and Tovey 2006), how can this be controlled, even when a sham intervention is provided?

Research on CAM has tended to reveal its complexity rather than enable it to be more clearly defined; however, this is not unusual in science, where objects of inquiry—'epistemic objects' for Knorr Cetina (2005)—typically begin to unfold and multiply in the very act of being studied. Knorr Cetina explains that:

> Objects of knowledge are characteristically open, question-generating and complex. They are processes and projections rather than definitive things. ... Since epistemic objects are always in the process of being materially defined, they continually acquire new properties and change the ones they have. (2005: 190)

Such characteristics seem to apply very well to CAM therapies, whose slipperiness in the face of scientific scrutiny reflects their multi-dimensionality and context dependence. Like other epistemic objects, CAM therapies can be understood as multiple, taking different forms and meanings in different places (Knorr Cetina 2005; see also Mol 2002; Zhan 2009).

An understanding of the various epistemic cultures that comprise science and how ontological and epistemological challenges are dealt with differently across different knowledge-making communities (Knorr Cetina 1999) may also benefit CAM research. Brosnan (2016) has highlighted contrasting epistemic cultures within Chinese medicine and osteopathic research, showing that, far from being a homogenous field, CAM is characterised by 'epistemic disunity' (Knorr Cetina 1999: 4). A small number of other studies have emerged in recent years, exploring the knowledge-making beliefs and practices of specific CAM practitioner and academic communities (Heirs 2015; Kim 2007; Lin 2017; Polich et al. 2010; Vuolanto 2015). Further work on the epistemic cultures that comprise CAM would result in a more nuanced understanding of this broad-ranging research field (Brosnan 2016: 184).

Another perspective that could enhance CAM studies is Jasanoff's (2004) concept of co-production, which encapsulates the idea that knowledge creation is both driven by, and constitutive of, social life. In the context of CAM research, this approach would draw attention to how CAM knowledge is not just influenced by, but *made through*, the apparatuses of scientific research within universities and industry. For instance, when CAM is tested through clinical trials, CAM practices often take on particular forms that can be studied through trial methodologies (Sagli 2010; Verhoef et al. 2005). Rather than viewing this as a top-down 'subjugation' or 'colonisation' of authentic CAM practice (cf Flatt 2012; Hollenberg and Muzzin 2010), co-production prompts us to study instead the new forms that CAM actually takes in these settings. Equally, it encourages consideration of how CAM is implicated in the production of new kinds of knowledge.[2] CAM in fact has the potential to drive the development of new kinds of science because of the problems it poses for RCT methodologies (MacPherson et al. 2016). Indeed, alternative study designs, such as pragmatic trials and whole systems research, have emerged in no small part from efforts in CAM research to better capture CAM's holistic aspects (MacPherson 2004; MacPherson et al. 2016; Verhoef et al. 2005). CAM studies have also led to new clinical interest in the placebo effect, while specific techniques and mechanobiological insights derived from CAM research are now being applied in biomedicine (MacPherson et al. 2016). Through the lens of co-production, we can study how science and CAM interact: scientific knowledge shapes CAM, and processes of scientific knowledge-making are *transformed by* CAM.

How CAM-related knowledge and technologies are understood and deployed is also influenced by the different 'civic epistemologies' found in different nation-states, that is, national cultures around the status of experts and expertise, knowledge-making, and public engagement (Jasanoff 2005). Homeopathy provides a case in point here: it is widely accepted in India, where it is used in a highly pluralistic healthcare context alongside a range of modalities with religious origins (Broom and Doron 2013); it is marginalised and largely discredited in Australia, particularly following a major review by the National Health and Medical Research Council (NHMRC 2015), whilst, in the UK, support from the royal family has probably helped to protect homeopathy's position as one of few CAM types included in the National Health Service (NHS) (Heirs 2015).

CAM can be involved in shaping civic epistemologies and the relationships between nations. For example, the state support of traditional Chinese medicine (TCM) in China is strongly bound to the project of nation-building. Under Mao Zedong, TCM was given official state recognition and promoted as a cultural export, explicitly framed as a vehicle for bringing Chinese expertise and healthcare to an 'international proletariat' (Zhan 2009: 36–40). In more recent times, now as part of the global flow of capital, TCM is deployed as a means of developing economic co-operation between China and other countries, for instance, through cross-national funding of education and research programmes or through inclusion in free-trade agreements (see Brosnan et al. 2016; Stöckelová and Klepal, this volume).

What these developments highlight is that, while CAM can be understood as paradigmatic of challenges to the authority of bioscientific frameworks, it is also increasingly *part of* the apparatus of contemporary bioscientific research. It is transformed by—and intervenes in—dominant modes of knowledge production, as well as other political and cultural domains. These complex epistemological configurations are explored in a range of empirical contexts in this volume.

Overview of the Volume

The volume is structured around three interrelated themes, each representing different dimensions of CAM's ongoing configuration. Part I, 'Defining CAM', explores how and why boundaries within CAM, and between CAM and other health practices, are being constructed, challenged, and changed and how such boundary work is implicated in wider social transformations. Stöckelová and Klepal's ethnographic study (Chapter 2) explores three different versions of Chinese medicine currently discernible in the Czech Republic, revealing how each reflects different eras and forms of engagement between Chinese and Western medicine and between China and the Central and Eastern European region. Not only is Chinese medicine a cosmopolitan modality that takes on local forms, the authors show that it is also cosmopolitical, transforming local settings and medical cultures.

In Chapter 3, Vuolanto focusses on a public controversy over research conducted in a Finnish university nursing department on therapeutic touch, examining how the therapy, nursing and nursing science, and patients—and the boundaries of science and technology more broadly— were constructed within various social worlds that responded to the debate. Also drawing on social worlds theory, Winiger looks at the discursive meanings given to *qigong* within the worlds of Chinese *qigong* practitioners, social science, and biomedical science. The gulfs between their different understandings of what *qigong* 'is', Winiger argues, may impede research on this modality's applications.

Part II, 'Doing CAM in different contexts', asks how CAM as material practice is shaped by politics and regulation in a range of different national settings. Comparing and contrasting the development and regulation of CAM in Portugal and Brazil, Almeida, Siegal, and Barros draw attention to CAM's 'glocalisation': modalities travel the globe and are shaped by local contexts. Their study is one of few to compare different CAM types, documenting the fates of homeopathy, acupuncture, and TCM in the two countries. Continuing with the glocalisation theme, in Chapter 6, Penkala-Gawęcka provides an ethnographic insight into the place of CAM in the Kyrgyz capital Bishkek, where popular therapies include a special bed and other technologies produced by a South Korean company. As she points out, while the globalisation of biotechnology has been well-studied, this is not true of CAM technology. Penkala-Gawęcka's chapter makes an important contribution to this area (as do Stöckelová and Klepal), drawing on ANT to trace the networks that coalesce around the 'miracle bed'.

Also taking an ANT approach, in a rather different context, Danell's chapter analyses CAM-related motions raised in the Swedish parliament over the past several decades, documenting how CAM understandings are translated in the political arena and how networks stabilise around certain issues. Ijaz and Boon also explore historical policy debates over CAM in Chapter 8, focussing on the regulation of acupuncture in Ontario. They show that 'safety' operated as a boundary object in the debates and was used ultimately to restrict Chinese-language-based practitioners and devalue traditional Chinese medical knowledge, constituting, according to Ijaz and Boon, the neo-colonial misappropriation of CAM knowledge.

Part III, 'Making CAM knowledge', looks at the ways CAM evidence is being classified, produced and used in various settings. In Chapter 9, Fournier and Oakley examine documents related to traditional medicine integration produced by the World Bank, WHO, and Health Canada. Tracing the discourses used to construct traditional medicine, they show that its knowledge base is often treated through a deficit model and as needing to be brought into alignment with biomedicine, even while these institutions recognise its importance in healthcare. Like Ijaz and Boon, Fournier and Oakley read this as a continuation of colonialism. In the next chapter, however, Ning observes that there is space for practitioners to both resist and align with dominant modes of knowledge-making. From her ethnography of TCM practice in Canada, she describes practitioners' nuanced clinical styles that preserve traditional approaches, suggesting that the encroachment of biomedical paradigms into CAM is not a linear or inevitable process and that its uptake can be understood as an example of epistemic hybridity.

Pedersen and Baarts also take us into clinical knowledge-making arenas in their chapter, which draws on several years of ethnographic research on CAM practice and use in Denmark and highlights the role of 'embodied expertise' in CAM clinical encounters, bringing to light the role of place, space, objects, and relationships in CAM knowledge production. Finally, in Chapter 12, Carpier and Cohen present a detailed document and interview-based analysis of the ways that dietary and herbal supplements have been categorised and evaluated by various federal agencies in the USA. Being designated as CAM has brought these supplements into an ambiguous regulatory space between 'food' and 'drugs', where the substances both challenge, and are challenged by, existing institutional and scientific norms.

Conclusion

By calling for new approaches in the sociology of CAM, we do not seek in this volume to dismiss the wealth of work that has been conducted in recent years and which has contributed to understanding the rise of

CAM as a social and cultural phenomenon. Nor do we wish to abandon the sociological understanding of the effects of medical dominance on CAM to which prior work has sensitised us. Indeed, analysis of the effects of social structure and power relations on practice is a strength of the sociological approach and a perspective that has sometimes lacked in STS (Curtis 2003; Inglis 2005). The chapters in this book have not entirely moved away from considering CAM in relation to biomedicine, but they also document empirical changes that make the binary less salient—from CAM's inclusion in national scientific research programmes to practitioners' engagement in epistemic hybridity—and show that its reproduction is specific to particular social worlds. Common across many chapters is an effort to make visible the multiplicity of actors that engage in defining CAM, science, and CAM-related technologies, including those marginal and less well known, as well as the more dominant.

Along with CAM's multiplicity, together the chapters highlight the transnational character of contemporary CAM, including the movement of CAM technologies and knowledge from one setting to another, between institutions, and into dialogue with different regimes of evidence. Several chapters explicitly highlight some of the institutional formations that impede research into the big question of whether and how CAM works. By drawing on perspectives that account for CAM's materiality, contingency, and interaction with processes of knowledge-making, we argue that sociology will be better equipped to study the evolution of this increasingly significant domain of healthcare and to engage more deeply with some of the big questions. In turn, these approaches, we hope, will begin to shift public and professional debates over CAM away from the dualisms and polarity that they reproduce to a more open-ended interpretation that sees CAM as a set of practices that continually undergo transformation.

Notes

1. We use the term 'complementary and alternative medicine' (CAM) throughout this introduction because of its common usage in sociology, yet we are aware that the name itself is a political and social construction (Gale 2014) that reinforces some of the dualistic thinking we seek to undermine. We have left other contributors to decide on the terminology most appropriate to their work, hence some chapters refer to traditional, complementary, and alternative medicine (TCAM), while others simply to alternative medicine.
2. Aside from transforming science, Lin (2017) has recently argued that engaging more symmetrically with CAM (specifically, Chinese medicine) also opens the door for CAM concepts to transform and potentially decolonise Science and Technology Studies (STS).

References

Adams, J., & Tovey, P. (Eds.). (2008). *Complementary and alternative medicine in nursing and midwifery: Towards a critical social science.* London and New York: Routledge.

Amsterdamska, O. (2005). Demarcating epidemiology. *Science, Technology and Human Values, 30*, 17–51.

Andrews, G. J., Evans, J., & McAlister, S. (2013). "Creating the right therapy vibe": Relational performances in holistic medicine. *Social Science and Medicine, 83*, 99–109.

Barnes, B. (1974). *Scientific knowledge and sociological theory.* London: Routledge and Kegan Paul.

Barry, C. A. (2006). The role of evidence in alternative medicine: Contrasting biomedical and anthropological approaches. *Social Science and Medicine, 62*(11), 2646–2657.

Bloor, D. (1976). *Knowledge and social imagery.* London: Routledge Direct Editions.

Blume, S. (2006). Anti-vaccination movements and their interpretations. *Social Science and Medicine, 62*(3), 628–642.

Brante, T., & Elzinga, A. (1990). Towards a theory of scientific controversies. *Science Studies, 2*, 33–46.

Broom, A. F., & Doron, A. (2013). Traditional medicines, collective negotiation, and representations of risk in Indian cancer care. *Qualitative Health Research, 23*(1), 54–65.

Brosnan, C. (2015). "Quackery" in the academy? Professional knowledge, autonomy and the debate over complementary medicine degrees. *Sociology, 49*(6), 1047–1064.

Brosnan, C. (2016). Epistemic cultures in complementary medicine: Knowledge-making in university departments of osteopathy and Chinese medicine. *Health Sociology Review, 25*(2), 171–186.

Brosnan, C., Chung, V., Zhang, A., & Adams, J. (2016). Regional influences on Chinese Medicine education: Comparing Australia and Hong Kong. *Evidence-Based Complementary and Alternative Medicine*, Article ID 6960207, 9 pages. https://doi.org/10.1155/2016/6960207.

Brossard, D. (2009). Media scientific journals and science communication: Examining the construction of scientific controversies. *Public Understanding of Science, 18*(3), 258–274.

Brown, N., & Webster, A. (2004). *New medical technologies and society. Reordering life*. Cambridge: Polity Press.

Brown, P., Zavestoski, S., McCormick, S., Mayer, B., Morello-Frosch, R., & Gasior Altman, R. (2004). Embodied health movements: New approaches to social movements in health. *Sociology of Health and Illness, 26*(1), 50–80.

Caldwell, E. F. (2017). Quackademia? Mass-media delegitimation of homeopathy education. *Science as Culture, 26*(3), 380–407.

Callon, M. (1986). Some elements of a sociology of translation: Domestication of the scallops and the fishermen of St Brieuc Bay. *Sociological Review, 32* (1_Suppl.): 196–233.

Callon, M. (1999). The role of lay people in the production and dissemination of scientific knowledge. *Science Technology and Society, 4*(1), 81–94.

Cant, S., & Sharma, U. (1996). Introduction. In S. Cant & U. Sharma (Eds.), *Complementary and alternative medicines: Knowledge and practice* (pp. 1–24). London: Free Association Books.

Chatwin, J., & Tovey, P. (2006). Regulation and the positioning of complementary and alternative medicine. In A. Webster (Ed.), *New technologies in health care* (pp. 224–231). Basingstoke: Palgrave Macmillan.

Clarke, A., & Montini, T. (1993). The many faces of RU486: Tales of situated knowledges and technological contestations. *Science, Technology and Human Values, 18*(1), 42–78.

Clarke, A., & Star, S. L. (2008). The social worlds framework: A theory/ methods package. In E. J. Hackett, O. Amsterdamska, M. Lynch, & J. Wajcman (Eds.), *The handbook of science and technology studies* (pp. 113–137). Cambridge, MA: MIT Press.

Collins, H. M. (1981). Son of seven sexes: The social destruction of a physical phenomenon. *Social Studies of Science, 11*(1), 33–62.

Curtis, B. (2003). Book review: *Science de la science et réflexivité. Cours du Collège de France 2000–2001*, by Pierre Bourdieu. *Science, Technology and Human Values, 28*, 538–543.

Danell, J.-A. B. (Forthcoming). "I could feel it!"—An actor network study on how users of complementary medicine experience and form knowledge about treatments.

Danell, J.-A. B., & Danell, R. (2009). Publication activity in complementary and alternative medicine. *Scientometrics, 80*(2), 539–551.

Derkatch, C. (2008). Method as argument: Boundary work in evidence-based medicine. *Social Epistemology, 22*(4), 371–388.

Derkatch, C. (2012). Demarcating medicine's boundaries: Constituting and categorizing in the journals of the American Medical Association. *Technical Communication Quarterly, 21*(3), 210–229.

Derkatch, C. (2016). *Bounding biomedicine: Evidence and rhetoric in the new science of alternative medicine*. Chicago and London: University of Chicago Press.

Dolby, R. (1979). Reflections on deviant science. In R. Wallis (Ed.), *On the margins of science: The social construction of rejected knowledge, Sociological review monograph* (pp. 9–47). Keele, UK: University of Keele.

Epstein, S. (1996). *Impure science: AIDS, activism, and the politics of knowledge*. Berkeley: University of California Press.

Fischer, F. H., Lewith, G., Witt, C. M., Linde, K., von Ammon, K., Cardini, F., et al. (2014). High prevalence but limited evidence in complementary and alternative medicine: Guidelines for future research. *BMC Complementary and Alternative Medicine, 14*(1), 1–9. https://doi.org/10.1186/1472-6882-14-46.

Flatt, J. (2012). Decontextualized versus lived worlds: Critical thoughts on the intersection of evidence, lifeworld, and values. *The Journal of Alternative and Complementary Medicine, 18*(5), 513–521.

Forstorp, P. A. (2005). The construction of pseudo-science: Science patrolling and knowledge policing by academic prefects and weeders. *VEST: Journal of Science & Technology Studies, 18*(3–4), 17–71.

Fries, C. (2013). Self-care and complementary and alternative medicine as care for the self: An embodied basis for distinction. *Health Sociology Review, 22*(1), 37–51.

Gale, N. (2014). The sociology of traditional, complementary and alternative medicine. *Sociology Compass, 8*(6), 805–822.

Gale, N., & McHale, J. (2015). Introduction: Understanding CAM in the twenty-first century—The importance and challenge of multi-disciplinary perspectives. In N. Gale & J. McHale (Eds.), *Routledge handbook of complementary and alternative medicine: Perspectives from social science and law* (pp. 1–9). London: Routledge.

Gerson, E. M. (1983). Scientific work and social worlds. *Knowledge: Creation, Diffusion, Utilization, 4*(3), 357–377.

Gieryn, T. F. (1999). *Cultural boundaries of science: Credibility on the line.* Chicago and London: The University of Chicago Press.

Givati, A., & Hatton, K. (2015). Traditional acupuncturists and higher education in Britain: The dual, paradoxical impact of biomedical alignment on the holistic view. *Social Science and Medicine, 131*, 173–180.

Goldner, M. (2000). Integrative medicine: Issues to consider in this emerging form of health care. In J. Jacobs Kronenfeld (Ed.), *Health care providers, institutions, and patients: Changing patterns of care provision and care delivery (research in the sociology of health care, volume 17)* (pp. 215–236). Bingley: Emeraldpp.

Goldner, M. (2004). The dynamic interplay between western medicine and the complementary and alternative medicine movement: How activists perceive a range of responses from physicians and hospitals. *Sociology of Health & Illness, 26*(6), 710–736.

Heirs, M. (2015). Research, evidence and clinical practice in homeopathy. In N. Gale & J. McHale (Eds.), *Routledge handbook of complementary and alternative medicine: Perspectives from social science and law* (pp. 321–340). London: Routledge.

Hess, D. (2004). Medical modernisation, scientific research fields and the epistemic politics of health social movements. *Sociology of Health & Illness, 26*(6), 695–709.

Hess, D., Breyman, S., Campbell, N., & Martin, B. (2008). Science, technology, and social movements. In E. J. Hackett, O. Amsterdamska, M. Lynch, & J. Wajcman (Eds.), *The handbook of science and technology studies* (pp. 473–498). Cambridge, MA; London: The MIT Press.

Hollenberg, D., & Muzzin, L. (2010). Epistemological challenges to integrative medicine: An anti-colonial perspective on the combination of complementary/alternative medicine with biomedicine. *Health Sociology Review, 19*(1), 34–56.

Inglis, D. (2005). Review: Pierre Bourdieu, *Science of Science and Reflexivity. European Journal of Social Theory, 8*(3), 375–382.

Jackson, S., & Scambler, G. (2007). Perceptions of evidence-based medicine: Traditional acupuncturists in the UK and resistance to biomedical modes of evaluation. *Sociology of Health & Illness, 29*(3), 412–429.

Jasanoff, S. (Ed.). (2004). *States of knowledge: The coproduction of science and social order.* London: Routledge.

Jasanoff, S. (2005). *Designs on nature: Science and democracy in Europe and the United States.* Princeton, NJ: Princeton University Press.

Johannessen, H. (2007). Body praxis and the networks of powers. *Anthropology & Medicine, 13*(3), 267–278.

Kelner, M., Wellman, B., Welsh, S., & Boon, H. (2006). How far can complementary and alternative medicine go? The case of chiropractic and homeopathy. *Social Science and Medicine, 63*(10), 2617–2627.

Keshet, Y. (2009). The untenable boundaries of biomedical knowledge: Epistemologies and rhetoric strategies in the debate over evaluating complementary and alternative medicine. *Health, 13*(2), 131–155.

Keshet, Y. (2010). Hybrid knowledge and research on the efficacy of alternative and complementary medicine treatments. *Social Epistemology, 24*(4), 331–347.

Kim, J. (2007). Alternative medicine's encounter with laboratory science: The scientific construction of Korean medicine in a global age. *Social Studies of Science, 37*(6), 855–880.

Knorr Cetina, K. (1999). *Epistemic cultures: How the sciences make knowledge.* Cambridge, MA: Harvard University Press.

Knorr Cetina, K. (2005). Objectual practice. In T. Schatzki, K. Knorr Cetina, & E. Von Savigny (Eds.), *The practice turn in contemporary theory* (pp. 184–197). London: Routledge.

Kuhn, T. S. (1970). *The structure of scientific revolutions. Second edition, enlarged.* Chicago and London: The University of Chicago Press.

Latour, B. (2005). *Reassembling the social: An introduction to Actor Network-Theory.* Oxford: Oxford University Press.

Latour, B., & Woolgar, S. (1979). *Laboratory life: The social construction of scientific fields.* London: Sage.

Law, J. (1992). Notes on the theory of the actor network—Ordering, strategy, and heterogeneity. *Systems Practice, 5*(4), 379–393.

Law, J. (1999). After ANT: Complexity, naming and topology. In J. Law & J. Hassard (Eds.), *Actor network theory and after* (pp. 1–14). Oxford: Blackwell.

Lee-Treweek, G., & Heller, T. (2005). Introduction: Change and development in complementary and alternative medicine. In G. Lee-Treweek, T. Heller, S. Spurr, H. MacQueen, & J. Katz (Eds.), *Perspectives on complementary and alternative medicine: A reader* (pp. xi–xv). Abingdon: Routledge.

Lin, W. Y. (2017). Shi (勢), STS, and theory: Or what can we learn from Chinese medicine? *Science, Technology, & Human Values, 42*(3), 405–428.

MacPherson, H. (2004). Pragmatic clinical trials. *Complementary Therapies in Medicine, 12*(2), 136–140.

MacPherson, H., Hammerschlag, R., Coeytaux, R. R., Davis, R. T., Harris, R. E., Kong, J. T., et al. (2016). Unanticipated insights into biomedicine from the study of acupuncture. *The Journal of Alternative and Complementary Medicine, 22*(2), 101–107.

Martin, B., & Richards, E. (1995). Scientific knowledge, controversy, and public decision making. In S. Jasanoff, G. E. Markle, J. C. Petersen, & T. Pinch (Eds.), *Handbook of science and technology studies* (pp. 506–526). London: Sage.

Martin, E. (2012). Grafting together medical anthropology, feminism and tech-noscience. In M. Inhorn & E. Wentzell (Eds.), *Medical anthropology at the intersections: Histories, activisms and futures* (pp. 23–40). Durham, NC: Duke University Press.

Mellor, F. (2003). Between fact and fiction: Demarcating science from non-science in popular physics books. *Social Studies of Science, 33*(4), 509–538.

Meurk, C., Broom, A., Adams, J., & Sibbritt, D. (2012). Bodies of knowledge: Nature, holism and women's plural health practices. *Health, 17*(3), 300–318.

Mizrachi, N., & Shuval, J. T. (2005). Between formal and enacted policy: Changing the contours of boundaries. *Social Science and Medicine, 60*(7), 1649–1660.

Mizrachi, N., Shuval, J. T., & Gross, S. (2005). Boundary at work: Alternative medicine in biomedical settings. *Sociology of Health & Illness, 27*(1), 20–43.

Mol, A. (2002). *The body multiple: Ontology in medical practice*. Durham, NC: Duke University Press.

Myers, S. P., Xue, C. C., Cohen, M. M., Phelps, K. L., & Lewith, G. T. (2012). The legitimacy of academic complementary medicine. *Medical Journal of Australia, 197*(2), 69–70.

Nelkin, D. (Ed.). (1979). *Controversy: Politics of technical decisions*. Beverly Hills and London: Sage Publications.

NHMRC. (2015). NHMRC statement: Statement on homeopathy. Canberra: Australian Government, National Health and Medical Research Council. Retrieved July 2016, from https://www.nhmrc.gov.au/_files_nhmrc/publications/attachments/cam02_nhmrc_statement_homeopathy.pdf.

Ning, A. M. (2013). How "alternative" is CAM? Rethinking conventional dichotomies between biomedicine and complementary/alternative medicine. *Health, 17*(2), 135–158.

Nowotny, H. (1975). Controversies in science: Remarks on the different modes of production of knowledge and their use. *Zeitschrift für Soziologie, 4*(1), 34–45.

Owens, K. (2015). Boundary objects in complementary and alternative medicine: Acupuncture vs. Christian Science. *Social Science & Medicine, 128*, 18–24.

Polich, G., Dole, C., & Kaptchuk, T. J. (2010). The need to act a little more "scientific": Biomedical researchers investigating complementary and alternative medicine. *Sociology of Health & Illness, 32*(1), 106–122.

Popper, K. (1990). *The logic of scientific discovery*. 14th impression [Originally published in 1934/Logik der Forschung]. London: Unwin Hyman Ltd.

Rayner, L., & Easthope, G. (2001). Postmodern consumption and alternative medications. *Journal of Sociology, 37*(2), 157–176.

Sagli, G. (2010). The contested reality of acupuncture effects: Measurement, meaning and relations of power in the context of an integration initiative in Norway. *Anthropological Notebooks, 16*(2), 39–55.

Saks, M. (1995). *Professions and the public interest: Medical power, altruism and alternative medicine*. London: Routledge.

Saks, M. (1996). From quackery to complementary medicine: The shifting boundaries between orthodox and unorthodox medical knowledge. In S. Cant & U. Sharma (Eds.), *Complementary and alternative medicines: Knowledge in practice* (pp. 27–43). London: Free Association Books.

Scott, A. L. (1998). The symbolizing body and the metaphysics of alternative medicine. *Body and Society, 4*(3), 21–37.

Shuval, J. T., Gross, R., Ashkenazi, Y., & Scharchter, L. (2012). Integrating CAM and biomedicine in primary care settings: Physicians' perspectives on boundaries and boundary work. *Qualitative Health Research, 22*(10), 1317–1329.

Siahpush, M. (2000). A critical review of the sociology of alternative medicine: Research on users, practitioners and the orthodoxy. *Health, 4*(2), 159–178.

Sismondo, S. (2004). *An introduction to science and technology studies.* Oxford: Blackwell.

Sismondo, S. (2008). Science and technology studies and an engaged program. In E. Hackett, O. Amsterdamska, M. Lynch, & J. Wajcman (Eds.), *The handbook of science and technology studies* (3rd ed., pp. 13–31). Cambridge, MA: The MIT Press.

Star, S. L. (2010). This is not a boundary object: Reflections on the origin of a concept. *Science, Technology and Human Values, 35*(5), 601–617.

Star, S. L., & Griesemer, J. R. (1989). Institutional ecology, "translations" and boundary objects: Amateurs and professionals in Berkeley's Museum of Vertebrate Zoology, 1907–39. *Social Studies of Science, 19*(3), 387–420.

Taylor, C. A. (1996). *Defining science. A rhetoric of demarcation.* Madison: University of Wisconsin Press.

Verhoef, M. J., Lewith, G., Ritenbaugh, C., Boon, H., Fleishman, S., & Leis, A. (2005). Complementary and alternative medicine whole systems research: Beyond identification of inadequacies of the RCT. *Complementary Therapies in Medicine, 13*(3), 206–212.

Villanueva-Russell, Y. (2009). Chiropractors as folk devils: Published and unpublished news coverage of a moral panic. *Deviant Behavior, 30*(2), 175–200.

Vuolanto, P. (2015). Boundary work and power in the controversy over therapeutic touch in Finnish nursing science. *Minerva, 53*(4), 359–380.

Webster, A. (1979). Scientific controversy and socio-cognitive metonymy: The case of acupuncture. In R. Wallis (Ed.), *On the margins of science: The social construction of rejected knowledge, Sociological review monograph* (pp. 121–137). Keele, UK: University of Keele.

Webster, A. (2002). Innovative health technologies and the social: Redefining health, medicine and the body. *Current Sociology, 50*(3), 443–457.

Webster, A. (2006). Introduction: New technologies in health care: Opening the black bag. In A. Webster (Ed.), *New technologies in health care* (pp. 1–8). Basingstoke: Palgrave Macmillan.

Webster, A. (2007). *Health, technology and society: A sociological critique.* New York: Palgrave Macmillan.

Wieland, L. S., Manheimer, E., & Berman, B. M. (2011). Development and classification of an operational definition of complementary and alternative medicine for the Cochrane collaboration. *Alternative Therapies in Health and Medicine, 17*(2), 50–59.

Willis, E. (1983). *Medical dominance: The division of labour in Australian health care*. Sydney: George Allen and Unwin.

Zhan, M. (2009). *Other-worldly: Making Chinese medicine through transnational frames*. Durham: Duke University Press.

Zhan, M. (2014). The empirical as conceptual: Transdisciplinary engagements with an "experiential medicine". *Science, Technology and Human Values, 39*(2), 236–263.

Part I

Defining CAM: Boundaries Between and Within CAM and Biomedicine

2

Evidence-Based Alternative, 'Slanted Eyes' and Electric Circuits: Doing Chinese Medicine in the Post/Socialist Czech Republic

Tereza Stöckelová and Jaroslav Klepal

In June 2015, 'The Health Ministers Meeting' held in Prague brought together a dozen ministerial delegations from Central and East European (CEE) countries and one from China. During the three-day summit, hundreds of politicians, representatives of the World Health Organization (WHO), entrepreneurs from various medical industries, health managers, experts on public health and physicians discussed ways of furthering cooperation between China and the CEE region in the field of healthcare, including the use of 'Traditional Chinese Medicine' (TCM). The summit was sponsored by corporate businesses, primarily by the PPF investment group, majority-owned by Czech billionaire Petr Kellner, and a private conglomerate, CEFC China Energy, and it was co-organised by the Czech-Chinese Chamber of Collaboration. It was also accompanied by, on the one hand, protests from a group of supporters of the Falung Gong movement against the Chinese state's civil right abuses and, on the other hand, by strong criticism voiced in public media by

T. Stöckelová (✉) • J. Klepal
Institute of Sociology of the Czech Academy of Sciences,
Prague, Czech Republic

© The Author(s) 2018
C. Brosnan et al. (eds.), *Complementary and Alternative Medicine*, Health,
Technology and Society, https://doi.org/10.1007/978-3-319-73939-7_2

representatives of the Czech Medical Chamber (an organisation with the obligatory membership of all roughly 40,000 physicians practising in the country) who view the planned introduction of TCM to the Czech Republic (CR) as an attack on the evidence-based and scientific nature of the country's medicine and public healthcare system.

In the midst of speeches, panel discussions, closed bilateral meetings, signing of agreements and celebration dinners, you could hear, read, and even experience on your own body a great deal about TCM. The Czech prime minister stressed that 'in the world TCM is getting wider popularity and it is supported by the WHO', adding that he believes that 'like in China we will succeed in integrating our Western conception of medicine and its modern diagnostic and medical procedures with the thousand-year-old knowledge and experience passed down by generations' (field notes, June 2015). An integral part of the summit was the 'TCM exhibition', organised by the Chinese side. On the walls, you could read posters titled, for instance, 'Combining Modern Technology with Traditional Classics to Form New Models of TCM Healthcare'. Century-old acupuncture needles were shown side by side with high-tech electropuncture devices and diagnostic computer software. There were also practitioners of Chinese medicine (CM) present as a living exhibit, who could perform diagnosis either by examining your tongue and pulse or by connecting you to their computers. On the third day of the summit, top-ranking officials in the Czech and Chinese delegations, together with a representative of the WHO, went from Prague to a regional university hospital where the opening ceremony of the Czech-Chinese Centre for TCM took place. Two discussion panels at the summit explicitly dealt with issues of TCM. One of them, titled 'TCM Goes Global', sought to introduce TCM as a form of medicine that transcends boundaries in the world; that has found its way into diverse places, such as North Korea, Western Europe, and Cuba, and has attracted a relentless flow of internationals who come to China to study it. As the vice-president of a university of CM summed it up during the panel discussion: 'TCM has a talent for globalisation' (field notes, June 2015).

Indeed, CM has in its different versions been a tireless traveller of the globe and has become a cosmopolitan reality.[1] In recent decades, CM has moved through the vast mainland of China and spread to the wider region of Asia and even beyond, transforming itself into a 'world medicine' (Scheid 2007). It has cut its way through the United States (Baer et al. 1998; Barnes 2003; Flesch 2013; Pritzker 2010; Zhan 2009), Australia and New Zealand (Baer 2007; Dew 2000), Western Europe (Anderson 2010; Candelise 2011; Lieber 2012; Sagli 2010) and the global south (Pokam 2011; Hsu 2009, 2015; Langwick 2010). As Scheid suggested, CM has become 'widely welcomed and globally successful precisely because it is easy to produce, and easy to insert into widely different local contexts, but also because it subtly adjusts itself to differences in local demands' (2007: 392).

In this chapter, drawing on ongoing ethnographic research on 'the interfaces between biomedicine and alternative therapeutic practices' that we began in January 2015, we follow CM in the CR.[2] We thus set out to further investigate CM's 'talent for globalisation'. However, we approach CM not only as a cosmopolitan medicine that inserts itself into and adjusts to the local setting but also as a *cosmopolitical* (Stengers 2010) medicine that actively remakes, reorders, and challenges the particular local setting with its (biomedical) bodies, technologies, and reasoning.

CM has not, however, just travelled through space. Consider CM's time travels from ancient times up to the present day, made possible by its ability to invent or live through diverse versions of itself (Hanson 1998; Scheid 2007; Zhan 2009). Take the various engagements and disengagements of CM with political and economic regimes, ranging from colonialism and Maoism to global capitalism (Scheid 2002). Let's not forget the recurring occasions on which CM has tied in with the clinical and research practices of biomedicine (Andrews 2014; Chan and Lee 2002), which have even been altered by CM (MacPherson et al. 2016). The travels and transitions of CM through these heterogeneous interconnected settings have contributed to its becoming something intrinsically plural (Scheid 2002), syncretic (Zhang 2007), and correlative (Lin and Law 2014).

Along with CM's travel in the CR and wider Central and Eastern Europe we also discuss in this chapter its journey to and through post/socialism. Contrary to the claims strongly asserted at the Health Ministers Meeting that CM was emerging in the region today as an innovation, we show that CM had already arrived and thrived in the CR in the time of state socialism and postsocialism. We argue that the TCM *enacted* (Mol 2002) as part of the official Czech-Chinese initiative and in relation to the changing global political economy and the rise of China in recent years is just one version of CM, and we trace the three most visible versions of CM present in the CR since the late 1950s. Foregrounding post/socialism in these enactments of Chinese medicine sensitises our analysis to the issues of temporality. While much attention has been paid in STS to the study of the spatial arrangements of technologies and medicine (e.g. de Laet and Mol 2000; Mol and Law 1994; Law and Singleton 2005) in between the First and Third Worlds, there has been a lack of attention paid to the various *politico-temporal* continuities and disconti-nuities of post/socialism in the Second World.

In this chapter we do not follow CM as a clear-cut object, system, or package that travels smoothly from region to region or era to era. What CM is and what travels are empirical questions for us. Also, we do not consider the widespread existence of CM in many corners of the world as the result of disseminated knowledge about the cosmos, body, health and disease only. We try to understand the specific social, economic, and political relations and cleavages which shape particular versions of CM, and we foreground the particular constitutive practices and materialities of CM—herbs, needles, body techniques, educational curricula, states' regulations, and the standards of healthcare—through which three differ-ent, yet partially connected (Strathern 1991) versions of CM have been forming in the post/socialist CR. In the following sections we discuss 'medical acupuncture', 'traditional CM' and 'TCM', as they successively emerged and today coexist in the Czech medical field.

Medical Acupuncture: Biomedicalising CM During Socialism

In September 2015 the opening of an outpatient department at the Czech-Chinese Centre for TCM and its continued visibility in the media prompted a meeting between the scientific committee of the Czech

Medical Chamber and representatives of the Czech Medical Acupuncture Society (CMAS).[3] In the meeting the current and former heads of CMAS tried to debunk the claims of the proponents of the Czech-Chinese project that Chinese medicine was something new and innovative for Czech patients and that 'acupuncture never existed here before' (presentation 2015; research interviews, January and April 2016). In their presentation they pointed out that acupuncture has a more than 50-year history in the CR. Around 7000 physicians had been trained in acupuncture since the 1970s and hundreds of them had practised it with quality results comparable to other EU countries, the United States, or Australia, which can be demonstrated by the work that physicians practising acupuncture had published in medical journals. Thus the representatives of CMAS were ready to join the Czech Medical Chamber in critiquing the celebration of 'TCM' in the Czech-Chinese project because it seemed to have the effect of erasing the tradition of medical acupuncture they had been building since socialist times and of undermining the legitimate position in the Czech medical community that they had worked hard to negotiate for themselves over the course of years of practice, research, teaching and manufacturing acupuncture 'on a scientific basis'. They were ready to fight the current political and medical establishment enchanted by 'Chinese money' in the name of their stubborn predecessors, on behalf of the years spent studying acupuncture after getting their medical degrees, and on behalf of the patients in whose bodies they had been inserting acupuncture needles for decades (research interview, April 2016).

According to CMAS, acupuncture was brought to then Czechoslovakia by a military physician and active member of the Communist Party, Richard Umlauf, who learnt it first-hand when he was sent with other military and civilian medical professionals on a mission to North Korea after the war in the late 1950s. After returning to Czechoslovakia, he became an enthusiastic promoter and practitioner of acupuncture in the 1960s. In 1965, the first Czech book on acupuncture was published. It provided an account of acupuncture's philosophical-theoretical background in 'Chinese folk medicine', its uses for treating various neurological illnesses, and the 'scientific explanation' for its possible effectiveness based on the theories of Soviet neurophysiology (Vymazal and Tuháček 1965). In the same year, the first conference on acupuncture was organised by Umlauf at a military hospital in Slovakia under the official patronage of what at that time was called the Czechoslovak Medical Association of J. E. Purkyně, whose past- and present-day mission includes focusing on 'the use of only such diagnostic, preventive and medical methods whose nature and effects are based on currently acknowledged scientific evidence' (CMA JEP 2015: 3). Thus, in the 1960s, a group of medical professionals interested in CM was formed, and they soon after sought to obtain professional recognition: the first independent and official department of acupuncture was established by the Ministry of Health in a university hospital in Brno in 1975; in 1976, two physicians, one of them Dr Umlauf, obtained medical certification in acupuncture; and gradually dozens of papers written by acupuncturists started to appear in the country's main medical journals such as *Praktický lékař* (General Practitioner) and *Časopis lékařů českých* (Journal of Czech Physicians). Umlauf's effort to build a community of medical acupuncturists in Czechoslovakia and to integrate it into the international community bore fruit in 1988 when the third congress of the International Council of Medical Acupuncture and Related Techniques (ICMART) was held for the first time in the capital of an Eastern bloc country, Prague, and Umlauf became ICMART's president (Pára and Barešová 2006; Pára 2006a, 2006b, 2015).

Medical acupuncture seemed to thrive and spread from the 1970s. At that time, it was not uncommon, as we were told in the interviews, for some Communist Party members including high-ranking apparatchiks and their families to seek acupuncture treatment. An important step in the enactment of medical acupuncture was not only its translation into the logic of the state's 'scientific materialism' but also its integration into the system of socialist healthcare. In 1977, the Ministry of Health issued the first decree defining the methodological guidelines for using acupuncture and established it in law as an 'interdisciplinary method' of medicine (Pára 2006a: 3) to be practised by physicians licensed by the Institute for Postgraduate Medical Education, which began to teach courses in acupuncture. It is important to note that this same decree (amended in 1981) is still in force, and it defines in legal terms who is allowed to practise acupuncture in the CR today. When the Ministry of Health was drafting its methodological guidelines in 1976, its 'Statement of Justification' for the official introduction of acupuncture into the socialist healthcare system argued that acupuncture was being used worldwide at that time (in Asian countries, Western countries, the Soviet Union), that this 'medical method' could be used to effectively reduce 'pain on various levels of the central nervous system' or to restore 'some disturbed motor functions', and that it could have a positive impact on the state's planned economy by 'reducing periods of incapacity to work' and reducing expenditures on 'pharmaceuticals ranging from analgesics and sedatives to hypnotic drugs, etc.' (Ministerstvo zdravotnictví 1976: 1–2). Interestingly, the same argument regarding the financial efficiency of acupuncture, or of CM in general, is now being used as an argument by the proponents of the Czech–Chinese project 40 years later.

Another vital way of enacting medical acupuncture was by linking it to the state's technological research and industry. Years of experimental research on the objectification of acupuncture points (their morphology, electric impedance, and relations to body organs), including studies on animals, were translated into innovative devices. After the development of a prototype for an acupuncture point detector—a device called the AKD 401, built by the state firm Prema in Stará Turá and 'based on Japanese and French inspiration', as was explained to us by the former head of CMAS who owns one of the surviving devices (research interview, April 2016)—in 1978, the state granted a patent for something called an Acudiast (Fig. 2.1), an electric 'arrangement for the identification, measurement, and stimulation of reflexive processes on the surface of the body' (Úřad pro vynálezy a osvědčení 1982: 1). This electropuncture device for physicians was manufactured by what was then the state firm Metra Blansko, which produced various electrical measurement instruments.

In 1982, another state company, Tesla, introduced an electropuncture device called Stimul onto the domestic market that with the aid of 'modern electronics replaces [acupuncture] needles and allows a layperson to apply proven experience and knowledge and to do so painlessly' (Tesla 1982: 5). Thus, compared to Acudiast, Stimul was designed to be used— after consultation with a doctor—by every citizen, whether at her home or workplace, to help restore her body, which was afflicted with diseases of affluence ranging from tobacco addiction to arthritis.[4] By the time Tesla was privatised in the 1990s, it had manufactured more than one

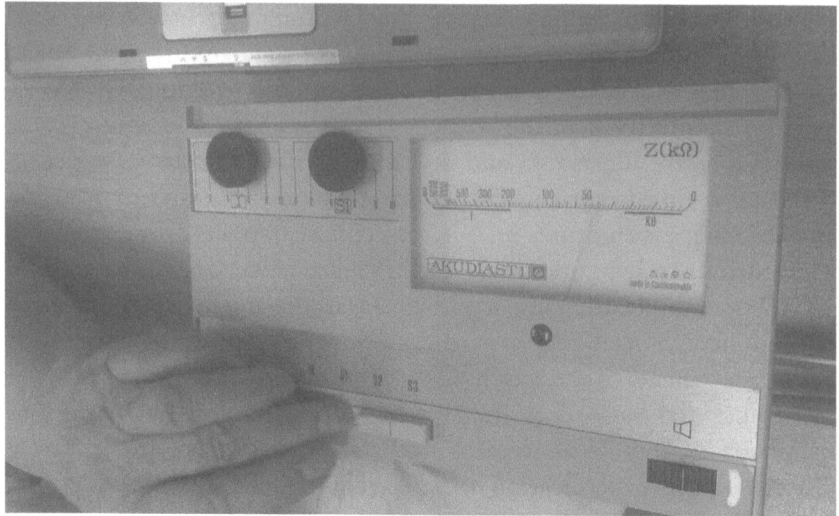

Fig. 2.1 A surviving (and working) Acudiast I in the hands of one of its inventors (photo: authors)

million Stimuls in two product lines (Pára and Barešová 2006), and a significant number of these devices were marketed late in the state-socialist period to the Middle East (research interview, April 2016).

Those medical acupuncturists who favoured doing acupuncture with needles instead of new devices were supplied by Chirana, a Czechoslovakian firm that produced medical instruments. As we were told by then acupuncturists, Chirana's needles were expensive during the socialist period. They also broke easily, were thick and allegedly painful, and they had to be sterilised and re-sharpened after each use. However, there are still acupuncturists today who use them occasionally because Chirana's needle 'is long, strong, and flexible enough and has a handle that is heavy enough that when you insert the needle and make it vibrate, you produce a [electric] current with a particular frequency that starts to affect the patient's neurotransmitters', which is something that 'cheap needles imported from China cannot do' (research interview, December 2015).

Medical acupuncture has managed to become a relatively stable element in the post/socialist healthcare system in the CR, although it has had to struggle for its legitimacy within biomedicine. By adopting the Soviet reflex theory, putting it in the hands of physicians only, practising it in response to biomedical diagnoses, and linking it to the socialist state's technology and industry, its practitioners enacted medical acupuncture in recent decades as an 'interdisciplinary medical method' in which realities such as *qi*, *yin* and *yang*, or *shen* have no place. We were told many times by our CMAS interlocutors that 'what we do is not Chinese medicine or TCM, it is the Euro-American way of doing acupuncture'. And as one of the leading medical acupuncturists in the country argued with reference to a recent investigation of tattoos on the mummified body of Ötzi, a Neolithic man from Central Europe, acupuncture might not be Chinese but rather European in origin and its history might need to be substantially revised (Fiala 2010).

Traditional CM: Cultivating Autonomy and Care with 'Slanted Eyes'

The liberalisation, marketisation, and partial privatisation of healthcare after the regime change in 1989 brought various complementary and alternative medicine (CAM) approaches and techniques to the attention of the wider public in the CR (Křížová 2004, 2015). It was in these changing circumstances that another version of CM was able to consolidate and strengthen itself. The two main schools of 'traditional CM' in the CR were established in 1990 and 2006, and in 2012, the Chamber of Traditional Chinese Medicine was set up to define professional standards in the field and to represent traditional CM in public and policy debates. While the role of biomedical doctors has been pivotal in these developments, the relationship between traditional CM and biomedicine has been significantly different than in the case of medical acupuncture. As we will show in detail, CM and its techniques were not in this case to be subsumed under biomedicine but cultivated as an autonomous practice with its own theory of body and health, diagnostic repertoire, and treatment approaches and only partially connected to biomedicine.

While this version of CM was only able to thrive after the regime change in 1989, its roots run deep into socialist times. To illustrate this, let's take a quick look at the trajectories of two important figures in 'traditional' CM—Dr Kapka and Dr Bylinná. Even though they were working in biomedical facilities, both of these physicians also started to develop a separate, dissident medical practice involving CM, aimed at acquiring a certain amount of autonomy from—and in some respects even opposition to—biomedicine. Dr Kapka was a psychiatrist who worked in the environmentally and socially deprived region of former Sudetenland and had been experimenting since 1960 with CM in his medical care. He was even able to visit some alternative clinics in Western Germany during the 1960s and in 1988 wrote the highly popular book *The Puzzle of Life* explaining key principles and practices of Eastern medical systems. Although he practised acupuncture based on the theories of *qi* and the *Five Phases* and he learnt to use herbal remedies and experimented with dieting and meditation to combat the iatrogenic effects of socialist biomedicine, he didn't encounter any major obstacles to his endeavours because he was working in northern Bohemia, which was geographically remote from the centre of power (interview, March 2015).

Dr Bylinná, who was employed at a major university hospital in Prague, by contrast was subject to surveillance from the state secret police for 'subversion of the system of socialist nutrition' (she experimented with vegetarianism) and disciplinary measures from her superiors. Even before 1989, she had some contacts with French CM practitioners, which would soon after intensify, while she only made her first contacts in China later on, in the 1990s, and most of her contacts were Chinese scholars who had resisted the integration of CM with biomedicine (interview, February 2015).

Both Kapka and Bylinná took advantage of the possibility to open a private practice and private schools after 1990. Kapka delved into 'information medicine', inventively mixing together various alternative approaches—CM, electroacupuncture, homeopathy, and the results of 'secret Soviet cosmic research' (interview, March 2015). He developed his own diagnostic devices and marketed a growing portfolio of information medicines, which are used by thousands of his patients. Bylinná focused on traditional CM and established the first school of CM in the country, which offers a four-year curriculum in CM, and over the years has produced a junior generation of CM practitioners. However, because the 1977 decree issued by the Ministry of Health is still in force, graduates of this school who do not also have a biomedical education (and subsequent certification in medical acupuncture from the Institute for Postgraduate Medical Education) are significantly restricted in their legal right to provide medical services in the field of CM without the direct supervision of a medical doctor.[5] Although there are practitioners with no biomedical education who still provide CM treatment, including acupuncture, they are working in a grey area of the law.

As we learnt at the traditional CM clinic Zdraví (the head of which has strong ties with one of the traditional CM schools and has a student practice at the clinic where future medical acupuncturists licensed by the Institute for Postgraduate Medical Education can work), where we have been conducting participant observation since 2015, this version of CM has an ambivalent relationship to biomedicine. On the one hand, the Zdraví clinic visibly performs a different physical and social space to an ordinary biomedical one. Upon entering, you find yourself in a reception area next to a 'health food' restaurant that is run by the clinic and offers lunches for the clinic's practitioners, patients, and the public. The clinic has 12 examination rooms, which are bright and warm, and the corridors are filled with calm, meditative music and furnished with medical and non-medical items that evoke China and CM: posters of human anatomy with meridians, figures of Buddha and dragons, and Chinese landscape drawings. The first thing your body interacts with upon arriving in the examination room is a cup of tea. All ten practitioners, who are all native Czechs, are dressed not in white coats but in their civilian clothes, and one of the two male practitioners sometimes wears a shirt with a slightly oriental look to it. Patients rarely have to wait for their appointments—even on very busy days, appointments start on time. This is a rather different setup from that of a usual biomedical facility— the public facilities in most cases do not create such a welcoming impression (the patients usually have to wait for quite some time to see the doctor they have an appointment with), and the private ones (such as dental surgeries) would usually have its attachment to biomedicine clearly on display (white coats, biomedical posters, and advertisements on walls).

The difference of this clinic from a biomedical facility is also enacted in the way it foregrounds the practitioners' corporeality. Not only do the practitioners discuss their own (or their family members') health and bodily conditions during treatment sessions with patients but the practitioners' own bodies are also sites of CM interventions (they use CM treatments too) and could serve as proof of the effectiveness of CM. The personalisation of care is thus achieved not by simply attending to the specific nature of the patient's condition but rather by means of building of a relationship between the practitioner and the patient, a relationship in which the practitioners are involved not just as care professionals but also in terms of their own (vulnerable) corporeality. The bodies of clients and practitioners are enacted as fundamentally comparable and mutual. In nearly every therapeutic session we attended, the affectivity was affirmed and enhanced at least by the practitioner touching the patient (with her hand) in a brief, non-instrumental way before the patient was left in a quiet room with the acupuncture needles in her body. As one woman commented: 'This is a very pleasant touch' (field notes, July 2015).

When we asked the head of the Zdraví clinic how they relate to biomedicine in their everyday practice, she replied that 'you have to forget biomedicine to some extent. This is a totally different way of looking at a human' (research interview, February 2015). This is also what all patients are instructed to do during their second session, when they are told what their CM diagnosis is: 'Forget everything you know about Western medicine'. Critical comments about biomedicine were also made relatively frequently during the therapeutic sessions that we were able to observe. Interestingly, a significant portion of the reservations that practitioners have about biomedicine also applies to Chinese medicine as practised in contemporary China. While these practitioners have been travelling to study in China since the 1990s, they are critical of the 'integrated approach' that is typically applied in established Chinese hospitals (cf. Zhan 2009). As another leading Czech practitioner told us, this integrated approach to medicine 'is a mule that won't be led'. He personally practises traditional CM in an approach that he calls doing CM with 'slanted eyes', by which he means mentally, bodily, and spiritually switching from the biomedical mode to that of Chinese medicine, in which figure, for example, the realities of souls and analogical reasoning that biomedicine does not recognise (research interviews, July 2015 and April 2016). Similarly, on a recent trip to China, the head of the Chamber of Traditional CM was visiting a 'dissident' practitioner in order to learn the traditional and 'authentic' approach to acupuncture that he was unfamiliar with that had been passed down within one particular family (field notes, December 2015), in contrast to the biomedicalised TCM that is supported by the Chinese state. All these practices aim to purge CM of biomedicine and foster its ontological and epistemological autonomy.

This, however, is not the end of the story, and the relationship to biomedicine that we were able to observe at Zdraví is more complicated in practice. Take diagnostics for example: the practitioners at the clinic perform a CM examination of the patient's pulse and tongue, but during the patient's first visit, in addition to these techniques, the patient also fills in a detailed questionnaire on her medical history, any medication she uses, and various bodily habits and preferences (including food, sleep, and secretion). This questionnaire was compiled by the head of the clinic, 'drawing on what we had in internal medicine and adding CM to it' (field notes, April 2015). The questionnaire thus puts the realities of biomedicine and CM side by side. It draws the practitioners' attention (especially in the case of more serious conditions) to the biomedical reports that the patients can bring with them and in some cases to the need to persuade the patients to (also) get a biomedical examination—which was the case of one patient who had internal gynaecological problems but refused to go for an ultrasound (field notes, April 2015). When we asked a year later how the treatment had progressed, the head of the clinic told us that she had terminated working with the patient because the woman refused to undergo a biomedical diagnostic procedure (research interview, April 2016). All the clinic practitioners without a biomedical education are also currently trying to get one. Not only will doing so strengthen their position under the current law but such an education is considered at the clinic to also be a potentially useful resource for the care they offer.

Thus, technology and biomedicine are not simply absent from the clinic but are rather *absent present* (Law and Singleton 2005) in the clinic. In the examination rooms, there are no computers and no electrical medical technology. But in the staffroom, practitioners sit behind computers and a sophisticated online system is used to organise and run the clinic (scheduling sessions, distributing work among the practitioners). And we were able to observe that they also make use of, take into account, and sometimes suggest the patient seek a biomedical diagnosis.

The Czech traditional CM practitioners we observed have an ambivalent relationship to contemporary China. As the earlier quotation shows, they are suspicious of 'integrated medicine', which in their view suffers from drawbacks similar to those of European biomedicine, namely 'a factory approach' to patients. If they travel to China, they often search for 'traditional' diagnostic and therapeutic techniques and know-how that have been passed down over many generations within a family, avoiding more biomedicalised forms. They cultivate ties with practitioners in the United States and Western Europe (e.g. by regularly attending the international CM congress in Rothenburg, Germany), whom they often regard as being truer to the original Chinese tradition than CM in contemporary China.

TCM: Establishing an 'Evidence-Based' Alternative

After the regime change in 1989, the CR (then still Czechoslovakia) embraced the West, in both political and economic terms. In biomedicine, too, it was the ideal of Western healthcare that dominated postsocialist governmental and institutional policies and from which many new elements were introduced into the national healthcare system. To name just a few that have been introduced since the early 1990s: the privatisation of some parts of the healthcare system, mainly outpatient care (Saltman and Figueras 1997; Háva and Mašková-Hanušová 2009); new high-tech diagnostic machines have been acquired with the help of EU funds; and the introduction of 'informed consent forms', which supposedly turn patients patronised by the state into rational consumers of health services. Despite the many continuities within the system, anything depicted as 'Eastern' and 'socialist' was largely associated with backwardness.

This geopolitical imaginary started to be gradually dismantled after 2008 with the impact of the economic and political crises of the EU and with the rise of aspiring new powers in the global arena such as China (Shambaugh 2013). Both the Czech conservative government that was in office between 2010 and 2013 and the centre-left government that has been in power since 2013 have significantly strengthened political and economic collaboration beyond Western Europe and the United States, and the CEE region has also begun to be much more actively sought out by Chinese investors (Fürst 2015). Yet the recent (re)turn to the 'East' by Czech political elites would have been inconceivable without Czech capitalists such as Petr Kellner, who discovered China first at the turn of the millennium for the company he owns that offers consumer loans and later for his biotechnological company Sotio, which focuses on the development of therapeutic cancer vaccines. In order to penetrate the Chinese healthcare market, Sotio had to be officially backed by the Czech state, and this was achieved by reviving the agreements based on 'friendship and cooperation' in the field of healthcare that existed between Czechoslovakia and China in socialist times. If vaccines, laboratory equipment, clinical trials, or medical beds were moving in one direction, then pharmaceuticals, spa patients, and TCM, China's 'national treasure', had to be moving 'reciprocally' in the other direction.

It is in this new geopolitical mosaic that the Health Ministers Meeting was held in Prague in 2015 and the Czech-Chinese Centre for TCM was established in the regional university hospital. Currently, one practitioner from China works in the centre on the basis of a special decision issued by of the Ministry of Health in August 2015 that allows him, under the supervision of a certified Czech physician, to provide medical services 'in the diagnostic field: in TCM diagnostics—general objective findings, objective findings on tongue, and objective findings relating to pulse; in the field of therapy—non-surgical specialised treatments in the form of acupuncture, cupping and Tui Na massage' (Mach 2016: 16). In 2018, a brand-new TCM clinic is scheduled to open as part of that same regional university hospital, and it is supposed to be fully funded by CEFC China Energy Company at an estimated cost of EUR 10 million. The new clinic is expected to become a flagship project for the spread of TCM into the official healthcare systems of states across the CEE region.

The Czech-Chinese project provoked a sharp response from the Czech Medical Chamber, which declared TCM to be charlatanism, a product of Chinese Maoism, and a threat to local, modern, evidence-based medicine (EBM) (Cikrt 2015). The Chamber even filed a lawsuit—so far unsuccessful—challenging the legality of practising TCM on university premises (Mach 2016: 16–17). The Ministry of Health and the director of the university hospital that hosts the centre, who is known in the community as a respected vaccinologist, have framed their defence strictly in the terms of EBM: they cite controlled clinical studies with positive outcomes for the use of acupuncture in selected biomedical diagnoses, most notably the treatment of pain. They also refer frequently to the use of CM in established clinics in the United States and Western Europe. The diagnostic and therapeutic practices in the TCM centre are claimed to be not only complementary to biomedicine but also fully founded in biomedicine. Any patient entering the centre is first given an examination using 'Western' methods, the results of which are evaluated by a Czech physician, and only then is the patient, along with the results of the examination, referred to a Chinese practitioner (DVTV 2015). In the words of the centre's chief physician, 'biomedical insight into the body will help the Chinese acupuncturist to determine where to put his acupuncture needle' (Radioforum 2016). In this depiction of the centre's work, the acupuncture practised there is fully accounted for in biomedical terms and is enacted as a technique that can be used to treat only selected biomedical conditions. It is no surprise in this context that the Chinese partner organisation in the project is the Shuguang Hospital, affiliated with the Shanghai University of Traditional Chinese Medicine, which is known as a key proponent of 'integrated Chinese and Western medicine' in China (Zhan 2009).

A similar motive can be observed in the negotiations over importing Chinese herbal remedies to the CR. Currently, Chinese herbs and herbal remedies for sale in the CR are classed as food supplements. Chinese pharmaceutical businesses are now interested in getting the classification of herbal remedies changed to *medicinal products*, which would allow them to be more widely covered under the system of public health insurance.[6] Through the CR, they could also enter the broader EU market. During the negotiations related to the Health Ministers meeting, we were able to observe Chinese entrepreneurs insisting that their medical remedies already have many 'Western' features. And indeed, the TCM pills they literally brought with them to the negotiation table looked little like a 'natural' alternative and were instead indistinguishable from painkillers produced locally by a Czech pharmaceutical company (field notes, 2015).

If spatially the project is a fluid mixture of Chinese, Czech and Western elements and references, its temporal aspect is no less intriguing. Firstly, it breaks with the modernisation narrative, which is a linear account of medical progress out of medieval darkness into the light of modern science. On the contrary, as the speech by the Czech prime minister quoted in the opening of this chapter reveals, ancient wisdom should be seamlessly combinable with modern medicine for the benefit of patients. Secondly, while 'friendship cooperation and reciprocity' in the field of healthcare are a revival of the ethos that was part of the shared socialist past of the two countries, the Czech proponents also highlight the contemporary capitalist character of China. As the head of the foreign department of the Office of the Czech President stated in an interview after the Chinese president's visit to the CR in April 2016, 'the Chinese communist today looks more like a businessman from Wall Street rather a Stalinist from the 1950s', and 'by their fruit you will recognise them' (DVTV 2016). He implied that Communist Party rule in China does not necessarily mean communism in practice. Critics of the project have tried without much success to use the narrative of medical progress and the threat of communist China in their efforts to delegitimise the new TCM centre and related planned activities. The project continues to benefit from strong political support and the interest from patients is reportedly extremely high (Radioforum 2016).

Conclusion

In this chapter, we traced the multiple and somewhat unstable and changing versions of Chinese medicine that have been enacted in the post/socialist CR. We showed that 'medical acupuncture', the use of which was established in the official healthcare system in the socialist period, has been established as an interdisciplinary method of biomedicine through experimental research, institutionalisation and professionalisation, tech-nologisation and industrialisation, and by purging it of its embeddedness in Chinese culture and medicine. Another version of Chinese medicine, conceived as 'traditional CM' by Czech practitioners, which benefited from both the westward and eastward ties it formed during and after socialism, has been practised as a set of therapeutic techniques (acupuncture, herbal therapies, dieting, exercise, and massage) that are (and should remain) autonomous from biomedicine. And finally, the most recent version of CM—the integrative 'TCM' of the Czech-Chinese project—has arrived in the CR as part of the shifting global political economy and is being 'introduced' as an innovation that could significantly transform the healthcare system of the Czech state (and possibly those of other countries in the CEE region), in which TCM would play the role of an 'evidence-based' alternative and supplement to biomedicine.

In all three versions, we were able to see how cosmopolitan, plural, and syncretic Chinese medicine can be. Yet in this chapter, we also showed that these versions of CM may produce various cosmopolitical (Stengers 2010) and economic effects. The TCM that the Czech-Chinese project has brought to the country seeks to substantially reorder the provision of public healthcare and the legislative context that defines the medical profession and medicinal products. Medical acupuncture, which recasts elusive meridians and acupoints as electric circuits, made the production lines of the socialist state churn out electropuncture diagnostic and therapeutic devices for use in both therapists' offices and households. And the local practitioners of traditional CM challenge biomedicine in their everyday practices, for example, in the way they share their knowledge of vulnerable corporeality with each other and with their patients, and in how they embody traditional CM's ontological difference from biomedicine.

While foregrounding post/socialism in these versions of CM, we also dealt here with various politico-temporal continuities and discontinuities. On the one hand, all the studied versions perform *their own* temporality: integrative TCM disrupts the linear account of medical progress by mixing the traditional and the modern; the 'spatialised time' (Fabian 1983) of local practitioners' traditional CM enables this version of CM to distance itself from modernised and industrialised CM in contemporary China and at the same time to tie in with the 'authentic' CM of ancient

China (and its survival as passed down in family lines and through apprenticeships both in the East and the West); and medical acupuncture has recently been struggling to free itself of the residue of 'pre-scientific' CM and to redefine the origins of CM.

On the other hand, these versions of CM are performed *in* different (and often overlapping and conflicting) political temporalities. Even though the TCM introduced by the Czech-Chinese project echoes the socialist rhetoric of friendship and cooperation (declared in agreements between Czechoslovakia and China in the 1950s), it is rather business interests and the power of the yuan that breathes life into this version of CM. The traditional CM of local practitioners (with biomedical degrees) benefited from the change in regime, after which it was able to move out of the dissident or unofficial shadows and into state healthcare institutions and private clinics. But having still not fully obtained official and legal recognition, traditional CM has become trapped (together with a new generation of practitioners without biomedical degrees) in another grey zone. Finally, the continuing marginalisation of medical acupuncture, which representatives of CMAS are currently trying to resist, seems to be an effect of the close coexistence it used to have with the former socialist state and its system of healthcare, scientific research, and planned economy.

These versions of CM and their enactments do not, however, exist independently of each other. We have seen both conflicts and alliances between them. We showed that leading Czech practitioners of traditional CM are suspicious of the TCM imported by the Czech-Chinese project, as it is overly integrated with biomedicine (and with the current Chinese state), and the future mainstreaming of this version could dilute the ontological and epistemological autonomy of CM that these practitioners have been cultivating. Interestingly, the older generation, such as Dr Kapka and Dr Bylinná, criticised and left medical acupuncture during socialism for very similar reasons. At the same time, at least some Czech practitioners of traditional CM acknowledge that the integrated TCM of the Czech-Chinese project serves as a 'lightning rod' for traditional CM, which means that the biomedical establishment's outrage at CM has been directed more towards the Czech-Chinese project and the centre than at the hundreds of Czech practitioners who treat patients without having any certified biomedical education (research interview with one of the leading figures of traditional CM, April 2016). The support from political and business elites for the Czech-Chinese project—the form of support that the Chamber for Traditional CM has lacked—which will probably bring about significant changes in legislation and the healthcare system has also been welcomed by traditional CM practitioners. The partial alliance between these two versions of CM has led to the appearance of Chinese herbal remedies in the centre that operates in the regional university hospital, which are supplied by the private business of a leading Czech practitioner of traditional CM.

As for the medical acupuncturists, we noticed that they redirected their critique away from Czech practitioners of traditional CM who didn't have medical degrees and towards the Czech-Chinese project, on the grounds that the project supposedly erases everything they have achieved in the past with their own scientific research and evidence-based clinical practice. While the experiment protocols, publications, and patents on the devices used by the earlier generation of medical acupuncturists lie in dusty boxes stored in attics and basements, representatives of CMAS, siding with the Czech Medical Chamber in critiquing the Czech-Chinese project, hope that medical acupuncture will regain official support and will be redefined not as a 'method' but as a 'branch' of biomedicine that could be included in the curricula of medical schools, and make the argument for inviting experts from China redundant.

Instead of understanding CM as a clear-cut object or system that, owing to its 'talent for globalisation', smoothly travels from region to region and era to era, we showed in this chapter how, in its different versions, CM has been brought to life in the changing socio-material, economic, and political conditions of the post/socialist CR, while partly also reconfiguring them. It is all three complex, partially connected but at times conflicting versions that have made CM a vivid reality in the country.

Acknowledgements Work on the chapter was supported by grant no. 15-16452S awarded by the Czech Science Foundation. We would like to thank the editors of this volume for their invaluable comments on earlier versions of this chapter.

Notes

1. A note on terminology. In this chapter, we use the term Chinese medicine (CM) to mean the generic notion most often used in scholarly literature. We talk about 'TCM' (from 'Traditional Chinese Medicine') to refer to the version of CM exported currently worldwide by the Chinese state. Later, we will introduce 'traditional CM' and 'medical acupuncture' to denote two other versions of CM in the CR that we will extensively discuss in this chapter. As we will show these versions are to some extent related but are also significantly different in some respects.

2. Our fieldwork involves participant observation in a thriving private CM clinic that we refer to here as 'Zdraví' and in the private surgery of a GP who uses various CAM treatments including CM in her practice. We also participated in a number of meetings and events connected with the Czech-Chinese initiative in the current top-down introduction of TCM into the CR. We attended a two-semester course in CM for medical students at a public university, and we conducted over 30 interviews with Czech CM practitioners, representatives of the Czech Chamber of TCM, healthcare managers and officials involved in the Czech-Chinese initiative, and CM patients. Our efforts to grasp current developments also include a close reading of relevant legal and policy documents and of the debates on the subject in the media. We present data from observation and research interviews in anonymised form.

3. Originally part of the Physiatrist Society during socialism, Czech Medical Acupuncture Society (CMAS) was granted an independent status within the Czech Medical Association of J. E. Purkyně, the main self-governing and voluntary association of professional societies in Czech biomedicine, shortly after 1989. In the first half of the 1990s, with a few thousand members, it was one of the five largest societies within the Association. With the new law in 1997 that removed acupuncture from the services covered under public health insurance, together with various criticisms from within the Czech Medical Association and also from outside (mainly from an influential club of 'sceptics' called 'Sisyfos', combating 'irrationality' and 'pseudoscience' in Czech science and medicine), CMAS was forced in 2002 to close two of its most scientifically contentious divisions: for electroacupuncture and auriculotherapy. In their place, CMAS established a new department for 'the study of diagnostics and therapy in acupuncture and related techniques using research based on EBM'

(Pára 2006b: 6). After that, the number of members of the CMAS dropped significantly; currently, CMAS has around 500 members.

4. See also the Czechoslovak public television commercial from 1982 promoting the home use of Stimul 3 and providing information about its production on an industrial scale, available at http://www.ceskatelevize.cz/ivysilani/10116288585-archiv-ct24/215411058210004/obsah/376504-stimul-3-elektroakupunktura-1982 (accessed on 5 February 2017).

5. In addition, Act No. 95/2004 Coll., on the Conditions for the Acquisition and Recognition of the Professional Qualifications of Doctor, Dentist, and Pharmacist, and Act No. 96/2004 Coll., on the Conditions for the Acquisition and Recognition of the Professional Qualifications of Non-Medical Healthcare Professions, both stipulate that only a person with a biomedical degree can provide medical services that puncture the surface of the skin (such as acupuncture).

6. In January 2017, Pojišťovna VZP, a. s., established in 2004 as a subsidiary company of the biggest public health insurance company in the country, offering commercial insurance of foreigners, announced it would newly cover TCM services provided by Beijing Tong Ren Tang Czech Republic SE (Pojišťovna VZP, a. s. 2017). This might be seen as a pilot step testing the possibilities of TCM coverage by the public health insurance.

References

Anderson, K. T. (2010). Holistic medicine not "torture": Performing acupuncture in Galway, Ireland. *Medical Anthropology, 29*(3), 253–277.

Andrews, B. (2014). *The making of modern Chinese medicine, 1850–1960.* Vancouver: University of British Columbia Press.

Baer, H. A. (2007). The drive for legitimation in Chinese medicine and acupuncture in Australia: Successes and dilemmas. *Journal of Evidence-Based Complementary & Alternative Medicine, 12*(2), 87–98.

Baer, H. A., Jen, C., Tanassi, L. M., Tsia, C., & Wahbeh, H. (1998). The drive for professionalization in acupuncture: A preliminary view from the San Francisco Bay area. *Social Science and Medicine, 46*(4–5), 533–537.

Barnes, L. L. (2003). The acupuncture wars: The professionalizing of American acupuncture—A view from Massachusetts. *Medical Anthropology, 22*(3), 261–301.

Candelise, L. (2011). Chinese medicine outside of China: The encounter between Chinese medical practices and conventional medicine in France and Italy. *China Perspectives, 3*, 43–50.

Chan, K., & Lee, H. (Eds.). (2002). *The way forward for Chinese medicine*. London and New York: Taylor and Francis.

Cikrt, T. (2015). *Protestuji proti invazi čínského šarlatánství do českého zdravotnictví* [I protest against the invasion of charlatanism to the Czech healthcare system]. *Zdravotnický deník, 17*(6). Retrieved February 5, 2017, from http://www.zdravotnickydenik.cz/blog/protestuji-proti-invazi-cinskeho-sarlatanstvi-do-ceskeho-zdravotnictvi.

CMA JEP. (2015). *Articles of association, rules of procedures, election regulations of Czech Medical Association of Jan Evangelista Purkyně*. Prague: CMA JEP. Retrieved February 5, 2017, from http://www.cls.cz/bylaws-of-association.

De Laet, M., & Mol, A. (2000). The Zimbabwe bush pump: Mechanics of a fluid technology. *Social Studies of Science, 30*(2), 225–263.

Dew, K. (2000). Deviant insiders: Medical acupuncturists in New Zealand. *Social Science and Medicine, 50*(12), 1785–1795.

DVTV. (2015). *Čínská medicína funguje proti bolesti, léčí celek, výhrady pramení z neznalosti, říká lékař* [Chinese medicine works against pain, it is holistic, reservations stem from ignorance]. *DVTV*, 6 November. Retrieved February 5, 2017, from http://video.aktualne.cz/dvtv/cinska-medicina-leci-celek-funguje-proti-bolesti-vyhrady-pra/r~c7e1308283ed11e5b286002590604f2e.

DVTV. (2016). *Kmoníček: Státy EU nám chtěly zabránit získat čínské investice, Čína předefinovala slovo komunista* [Kmoníček: EU countries wanted to prevent us from gaining Chinese investments. China redefined the word the communist]. *DVTV*, 1 April. Retrieved February 5, 2017, from http://video.aktualne.cz/dvtv/kmonicek-cina-zcela-predefinovala-obsah-slova-komunista-komu/r~157b2d04f76911e5a652002590604f2e.

Fabian, J. (1983). *Time and the other: How anthropology makes its object*. New York: Columbia University Press.

Fiala, P. (2010). Přepsané dějiny akupunktury? [Rewritten history of acupuncture?]. *Acupunctura Bohemo Slovaca, 2–3*, 4–8.

Flesch, H. (2013). A foot in both worlds: Education and the transformation of Chinese medicine in the United States. *Medical Anthropology, 32*(1), 8–24.

Fürst, R. (Ed.). (2015). *Čína znovu objevuje bývalou východní Evropu: Důvod k radosti či obavám?* [China rediscovers the former Eastern Europe: A reason for joy or worry?], Policy Paper. Prague: The Institute for International relations.

Hanson, M. (1998). Robust northerners and delicate southerners: The nineteenth-century invention of a southern *wenbing* tradition. *Positions: East Asia Cultures Critique, 6*(3), 515–549.

Háva, P., & Mašková-Hanušová, P. (2009). Zdravotní politika visegrádských zemí (1) [Healthcare policy in Visegrad Group countries (1)]. *Zdravotnictví v České republice, 12*(1), 12–21.

Hsu, E. (2009). Chinese propriety medicines: An "alternative modernity?" The case of the anti-malarial substance artemisinin in East Africa. *Medical Anthropology, 28*(2), 111–140.

Hsu, E. (2015). From social lives to playing fields: 'The Chinese antimalarial' as artemisnin monotherapy, artemisinin combination therapy and qinghao juice. *Anthropology & Medicine, 22*(1), 75–86.

Křížová, M. (Ed.). (2004). *Alternativní medicína jako problém* [Alternative medicine as a problem]. Praha: Karolinum.

Křížová, M. (2015). *Alternativní medicína v České republice* [Alternative medicine in the Czech Republic]. Prague: Karolinum.

Langwick, S. (2010). From non-aligned medicines to market-based herbals: China's relationship to the shifting politics of traditional medicine in Tanzania. *Medical Anthropology, 29*(1), 15–43.

Law, J., & Singleton, V. (2005). Object lesson. *Organization, 12*(3), 331–355.

Lieber, M. (2012). Practitioners of traditional Chinese medicine in Switzerland: Competing justifications for cultural legitimacy. *Ethnic and Racial Studies, 35*(4), 757–775.

Lin, W., & Law, J. (2014). A correlative STS: Lessons from a Chinese medical practice. *Social Studies of Science, 44*(6), 801–824.

Mach, J. (2016, April). ČLK k působení čínských lékařů v české nemocnici [Czech medical chamber on the practice of Chinese physicians in a Czech hospital]. *Tempum medicorum*, 16–17.

MacPherson, H., et al. (2016). Unanticipated insights into biomedicine from the study of acupuncture. *The Journal of Alternative and Complementary Medicine, 22*(2), 101–107.

Ministerstvo zdravotnictví. (1976). *Návrh metodického opatření k zabezpečení jednotného postupu při provádění akupunktury: Důvodová zpráva* [Proposal of methodological guidelines for the unified procedure of acupuncture application: Statement of Justification]. Prague: Ministry of Health.

Mol, A. (2002). *The body multiple: Ontology in medical practice*. Durham: Duke University Press.

Mol, A., & Law, J. (1994). Regions, networks and fluids: Anaemia and social topology. *Social Studies of Science, 24*(4), 641–671.

Pára, F. (2006a). Historie České lékařské akupunkturistické společnosti ČLS JEP (org. č. 60)—Část II [History of Czech Medical Acupuncture Society CMA JEP—II. part]. *Acupunctura Bohemo Slovaca, 3*, 2–3.

Pára, F. (2006b). Historie České lékařské akupunkturistické společnosti ČLS JEP (org. č. 60)—Část III [History of Czech Medical Acupuncture Society CMA JEP—III. part]. *Acupunctura Bohemo Slovaca, 3,* 4–6.

Pára, F. (2015). *Historie vzniku a rozvoje akupunktury v České a Slovenské republice I., II* [History of the birth and genesis of acupuncture in the Czech and Slovak Republic, I, II]. Unpublished presentation.

Pára, F., & Barešová, M. (2006). Historie České lékařské akupunkturistické společnosti ČLS JEP (org. č. 60)—Část I [History of Czech Medical Acupuncture Society CMA JEP—I. part]. *Acupunctura Bohemo Slovaca, 1-2,* 3–4.

Pojišťovna VZP, a.s. (2017). *Pojišťovna VZP, a. s. nově hradí i Tradiční čínskou medicínu* [Pojišťovna VZP, a. s. starts covering also Traditional Chinese medicine]. Press release, 27 January. Retrieved February 5, 2017, from https://www.pvzp.cz/cs/tiskova-zprava/pojistovna-vzp-a-s-nove-hradi-i-tradicni-cinskou-medicinu.

Pokam De Prince, H. (2011). Chinese medicine in Cameroon. *China Perspectives, 3,* 51–58.

Pritzker, S. E. (2010). The part of me that wants to grab: Embodied experience and living translation in U.S. Chinese medical education. *Ethos, 39*(3), 95–413.

Radioforum. (2016, April 6). *Czech public broadcast.*

Sagli, G. (2010). The establishing of Chinese medical concepts in Norwegian acupuncture schools: The cultural translation of jingluo ('circulation tracts'). *Anthropology & Medicine, 17*(3), 315–326.

Saltman, R. B., & Figueras, J. (1997). *European health care reform. Analysis of current strategies.* Copenhagen: WHO Regional Publications.

Scheid, V. (2002). *Chinese medicine in contemporary China: Plurality and synthesis.* Durham: Duke University Press.

Scheid, V. (2007). *Currents of tradition in Chinese medicine, 1626–2006.* Seattle: Eastland Press.

Shambaugh, D. (2013). *China goes global: The partial power.* Oxford: Oxford University Press.

Stengers, I. (2010). *Cosmopolitics I.* Minneapolis: University of Minnesota Press.

Strathern, M. (1991). *Partial connections.* Savage, MD: Rowman and Littlefield.

Tesla. (1982). *Stimul 3, přenosné kapesní zařízení pro aplikaci elektroakupunktury: Návod na použití* [User manual for a portable pocket device for the application of electroacupuncture Stimul 3]. Liberec: Tesla.

Úřad pro vynálezy a osvědčení v Praze. (1982). *Autorské osvědčení 196653* [Patent authorship certification No. 196653]. Prague: The National Office for Inventions and Standardization.

Vymazal, J., & Tuháček, M. (1965). *Akupunktura: teoretická i praktická studie se zaměřením k neurologii* [Acupunture: Study of theory and practice with respect to neurology]. Prague: Státní zdravotnické nakladatelství.

Zhan, M. (2009). *Other-worldly: Making Chinese medicine through transnational frames*. Durham, London: Duke University Press.

Zhang, Y. (2007). *Transforming emotions with Chinese medicine: An ethnographic account from contemporary China*. Albany, NY: SUNY Press.

3

The Incompatibility Between Social Worlds in Complementary and Alternative Medicine: The Case of Therapeutic Touch

Pia Vuolanto

Introduction

This chapter scrutinises one local controversy over one modality of complementary and alternative medicine (CAM), the treatment or tradition of 'therapeutic touch' (TT). In TT, the practitioner does not touch the patient but holds his or her hands above them. The energy fields activated in this way are supposed to cure the patient. This treatment caused a controversy in the mid-1990s in Finland. A book based on a master's thesis in nursing science (Rautajoki 1996) promoted its use in nursing. The book's publisher received the Finnish Association of Sceptics' annual Humbug Award. The master's thesis had achieved a good grade at a Finnish university's department of nursing science. In the wake of the Humbug Award, scholars in the department reacted abruptly and officially banned certain books and theories that could be connected with TT. A lively debate followed in which complementary and alternative

P. Vuolanto (✉)
School of Social Sciences and Humanities,
University of Tampere, Tampere, Finland

© The Author(s) 2018
C. Brosnan et al. (eds.), *Complementary and Alternative Medicine*, Health,
Technology and Society, https://doi.org/10.1007/978-3-319-73939-7_3

therapies were both challenged and defended by many different actors. The debate started in late 1996 and gradually faded away after few months at the end of summer 1997.

TT could be characterised as a 'non-contact' healing intervention (Wirth et al. 1993) or a 'non-invasive' nursing technique (Daley 1997) because it is intrinsic to this treatment that the nurse does not touch the patient but holds his or her hands above them. It is described as starting with the nurse 'centring' on disturbances in the energy fields of the patient's body. Next, the nurse assesses the patient's body from a distance of five to ten centimetres and then makes the intervention, which 'repatterns' the patient's energy field (O'Mathúna et al. 2002: 164; Rosa et al. 1998: 1005; Krieger 1979). This treatment method originated in the work of Dolores Krieger, a Professor of Nursing, and Dora Kunz, who is referred to as a 'lay healer and clairvoyant' in literature that presents the treatment as speculative and questionable (O'Mathúna et al. 2002: 163).

The Finnish controversy, which occurred 20 years ago, is an example of debates that frequently erupt around CAM in universities, within the media in different countries, for example, Australia, the United Kingdom and Canada (Brosnan 2015; Givati and Hatton 2015; Derkatch 2016; Caldwell 2017). TT is associated with the category of CAM and is highly controversial. For example, in the mid-1990s, it was brought up in the *Journal of the American Medical Association* (JAMA) (e.g. Rosa et al. 1998; Carpenter et al. 1998: 1905). There was a lively discussion in JAMA, comprising a TT research article and responses to it by medical practitioners, nurses, therapists and researchers from different fields in the United States. One of the most prominent nursing research journals, the *Journal of Advanced Nursing*, also published a debate around the same time, including discussants from the Unites States, the United Kingdom and Ireland (Daley 1997; Turner et al. 1998; O'Mathúna 1998; Meehan 1998).

The significance of the debate over TT is indicated by the fact that it also took place in Finland, quite far from the centres where nursing theory and TT were being developed at the time. TT was discussed in Finland in the mid-1990s, in particular. In Finland, nursing was brought into universities from 1979 onwards.[1] The lack of domestic theory and research resulted in a lot of influence being imported from abroad, particularly from the United States (Ollikainen 1996a). Nursing theories were imported and discussed actively, including work by the US nursing scholars Rogers and Parse, both of whom are associated with TT. Parse's theoretical work synthesising Rogers' theory was especially popular in Finland. Parse visited Finland in 1996 and again in 1997, and courses on her theory were organised in polytechnics (e.g. Henttonen 1996). To further the interaction with American scholars, at least one Finnish polytechnic also organised a trip to the Parse Scholars Seminar in the United States.

In science and technology studies (STS), CAM has been seen as an 'escape from medicine' (Webster 2007: 147). It has also been connected with the changing role of patients, who bring lay knowledges based on 'social ideas, religious beliefs, situated experiences and specific worldviews' (Wilcox 2010: 55) into play alongside scientifically proven knowledge in order to care for themselves as responsible 'health consumers' (Wyatt et al. 2010). The intention of this chapter is to add greater nuance to the understanding of CAM controversies and to help to discern the meanings different societal actors attach to these debates. I analyse the TT controversy by using the social worlds framework from STS. I aim to identify the multiple social worlds involved in defining CAM. My starting point is that when social worlds define CAM in a controversy, they are simultaneously also expressing their perceptions of science and technology.

The focus of this chapter is on how different actors from different social worlds understood TT and other CAM modalities, and what these different understandings made of knowledge, science and technology. As the patients themselves were silent, the controversy can also shed light on how the role of patients was understood in the different social worlds. The research question is: how was CAM understood in different social worlds in the controversy over TT, and what do these understandings reveal about the perceptions of science, technology and the patient role in these social worlds?

Theoretical and Methodological Issues

Studies that follow the social worlds framework begin by identifying the key individuals and social groups that are active around a social issue (Clarke and Star 2008). Social worlds are formed by individuals, social groups or sides that care about the issue so much that they are prepared to act in a controversy situation (Clarke and Montini 1993: 44). These include not only established collective actors such as organisations, institutions or social movements but also distinguishable actors who have their own perspectives on the issue and who are in different ways committed to action on the controversy (Clarke and Star 2008: 116). They each form unique 'universes of discourse' (Clarke and Star 2008: 116; Shibutani 1955: 567). The focus is on the 'multiplicities of perspective' of these different social worlds (Clarke and Montini 1993: 45).

The identification of social worlds involves tracing the primary activity of those worlds and the aims they further in the controversy (Strauss 1978: 122). The next step is to analyse whether some of the social worlds intersect with others or are segmented into specifiable sub-worlds (Strauss 1978: 122–123). Social worlds are fluid by nature rather than being static groups (Shibutani 1955: 567; Strauss 1978: 123). They may be perceptible in one controversy situation, but in a different controversy the social worlds might be formed differently. Also, actors or groups that form a social world can participate in it from different perspectives. Some actors might be very focused on the issue and include the social world as a major component of their identity, whereas others might have only a basic understanding of the issue or might be sympathetic towards the social world without being fully engaged in it (Unruh 1979: 122).

Importantly, for CAM controversies, the social worlds framework attempts to find actors who are not 'present' in the sense that they will take action, but who are implicated through the actions of the other actors (Clarke and Montini 1993: 45; Clarke and Star 2008: 119). These 'silent implicated actors' do not necessarily voice their own opinions or otherwise take active part in the controversy (Clarke and Star 2008: 119; Christensen and Casper 2000: S95). Instead, the other actors make assumptions about their role and stakes in it.

I see the social worlds framework as an approach through which to understand the various views on science and technology that emerged during the controversy over TT: at the same time as making CAM understandable for themselves, the actors in this controversy were also making sense of science and were working the boundary between science and other knowledge systems (Vuolanto 2015), that is, doing boundary work

(Gieryn 1999). These debates also encompassed silent actors—the patients—whose role was implicated by the different social worlds in many different ways. The concrete and rhetorical actions taken during the controversy had consequences for patients in their everyday lives. I use the social worlds framework because it helps me to scrutinise CAM controversies, which involve multiple social worlds, each of which formulates its relationship to and understanding of CAM, evidence-based medicine, science and technology, and the patient role in different ways.

I have identified five social worlds in the TT controversy: scepticism, medicine, nursing research, nursing and TT—with patients as silent implicated actors. Scepticism will be the first social world analysed in this chapter, because the controversy was started by actors in this world. This social world was motivated to protect the scientific worldview, and for them the book on TT broke the boundaries of scientific medical knowledge. Next, I will analyse a social world closely connected with the first, namely medicine, for which the cure of patients and alleviation of suffering were the primary motivations for participating in the controversy. They started their action with evidence-based knowledge about cures, which intersected with the first social world. The third social world discussed will be nursing research, which was reacting to the initiative of the scepticism world because the master's thesis had come from within it. In this social world, I found one clearly specifiable sub-world, that of former university researchers in nursing.

The fourth social world, nursing, is the world of professionals who aimed to understand the knowledge produced by nursing research. This social world illustrates the fluidity of the social worlds: in another controversy situation, the nurses could perhaps have been identified with the same world as nursing research, but here I will demonstrate nurses' ambivalence towards 'their science' (Nieminen 2008) during the controversy. The last social world that I identified was that of TT. In my analysis, this social world demonstrates that one single actor can represent a broader social world if the actor in question is an insider to that social world. I will analyse the actions of a single therapist who was very committed to this social world and of whose identity it formed a major part.

The research material that I draw on here consists of documentary material (the evaluation statements on the master's thesis and minutes of meetings in the university department) and discussion material (discussions in newspapers and in popular, professional and scientific journals). I aimed to cover all the material from the controversy in 1996–1997, in all its forums. I identified the social worlds through deep reading of the material in the tradition of the rhetoric of science (Fahnestock 2009; Segal 2009). I have picked out some quotes from the material to illustrate the rhetoric of each social world. All the material was in Finnish, and I have translated it.

Social Worlds in the Controversy over Therapeutic Touch

Scepticism

I approached the social world of scepticism through sceptics' writings. The first of these was the Finnish Association of Sceptics' statement on their annual Humbug Award. The controversy started when a book promoting the use of TT in nursing was published (Rautajoki 1996). The book's publisher received the Humbug Award. This award is meant to be an indication of poor and unscientific research. The Association of Finnish Sceptics is an organised manifestation of the scepticism movement, which gathers together laypeople and university researchers and professors. In 1996, the association's advisory board contained at least one physicist, two philosophers, a biologist, two theologians and one medical specialist, to name just a few of the disciplines represented. Their statement on the decision to give the Humbug Award to the publisher of the book on TT was frank in style, as in this excerpt:

> The association considers that Kirjayhtymä [the publisher of the book on TT] has blurred the boundary between literature intended for healthcare education and pseudoscientific literature by giving a platform to this kind of work in a book series of education and professional literature aimed at social and healthcare professionals … The therapy described in the book is a typical alternative treatment which mixes ethereal energy flows, gem therapy, cosmic dimensions, telepathy, distance healing, vibration frequencies, and other concepts belonging to so-called New Age thinking. (Statement 1996: 10)

In addition to this statement, I used three texts from the secretary of the association for my analysis of this social world. The sceptics were concerned about the reputation of science, which in their view would be damaged by the publication of books on topics such as TT; this kind of activity would tarnish the authority of science.

The social world of scepticism conceptualised therapies such as TT as 'New Age thinking', 'mythical belief', 'mysticism' and 'pseudoscience' (Statement 1996: 10–11). TT, in the sceptics' world, was dissociated from science and conceived as fraudulent and unscientific knowledge. It was characteristic of such therapies that they were formulated by blending different knowledge traditions. Thus, the book on TT was identified as an 'incredible mixture of misapprehensions of concepts from physics and mystifications' (Statement 1996: 10), formulated out of 'evolutionary theories, system theories, oriental philosophies and quantum physics' (Ollikainen 1996b: 38). For the sceptics, the mixing of elements from these different and mismatched knowledge traditions was an indication of unscientific knowledge. The sceptics especially associated TT with nursing science because the book was based on a master's thesis in that discipline. The fact that the book also used theories familiar from nursing science, such as Rogers and Parse, strengthened this impression for them.

For the social world of scepticism, science was represented by biomedicine and natural science in their purest forms. According to the sceptics, 'constant vigilance and critical thought' (Statement 1996: 11) were needed to prevent unscientific knowledge from attacking the authority of science and staining its reputation. Nursing science should follow the same criteria as the other sciences and should use technologies and develop techniques based on scientifically reliable knowledge. The sceptics picked up Kirlian photography as an example of a technology used to support the efficacy of TT. They argued in their statement: 'It is claimed that the invisible energy field can be visualised by, among other things, Kirlian photography, even though in research this method has been proven invalid' (Statement 1996: 10). Unlike the STS frame (Webster 2007: 147), the scepticism world did not frame this technology as an escape from medicine, which would require a conscious choice between different technologies—in this case, presumably, old and new technologies. Rather, the scepticism world saw it as the result of unawareness of the knowledge produced in medicine and of the laws of natural science.

From the viewpoint of the social world of sceptics, this lack of awareness of modern technology required immediate popular enlightenment, and thus was connected to one of the core tasks of the scepticism movement: to keep the population informed of the latest scientific and technological developments (Forstorp 2005).

For the sceptics, patients were in a vulnerable position. They could be easily tricked by marketing and quackery into trying various potentially harmful health treatments. The sceptics' message was that patients should place their trust in science and medical professionals. They wondered 'what would happen to patient safety if this kind of treatment were to be put into operation in official healthcare, even on a small scale' (Ollikainen 1996a: 15). Responsibility for patient care lay with the professionals and purveyors of professional knowledge, that is, academic publishing houses; patients were to be protected by them. The patients themselves were to have limited responsibility for their own health and a restricted choice of treatments. The treatments that patients could choose should be dependent on the professionals' assessment and the endorsement provided by scientific knowledge. The sceptics took on the role of enlightening the population as to the superiority of the scientific worldview: the population must be told loud and clear what treatments one should choose, what the principles of good care are and on what basis the treatments can be trusted. The sceptics saw nurses as a vulnerable part of the population, likely to be tricked into practising TT if they were to buy this book from a supposedly reputable publisher.

Medicine

My analysis of the social world of medicine is based on the writings of two medical specialists. They wrote two articles together, one for the *Finnish Medical Journal* and one for the journal of the Finnish Association of Sceptics. They introduced their position in the controversy over TT as follows:

In healthcare, the official medication is based on medicine and its evidence as to the efficacy and safety of the treatment. Belief medication, comprised of different kinds of teachings from folklore cures to New Age therapies, works on different grounds. The boundary between official medication and belief medication is not always clear. TT is an example of this blurry boundary: it is a phenomenon containing many characteristics of belief medication and originating in the United States. However, there are claims that TT is based on science, especially on nursing science. (Saano and Puustinen 1997a: 2306)

The medical specialists were concerned that the work of medical practitioners would not be seen as grounded in the methods and principles of science. In this way, they stressed the connection between science and their practical work.

In this social world, the main conceptualisation of the group of therapies that includes TT was 'belief medication' in both of the texts by the medical specialists. They also used the concepts 'pseudoscience', 'nonscience' and 'philosophy of life', characterising the book on TT, for instance, as a 'philosophy-of-life book typical of the New Age ethos' (Saano and Puustinen 1997b: 30). In their writings, the medical specialists linked TT with Martha Rogers, the nursing theorist who for them represented a 'typical New Age framework' that lumps together 'incommensurate conceptual systems' (Saano and Puustinen 1997b: 30).

For the social world of medicine, evidence-based medicine was the ideal type of science. They emphasised the 'diagnostic and curative methods that are based on reliable evidence', and that there should be evidence of both the 'effect and safety' of treatments (Saano and Puustinen 1997a: 2306). Characteristics of science in this social world included 'modern technology, effective products, or precise physiological and biochemical effectiveness' (Saano and Puustinen 1997a: 2306). This was confirmed by presenting examples from the book on TT:

Rautajoki states: 'Clear-sighted people can see the colourful radiation of the human being, which, with practice, is clearly identifiable even at a metre's distance from the body surface.'

On the other hand, the concept of energy in TT is connected with medicine: 'Energy can also be measured with electroencephalography (EEG), electrocardiography (EKG) and electromyography (EMG), which reveal electronic currents in the brain, heart and muscles.' Rautajoki and the theorists of TT clearly do not understand what they are talking about here, but the content and context do not matter as long as belief medication's current favourite term, 'energy', is the same. (Saano and Puustinen 1997b: 32)

In this excerpt, a lack of knowledge about technology in the book on TT is demonstrated and used to identify the characteristics of science. The quotations critique Rautajoki for trying to sound medical and techno-logical, and for making mistakes in her attempt to use the natural-scientific knowledge base to support the claims of TT. Proponents of TT such as Rautajoki are being pushed out of science by this boundary work. In the social world of medicine, this boundary work generates the impres-sion that practising TT is an escape from medicine and medical technol-ogy, in the same way as Webster (2007: 147) interprets CAM within the STS frame.

So how was the role of patients implicated in this social world? The medical specialists emphasised the role of responsible service providers in the care of patients. Responsible service providers rely on 'modern tech-nology, effective products, or the effectiveness of precise physiological and biochemical processes' (Saano and Puustinen 1997a: 2306). The medical specialists implied that patients must be protected from treat-ments that did not use these starting points of evidence-based medicine. According to this view, patients must be shielded from all curative mech-anisms on the market that are not verified through randomised controlled trials and repeatable empirical research. Responsible service providers think about the benefit to patients:

The patients' benefit requires professionals to exercise criticality and be able to take the patient's side against various health teachings and devices. Professionals also recognise marketing strategies and see them coming from behind a smokescreen. (Saano and Puustinen 1997b: 35)

The role of patients here is to rely on expertise, science and medical treat-ments proven by medical research, stressing the role of technology and scientific knowledge. The patient's freedom of choice seems to be subor-dinated to medicine and its proofs of effective treatment. Responsibility for care seems to lie with experts.

Nursing Research

My analysis of the social world of nursing research is based on the writings of three nursing academics (all departmental committee members) at the University of Tampere (UTA), a professor of nursing science at the University of Helsinki and a professor of nursing science at University of Turku, all of whom put forward their views in journal and newspaper articles. In their announcement of the Humbug Award, which was published in major newspapers in Finland, the sceptics emphasised that the roots of the book could be traced to a master's thesis which had been completed at the department of nursing science at UTA. Following this, the nursing scholars on the nursing science departmental committee at UTA discussed the quality of their own teaching:

> The departmental committee decided that from now on any nursing science theses that contain mentions of or references to New Age ideology or Parse's theory will not be accepted.
> The departmental committee also decided that it is necessary to reinstate evaluators'. statements in master's theses before publication, so that the assessment and evaluation of the level of the work will be easier. The evaluators must also pay more attention than previously to the evaluation forms for master's theses. (Nursing Science Departmental Committee 1996)

The Humbug Award and the departmental committee's decision meant that, for a short while, the department became an arena of public controversy. Students in the department were perplexed by the decision to ban some books and theories, and the incumbent nursing scholars were forced to clarify the principles of nursing science to the sceptics, the general public and the students. The banning of books and theories served as a tool to protect science in a situation where the reputation of nursing science had become vulnerable; 20 years later, it is no longer officially in effect (Vuolanto 2013).

The incumbent nursing scholars conceptualised TT as an 'alternative therapy', 'New Age-based teaching' and 'flimflam' (Ollikainen 1996a: 14–15). In the views of the nursing scholars, the theoretical basis of TT was associated with Parse, whose work was labelled poor science and unscientific knowledge, as in this example:

Parse's own theory therefore emerges from a soup cooked up with the following ingredients: some existential-phenomenological concepts understood in the Parse way, some of Roger's concepts, and some of Parse's own thoughts, the philosophical origin of which is impossible to trace. (Nieminen 1996: 160)

In the social world of nursing research, the field of science to be discussed was nursing science. It appears that the position of the incumbent nursing scholars was to defend the reputation of nursing science, as is evident in this answer given by the UTA professor of nursing science during an interview: 'Scientific university teaching and research in nursing science in Finland is not on any level involved with astral planes, energy fields or energy exchange, and it completely dissociates itself from these' (Ollikainen 1996a: 13). These nursing scholars were worried about the reputation of their discipline. They were also concerned that the academic status of nursing science would be lowered in the eyes of scholars from other disciplines, particularly medicine. Their view of science was that it should be autonomous, free of beliefs and influence from outside. The professor of nursing science from the University of Helsinki drew a clear boundary between scientific knowledge and 'teachings' such as TT, and stated: 'What people believe in as the highest force of life is a totally different thing. It has nothing to do with science' (Ollikainen 1996b: 39). The incumbent nursing scholars had a protective view of science. In order to defend the position of academic knowledge production, they maintained that science was recognisable through specific technical procedures of research and technologies that used the principles of scientific knowledge-making.

The role of patients in the social world of nursing research was to have trust in scientific knowledge. Trust in scientific knowledge here was intended to protect the patient from being tricked into different kinds of therapy such as TT. The professor from the University of Helsinki stated: 'The whole concept of "TT" is misleading people. It does not imply energy fields, which in fact are in question here' (Ollikainen 1996b: 39). Thus, the role of patients was not to be part of knowledge production processes or to participate in research work but to passively absorb scientific knowledge and to trust treatments based on it. The professor from the University of Turku argued: 'In Finland all healthcare staff take as their starting point respect for patients and their individual needs' (Lauri 1996). Patients were therefore to entrust the decision-making to experts and their scientifically proven knowledge. In this social world, individual care and the importance of looking at the overall situation of patients were taken as self-evident principles of nursing, but authority over the patient lay with the experts.

In this social world, I also identified one sub-world represented by former university researchers in nursing. The controversy engaged some people who had formerly been university researchers but had moved on to other institutions or retired. In particular, it involved two nursing scholars who had formerly worked at UTA. One of them had retired a little before the controversy, giving up her administrative duties and professorial status. She had been the professor of nursing science at UTA when the master's thesis on TT was accepted but had not been actively involved in the process, either as a supervisor or as an examiner. After retirement, she wrote a great deal and participated in ethical discussions inside the nursing profession, for instance, by running a Q&A column in Finland's professional nursing journal. In this column, she commented as an outsider on the departmental committee's decision to ban certain books:

> Constructing such a vague norm for literature used in master's theses hints at an internal crisis in the department. The researchers who supervise the theses do not have the open discussion and enthusiastic scientific argumentation that is often found in a vibrant research community. Having an open discussion of the issues in this situation would be a better decision than setting a vague external norm. (Kalkas 1997: 32)

Another former university researcher had moved to a government research institute in order to conduct research that would be more focused on policymaking and more tied with everyday political action than university research. She had been the examiner of the master's thesis on TT. Due to this former role, she was asked to comment on the controversial book on TT in the University of Helsinki's newspaper.

This researcher conceptualised TT and other therapies very differently from the incumbent nursing scholars. She called them 'alternative treatments', but when we look at her comment, it seems that she regarded them quite open-mindedly, not giving them the connotations of 'flimflam' or 'New Age-based teaching' invoked by the incumbent nursing scholars:

> The official healthcare system has not cast much of an eye over these kinds of alternative treatment and they have not even been taken as topics for research in a serious way. Anyway, we who come from nursing science do encounter people who use these treatments. Therefore I think that additional knowledge should be acquired about them by means of research. Thus it should be investigated why people use these treatments and what they get from them that official healthcare cannot offer, she says. (Ollikainen 1996b: 39)

The retired professor aimed her critique at the departmental committee's decision and questioned the use of the term 'New Age' in relation to TT and other therapies:

> In this case, the decision, at least the part concerning the New Age movement, is hard to follow, because the concept does not have an unambiguous meaning ... The question at issue is a common term for a diversity of phenomena, the philosophical starting points and worldviews of which differ in one way or another from the established, for example, Christian mindset. New Age phenomena include, for instance, yoga, shamanism, different 'holistic' healthcare methods, some feminist views, vegetarianism etc. (Kalkas 1997: 32)

Inside this sub-world of nursing research, the conceptualisations of therapies such as TT seemed to be more inclusive and understanding than those of the incumbent nursing scholars. These conceptualisations also came with a different view of science: the former university researchers did not emphasise 'science' or 'scientific knowledge' in the same way as the incumbent nursing scholars, nor did they seek to defend nursing science's reputation. They talked more often of 'research'. It seems that from their point of view it was important to defend the diversity of perspectives in nursing research. They seemed to emphasise that it would be harmful for one view to emerge as the most important in research and for other views to be silenced by the departmental committee. The researcher from a research institute suggested that alternative treatments should be taken as topics for research 'in a serious way'.

Both of these former university researchers strongly emphasised the interaction between research and society. One of them suggested that research was needed on the different treatments used by patients, while the retired professor argued:

> Many issues of clinical nursing practice are problems that cannot be researched without recognising the researcher's own experiences and the personal experiences of the patient or long-term personal observations within nursing practice. (Kalkas 1997: 32)

Contrary to the views of the incumbent nursing scholars, in this sub-world of nursing research, the implicated silent patients had personal experiences and a diversity of worldviews that they used to make choices regarding their own health and well-being. The patients were understood as independently choosing from a variety of healthcare modalities. There was no authoritative position above the patients which could be given to some other actor such as a doctor or nurse. Thus, the patients' role was to take responsibility for their own healthcare, and in this task their own experiences were seen as valuable.

Nursing

My analysis of the social world of nursing is based on a variety of materials: (1) two book reviews in the journal of Finland's nursing trade union, (2) seven advertisements for books and seminars in the journal of the nurses' national professional association, (3) one article in a Finnish local newspaper, (4) one article in a health journal, and (5) one article in a UTA student newspaper. Many of the nurses involved were referred to anonymously. Even though they had been interviewed in journals, they had requested that their names should not be mentioned. Some of the nurses wrote under their own names, as in the case of the book reviews.

Some of the professionals involved had continued their studies by entering nursing science programmes at university after gaining their professional qualifications at polytechnics. This is typical of nurse education in Finland. As a kind of further education, there are also courses offered by different educational institutions, such as summer universities. Summer universities are located in regions that do not have a university, or else are directly tied to local universities. They are owned jointly by municipalities and universities, and organise both university-level courses and professional education courses. Professor Parse visited one of the summer universities in Finland in May 1996 and delivered professional education to nurses before the Humbug Award in December 1996. According to a local newspaper, approximately 600 nurses attended her lecture at a national conference of nursing (Henttonen 1996: 1). Her books were also translated into Finnish at that time, which is a sign of the popularity of her books and theories. In the year following the Humbug Award, Parse visited Finland again, but the conference did not attract much attention.

In the social world of nursing, TT and other therapies were conceptualised in many ways. Some of the nurses had not made the connection between TT and Parse, and they defended Parse's theory as one of those that could be used in professional work: 'I was listening to Parse last summer when she was introducing her theory and her research method at the national conference of nursing science. At that time, this was a question of one theoretical approach to patient care' (Kalkas 1997: 32; question by anonymous 'Perplexed bystander'). One nurse was ambivalent about how to conceptualise TT after reading the book:

> Meditating in the middle of a working day is relaxing and rewarding for sure, but in our care communities using this treatment would give one a reputation as a 'crazy person'. However, what the heck, the book paints a picture of a novel, brave and boundary-breaking nurse who trusts her own and especially her patients' abilities. Is TT complete humbug, or at last a truly concrete theory amid the fashions that are so popular in nursing science nowadays? Read and decide for yourselves! (Lyyra 1997: 40)

Another nurse was critical of TT and wrote in her book review:

> As the text proceeds, the boundary between physical and non-physical touch becomes blurred ... It is unclear when physical touch is classified as therapeutic and when not. As a reader, I am not completely convinced that TT is the kind of holistic nursing where a person is taken into account as a whole and unique individual. (Routasalo 1997: 38)

Thus, nurses' conceptualisations of TT are varied, and in part exemplify the difficulties they had connecting TT with Parse's popular theories.

In the social world of nursing, the field of science to be discussed was nursing science. For nurses, science was a continuation of nurse education. Science was to serve the professionals' work, give it ideas and nourish it. The nurses were concerned that nursing science might be in tension with the principles of nursing practice: 'How do I learn to understand patients if I cannot be scientifically interested in their ideologies, even if those be New Age—whatever that is?' (Kalkas 1997: 32; question by anonymous 'Perplexed bystander'). Science should preserve the principles of good nursing practice and take them as guidelines for research. Thus, science should follow nursing practice, respecting the ideologies and lifestyles of patients and conducting research on them. In this social world, techniques, not technologies, of nursing practice in relation to touching were discussed.

Regardless of its ambivalence about therapies such as TT, this social world unanimously emphasised the role of patients as independent individuals making decisions about their own health. According to the newspaper report on the conference where Parse was teaching, the 'patient [was] the main character in the care situation' who was 'elevated as a king' (Henttonen 1996: 1, 4). The care situation was to be filled with the 'genuine presence' of the nurse and patient, and it was to be based on an equal interaction. The 'patient's wishes and evaluation abilities were at the centre' (Venäläinen 1997: 9), and the nurse was not to 'impose advice' or 'judge the patients' lifestyle' (Rantala 1997: 52). Thus, this social world emphasised patients' freedom of choice and their participation in decision-making.

Therapeutic Touch

I analysed the social world of TT through the work of one therapist, the one who wrote both the master's thesis on TT and the book on the same topic. She had been trained as a laboratory technician and subsequently had practised on a radiotherapy ward (Rautajoki 1993: 1). Following that, she had started studies in nursing science at university. During her studies, she participated in a reiki course, which according to her was the only way of studying treatments such as TT in Finland at that time (Rautajoki 1993: 96). She wrote her master's thesis based on a literature review of 65 nursing articles. The main topic of the articles was TT. The master's thesis was a conceptual analysis of the main themes of TT. As a nurse, she had used TT in patients' pain management (Rautajoki 1993: 1–2). Later, she also worked as a teacher of nurses at a polytechnic institute. She wrote a book about TT in a prestigious book series targeted at professional nurses. After the publisher was awarded the Humbug Award, the therapist wrote one article for a local newspaper in response to the incumbent nursing scholars and another for the University of Helsinki's newspaper. She was also interviewed in the University of Helsinki's newspaper by the secretary of the Finnish Association of Sceptics.

In her master's thesis, the therapist conceptualised TT as 'holistic nursing', 'non-traditional' and 'soft' treatment (Rautajoki 1993: 2). This was the only therapy she conceptualised, and she mainly referred to it by name. She did not produce categories such as CAM or New Age unlike some of the other actors. She wrote in her thesis:

> In Finland TT is an unknown concept in the area of official healthcare and for that reason it has not been studied in nursing science, but here too reiki therapy courses are being organised outside healthcare. (Rautajoki 1993: 1)

She analysed the main concepts of TT, such as 'energy', 'interaction' and 'touch', and studied what it is like as a treatment and what the roles of patient and nurse are in the practice of TT.

For this social world, the role of science was to analyse therapies such as TT and other phenomena. These 'should be dispassionately and open-mindedly analysed and researched, and not banned because the issue of energy fields or energy changes cannot yet be measured with current measuring tools' (Rautajoki 1997: 30). Through research, these therapies could also be legitimated: 'From the material, it was evident that TT is an accepted treatment in healthcare in other parts of the world' (Rautajoki 1997: 30). In this social world, research could be used to cultivate the discussion of different therapies that are used and popular among patients. In relation to the concept of 'energy' in her analysis of the TT literature, the therapist mixed elements from modern physics and Eastern mysticism, relying on work that attempts to discover parallels between the worldviews of physicists and mystics. In the master's thesis, she mostly used the work of Capra (1975). This indicates that science in this social world was used to support syncretist thinking, respecting the traditions of both physics and mysticism. It can also be interpreted as boundary work aimed at balancing between different worldviews: the therapist was closely involved and trained in the world of TT, but simultaneously she was also completing her master's thesis at university, and she was conscious of the tensions between these worlds (Rautajoki 1993: 103).

The limits of modern technology arose as an issue in this social world. Technology was brought up in the context of measuring the energy exchange during TT. The phenomena of TT 'cannot yet be measured' (Rautajoki 1997: 30), which indicates that the writer expected that in future the energy flows would also be measurable with modern technology. I interpret this type of argumentation as a willingness to work with, and stay in parallel with, the development of modern technologies rather than as an escape from technology or 'escape from medicine' in Webster's (2007) terms. The writer was convinced that technologies to study these phenomena had not yet been developed. For her, these phenomena were beyond the reach of technology, but she expected this to change in the future as modern technology developed further.

In this social world, for the patients, the therapist was a companion in an interaction that was based on a feeling of 'closeness' on the part of the patient and 'emphatic listening' on the part of the nurse (Rautajoki 1993: 25). The patient was an independent being seeking 'harmonisation' in his or her life (Rautajoki 1993: 103). This could be interpreted as argumentation targeted at general well-being rather than medical intervention (Webster 2007: 159). The therapist aimed to make it possible for the patient to choose between different therapies: patients themselves choose what is best for them. The therapist in this social world was concerned about the labelling of TT as humbug and the over-charging of patients. The patient in this social world was an autonomous thinker, a being who must be taken seriously and not labelled a 'hypo-chondriac' (Rautajoki 1993: 103). The therapist attempted to give the patient a central role in the choice between different therapies and treat-ments. This is in line with STS research arguing that lay knowledge is becoming stronger than expert views in current healthcare settings (Wilcox 2010: 54).

Conclusion

This chapter demonstrates the usefulness of the social worlds framework to study the under-researched area of CAM in STS. Christensen and Casper (2000: S98) sum up the contributions that the study of the social worlds of a controversy can bring: it can be used to examine the commu-nities through which specific issues enter scientific and public debate, to look outside the walls of science to other social worlds and to reveal the multiple meanings of the issues and their impact on various stakeholders. The rich controversy over TT revealed many parties that expressed their concerns and fears about TT and other therapies, and at the same time exposed their perceptions of science, technology and the patient role in healthcare. My analysis demonstrates that to see CAM only in juxtaposi-tion with medicine is to oversimplify the situation by neglecting the vari-ety of actors involved in defining CAM and disregarding the multiple meanings of CAM controversies and their impact on various stakehold-ers. My analysis has started to uncover the multiple communities through which CAM controversies enter scientific, public and professional debate. The controversy over TT demonstrates that it is possible that most com-munities participating in CAM controversies lie outside the walls of sci-ence, such as former university researchers, medical specialists, therapists and nurses—not to mention patients, who were silent and yet present.

The social worlds approach brings insight into the professional com-munities that participated in the controversy. It is interesting how differently from the professional community of nurses the professional community of medical specialists viewed their closest science, medicine. The way in which nurses understood and talked about their nearest discipline, nursing science, appeared to be an attempt to mould nursing science, whereas medical specialists took the authority of medicine for granted and built their position in the debate upon that authority (cf. Brosnan 2015). This may be due to the fact that during the debate over TT nursing science was still an emergent discipline, which had been rapidly academised, but which in Finland had only partially moved into universities, making the field prone to controversy (Vuolanto 2017). However, the professionals' relationship with science and knowledge might help us to begin to understand, as Garrety (1997: 758) proposes, 'why some voices are heard more clearly and loudly than others'. In light of my analysis, I consider it important that STS should recognise the diversity of voices and not interpret CAM controversies only in relation to medicine. Medicine has a strong voice in CAM controversies, and it is supported by powerful actors, such as the scepticism movement, that also attract attention in the media. This chapter illustrates that STS frameworks such as the social worlds approach have the potential to reach other forms of knowledge production, and other health professions as well.

Weaving an analysis of views of science and the patient role through an analysis of social worlds was revealing of the dynamics of the different communities. In this respect the social worlds of medicine, nursing research and scepticism differed from the other worlds. They accorded science power over the individual's health. Professionals were seen in these social worlds as experts who have the authority to make decisions about treatments on the basis of their ownership of scientific knowledge. Their reactions to the controversy support Webster's (2007: 146) view of CAM users as contesting the role of experts. In the TT controversy, medical specialists, incumbent nursing scholars and sceptics took this contest seriously, defended their authority and gave patients a minor role.

In the other social worlds and sub-worlds—former university researchers, nurses and therapists—the personal experiences, choices and participation of patients were emphasised much more. It seems that the actors that were closest to the patients were more inclined to give patients a voice. In particular, the social world of nursing, the sub-world of nursing research and the social world of TT appeared more willing to give patients an independent role in healthcare. This might be because in these social worlds it was natural to be loyal to the reference group (Shibutani 1955: 568) of patients. The other social worlds were more loyal to science and the scientific worldview. Another possible interpretation, closely related to this one, is that the social world of nursing, the sub-world of nursing research and the social world of TT were in a position where they could make compromises (Shibutani 1955: 568) and thus move between different social worlds more flexibly than the other social worlds. They could be seen as boundary agents, understanding patients from the position of nurses that are close to the healing traditions and different cultural understandings of health in the patients' world.

Helga Nowotny (1975: 43) highlights the cognitive incompatibilities in controversies in science. In the controversy studied here, the sides who were willing to commit themselves to commenting on TT and other therapies seem to come from incompatible social worlds. However, to study the social worlds of CAM more deeply would need much more research and broader material. There is also room for analysis of the hybrid understandings and anomalies that might appear within each social world if there were more actors involved than in this small and local controversy. The limited Finnish material presented here gives ideas for much broader future work on CAM controversies to deepen our understanding of each social world found here and to find even more social worlds involved in defining CAM in different cultural contexts.

Note

1. During the 1980s, nursing was institutionalised in seven Finnish universities. This was soon reduced to five, which continue their nursing programmes today. A special characteristic of Finland compared with other countries (Spitzer and Perrenoud 2006) is that professional nurses are not educated at universities but at the lower-level polytechnic institutes. University nursing curricula are intended to provide further education for nurses to become teachers, administrators and researchers, and to develop nursing research (Laiho 2012).

References

Brosnan, C. (2015). "Quackery" in the academy? Professional knowledge, autonomy and the debate over complementary medicine degrees. *Sociology, 49*(6), 1047–1064.

Caldwell, E. F. (2017). Quackademia? Mass-media delegitimation of homeopathy education. *Science as Culture.* https://doi.org/10.1080/09505431.2017.1316253

Capra, F. (1975). *The Tao of physics: An exploration of the parallels between modern physics and eastern mysticism.* Boston, MA: Shambhala Publications.

Carpenter, J., Hagemaster, J., & Joiner, B. (1998). To the editor. An even closer look at therapeutic touch. *JAMA, 280*(22), 1905.

Christensen, V. A., & Casper, M. J. (2000). Hormone mimics and disrupted bodies: Social worlds analysis of a scientific controversy. *Sociological Perspectives,* (Suppl.),: S93–S120.

Clarke, A., & Montini, T. (1993). The many faces of RU486: Tales of situated knowledges and technological contestations. *Science, Technology & Human Values, 18*(1), 42–78.

Clarke, A., & Star, S. L. (2008). The social worlds framework: A theory/methods package. In E. J. Hackett, O. Amsterdamska, M. Lynch, & J. Wajcman (Eds.), *The handbook of science and technology studies* (pp. 113–138). Cambridge, MA; London: MIT Press.

Daley, B. (1997). Therapeutic touch, nursing practice and contemporary cutaneous wound healing research. *Journal of Advanced Nursing, 25,* 1123–1132.

Derkatch, C. (2016). *Bounding biomedicine: Evidence and rhetoric in the new science of alternative medicine.* Chicago and London: University of Chicago Press.

Fahnestock, J. (2009). The rhetoric of the natural sciences. In A. A. Lunsford, K. H. Wilson, & R. A. Eberly (Eds.), *The SAGE handbook of rhetorical studies* (pp. 175–195). Los Angeles, London, New Delhi, Singapore, Washington, DC: SAGE Publications.

Forstorp, P. (2005). The construction of pseudo-science: Science patrolling and knowledge policing by academic prefects and weeders. *VEST, 18*(3–4), 17–71.

Garrety, K. (1997). Social worlds, actor-networks and controversy: The case of cholesterol, dietary fat and heart disease. *Social Studies of Science, 27*(5), 727–773.

Gieryn, T. F. (1999). *Cultural boundaries of science: Credibility on the line.* Chicago and London: The University of Chicago Press.

Givati, A., & Hatton, K. (2015). Traditional acupuncturists and higher education in Britain: The dual, paradoxical impact of biomedical alignment on the holistic view. *Social Science & Medicine, 131,* 173–180.

Henttonen, I. (1996, May 28). Health terror debated in Hämeenlinna. "Parseans" defend patient-centredness. *Hämeen sanomat.*

Kalkas, H. (1997). Ethical dilemma column "What are the ethics of research and teaching in nursing science like?" *Sairaanhoitaja* [Nurse], *70*(2), 32.

Krieger, D. (1979). *The therapeutic touch: How to use your hands to help or to heal.* New York: Prentice Hall Press.

Laiho, A. (2012). The evolving landscape of nursing science in the 21st century—The Finnish case. In P. Trowler, M. Saunders, & V. Bamber (Eds.), *Tribes and territories in the 21st century: Rethinking the significance of disciplines in higher education* (pp. 107–117). London and New York: Routledge.

Lauri, S. (1996, June 20). Nursing respecting the patient not new. *Helsingin sanomat.*

Lyyra, T. (1997). Therapeutic touch? *Tehy, 2,* 40.

Meehan, T. C. (1998). Therapeutic touch as a nursing intervention. *Journal of Advanced Nursing, 28*(1), 117–125.

Nieminen, H. (1996). Phenomenology, Parse and nursing science. *Hoitotiede* [Nursing Science], *8*(3), 158–161.

Nieminen, P. (2008). Caught in the science trap? A case study of the relationship between nurses and "their" science. In J. Välimaa & O. Ylijoki (Eds.), *Cultural perspectives on higher education* (pp. 127–141). New York: Springer.

Nowotny, H. (1975). Controversies in science: Remarks on the different modes of production of knowledge and their use. *Zeitschrift für Soziologie, 4*(1), 34–45.

Nursing Science Departmental Committee. (1996). Meeting minutes, 17 December. Nursing Science Departmental Committee, University of Tampere.

Ollikainen, M. (1996a). Humbug Award 1996: Humbug does not belong in nursing science: Interview with Professor Marita Paunonen. *Skeptikko* [Sceptic], *4*(96), 12–15.

Ollikainen, M. (1996b). Spiritual healing for nurses? *Yliopisto* [University], *20*(96), 38–39.

O'Mathúna, D. (1998). Janforum: Feedback—Therapeutic touch. *Journal of Advanced Nursing, 27*(1), 230.

O'Mathúna, D., Pryjmachuk, S., Spencer, W., Stanwick, M., & Matthiesen, S. (2002). A critical evaluation of the theory and practice of therapeutic touch. *Nursing Philosophy, 3*(2), 163–176.

Rantala, S. (1997). Philosophical theory of nursing. Book review of parse: Illuminations. *Tehy, 13,* 52.

Rautajoki, A. (1993). An analysis and a redefinition of the concept Therapeutic Touch. Master's thesis. University of Tampere, Department of Nursing Science.

Rautajoki, A. (1996). *Therapeutic touch.* Helsinki: Kirjayhtymä.

Rautajoki, A. (1997). Does nursing science scuttle its own teachings? *Yliopisto* [University], *2*(97), 29–30.

Rosa, L., Rosa, E., Sarner, L., & Barrett, S. (1998). A close look at therapeutic touch. *JAMA, 279*(13), 1005–1010.

Routasalo, P. (1997). Book review on Anja Rautajoki: Therapeutic touch. *Sairaanhoitaja* [Nurse], *70*(2), 38.

Saano, V., & Puustinen, R. (1997a). Belief medication—The new direction for nursing? The example of therapeutic touch. *Suomen lääkärilehti* [Finnish Medical Journal] *18–19,* 2306.

Saano, V., & Puustinen, R. (1997b). Humbug-awarded nursing teaching from the United States. *Skeptikko* [Sceptic], *1*(97), 30–35.

Segal, J. Z. (2009). Rhetoric of health and medicine. In A. A. Lunsford, K. H. Wilson, & R. A. Eberly (Eds.), *The SAGE handbook of rhetorical studies* (pp. 227–245). Los Angeles, London, New Delhi, Singapore, Washington, DC: SAGE Publications.

Shibutani, T. (1955). Reference groups as perspectives. *American Journal of Sociology, 60*(6), 562–569.

Spitzer, A., & Perrenoud, B. (2006). Reforms in nursing education across Western Europe: Implementation processes and current status. *Journal of Professional Nursing, 22*(3), 162–171.

Statement. (1996). Humbug Award 1996 (Author unknown). *Skeptikko* [Sceptic], *4*(96), 10–11.

Strauss, A. (1978). A social world perspective. *Studies in Symbolic Interaction, 1,* 119–128.

Turner, J. G., Clark, A. J., Gauthier, D. K., & Williams, M. (1998). The effect of therapeutic touch on pain and anxiety in burn patients. *Journal of Advanced Nursing, 28*(1), 10–20.

Unruh, D. R. (1979). Characteristics and types of participation in social worlds. *Symbolic Interaction, 2*(2), 115–129.

Venäläinen, R. (1997). Theories are being argued over at the department of nursing science: Is the student's legal protection in danger? *Aviisi* [Student Journal], *3*(97), 9.

Vuolanto, P. (2013). Boundary-work and the vulnerability of academic status: The case of Finnish nursing science. Acta Universitatis Tamperensis 1867. Tampere: Tampere University Press.

Vuolanto, P. (2015). Boundary work and power in the controversy over therapeutic touch in Finnish nursing science. *Minerva, 53*(4), 359–380.

Vuolanto, P. (2017). The universities' transformation thesis revisited: A case study of the relationship between nursing science and society. *Science and Technology Studies, 30*(2), 34–52.

Webster, A. (2007). *Health, technology and society: A sociological critique.* New York: Palgrave Macmillan.

Wilcox, S. (2010). Lay knowledge: The missing middle of the expertise debates. In R. Harris, N. Wathen, & S. Wyatt (Eds.), *Configuring health consumers: Health work and the imperative of personal responsibility* (pp. 45–64). New York: Palgrave Macmillan.

Wirth, D. P., Richardson, J. T., Eidelman, W. S., & O'Malley, A. C. (1993). Full thickness dermal wounds treated with non-contact therapeutic touch: A replication and extension. *Complementary Therapies in Medicine, 1*(3), 127–132.

Wyatt, S., Harris, R., & Wathen, N. (2010). Health(y) citizenship: Technology, work and narratives of responsibility. In R. Harris, N. Wathen, & S. Wyatt (Eds.), *Configuring health consumers: Health work and the imperative of personal responsibility* (pp. 1–10). New York: Palgrave Macmillan.

4

Qigong in Three Social Worlds: National Treasure, Social Signifier, or Breathing Exercise?

Fabian Winiger

Introduction

Drawing on the social worlds perspective in science and technology studies (STS), this chapter uses the case of Chinese '*qigong*'—one of the most widespread East Asian techniques of self-cultivation in Europe and North America—to trace the multiple discourses of this practice as it is articulated (a) by practitioners of *qigong* during the height of the Chinese *qigong* movement in the 1980s and 1990s, as reflected in popular books and magazines from that period; (b) by anthropologists and religious studies scholars who have written on the phenomenon since the late 1980s, and (c) by biomedically trained scientists studying the effects of *qigong* with conventional methods. It is suggested that each constitutes a distinct social world which gives rise to a self-contained 'universe of discourse' where *qigong* is constituted as an '[assemblage] of language, motive, and meaning', and where what *qigong* 'is' is expressive rather of

F. Winiger (✉)
Hong Kong Institute of Humanities and Social Sciences, Hong Kong
University, Hong Kong SAR, People's Republic of China

© The Author(s) 2018
C. Brosnan et al. (eds.), *Complementary and Alternative Medicine*, Health,
Technology and Society, https://doi.org/10.1007/978-3-319-73939-7_4

the production of 'doable problems' than of a discrete set of bodily practices (Fujimura 1987).

Although the notion of vital energy is no stranger to conventional Western medicine (Ning 2013), complementary and alternative medicine (CAM) modalities based on breath-of-life concepts like *qi* or *prana* offer no point of convergence with mainstream biomedical epistemology, and the worlds of biomedical science and CAM practitioners starkly diverge in the study of therapeutic modalities based on such concepts. Whereas herbal medical doctors can in principle exchange institutional prestige for accepting a biomedical reconstruction of their practice—for instance, by reframing the efficacy of Tibetan medicine through the extraction of its 'active ingredients' (Adams 2002)—*qigong* revolves around the manipulation of an inextricable but vital energy with no apparent material basis.

Such practices thus expose the epistemological fault line between the realms of fact ('medical explanations') and belief ('philosophy') which demarcates acceptable CAM practices. Consequently, therapeutic modalities based on a vitalistic ontology are 'among the most controversial of CAM practices' and an easy target for accusations of 'immorality, quackery and fraudulence' (Keshet 2011: 13, 14). The discussion quickly deteriorates to polemical bottom-line arguments of the sort that alternate between empathic statements that *qi* cannot be 'knocked on' like evidently material things, such as furniture, and the grave moral consequences if the flood gates were opened to any truth-claim however tendentious (Edwards et al. 1995). Clinically oriented research tends to look for evidence of efficacy outside tangible physiological benefit (the domain of 'disease' reserved for biomedically legitimised practices), in the arbitrary and subjective realms of 'illness' (Kleinman 1988). Social science research likewise tends to stop short of examining the physiological and material effects of such therapies. As a result, as observed by Brosnan, Vuolanto, and Danell in the introduction to this volume, 'the actual content of CAM is often taken-for-granted, and the focus is on how CAM is perceived by, experienced by or mediates relationships between people' (p. 2).

Research Material and Methods

The following study of the three different social worlds of *qigong* is based on analysis of three distinctive sets of primary sources. For emic understandings of *qigong* practices, the present argument centres on the Chinese literature on the topic published during the second '*qigong* fever' (*qigong re*) which swept the People's Republic of China (PRC) between the early 1980s and the late 1990s and at its peak involved several hundred million practitioners (Palmer 2007). In 1999, in the wake of a crack-down on Falung Gong, a large group of *qigong* practitioners which had turned into a militant salvationist movement and was perceived by the Party-state as a rival and a threat to its power (Li 2014; Ownby 2008; Penny 2012), public *qigong* practice was banned in the PRC and almost all officially sanctioned activity came to a halt. *Qigong*-related books and magazines are still published in the PRC, but almost all have changed their focus to practices of 'nurturing life' (*yangsheng*), an extraordinarily broad category ranging from collective disco-dancing for the elderly in public parks, the playing of traditional instruments, and jogging backwards to keeping pet birds and learning foreign languages (Farquhar and Zhang 2012)—providing cover to the politically more problematic *qigong* practices. Moreover, since the abrupt end of the Chinese *qigong* fever, interest in traditional body-cultivation practices has been eclipsed in the PRC by a burgeoning interest in psychoanalysis (Huang 2013), yoga, and various imported self-help and New Age beliefs (Iskra forthcoming).

Despite the explosive proliferation of *qigong*-related literature during the *qigong fever* and the spread of widely popular charismatic *qigong* 'masters' who attracted millions of followers, insofar as the Chinese *qigong* fever is reflected in print publications, most practitioners shared a basic understanding of the term *qigong* and its role in Chinese history, and disagreements seem to have mainly occurred in regard to the specific beliefs and practice methods advocated by individual *qigong* groups. Five publications representing this social world are chosen for their comprehensiveness (Ji et al. 1993; Li 1988), institutional prestige, that is, through publication by state-sponsored publishing houses (Gao et al. 1991), or support by well-known pioneers or patrons of the *qigong* milieu (Tao and Yang 1981, 1982, 1984, 1989; Zhang 1995).

For representations of *qigong* practices in the social scientific literature, studies published on the phenomenon since the late 1980s are discussed. With the ban of public *qigong* practice following the crack-down on Falun Gong, research on *qigong* in the PRC has become difficult to conduct. Although the Chinese *qigong* fever was the 'largest contemporary expression of urban religiosity' (Chau 2010: 23) in the PRC in the first 20 years after the end of the Cultural Revolution, a relatively small number of articles, book chapters, monographs, and doctoral dissertations has been published. The present discussion refers to every major English-language publication known to the author, as well as a small number of works in French and German.

Notwithstanding the considerable ambiguity evident in the biomedical literature regarding exactly what constitutes *qigong*, new studies are published on a regular basis in both CAM journals and conventional specialist journals. The biomedical literature discussed here is based on a PubMed search of systematic reviews on *qigong* practices (371 results), narrowed to reviews published in the previous ten years (36 results).[1] Articles were chosen to capture a wide range of journal and publication styles, including systematic reviews and meta-analyses of Randomized Controlled Trials (RCTs) authored by well-known sceptics of CAM (Lee et al. 2007, 2009, 2011), a recent Cochrane review (Hartley et al. 2015), a systematic review and construct analysis of *qigong* in cancer care (Klein et al. 2016), and additional studies mentioned which illustrate the understanding of such practices within the biomedical world of *qigong*.

Qigong as National Treasure

After years of suppression during the Cultural Revolution, the beginning of the Opening and Reform period (1978–present) allowed *qigong* masters to teach in public for the first time in years. Typically, aspiring *qigong* masters presented themselves through the archetypical three-partite narrative trope of *chu shan le* ('coming out of the mountains'): the aspiring adept withdrew from society and embarked on intense meditative training in the seclusion of China's mythical shrouded mountains. There, he or she was initiated into an ancient lineage of spiritual seekers, underwent rigorous ascetic training in secretive techniques of self-cultivation, triumphed over internal or external adversaries, and eventually climbed to new heights of spiritual insight. After completing this transformation, the ascended master returned to society to found his or her own group of disciples.

A great variety of Chinese-language literature on *qigong* was produced during the 1980s and 1990s, propagated by an even greater number of 'masters' and 'grandmasters': the *Complete Book of Contemporary Chinese Qigong* counted 182 different *qigong* groups and 161 types of *qigong* (Ji et al. 1993)[2]. The authors in this literature generally agree on the basic premise of *chu shan le*: that *qigong* has for millennia formed an integral component of the vast treasure trove of China's mythical national history but has been lost to the public at large. *Qigong* is typically understood as an emblematic, trans-historical carrier of an intangible Chinese national essence linked, tenuously, to key figures in Chinese history.

In this vein, the authors of the *Treasure Collection of Taoist Qigong* (Feng and Zhou 1990) attributed the origin of *qigong* to the Yellow Emperor, the mythical founding figure of Chinese medicine (Penny 1993: 170). Similarly, the *Complete Book* traced the origin of *qigong* to the legendary Pengzu, who lived to 800 years due to his practice of *qigong* and whose time is sometimes cited as the starting point of Chinese culture. Such accounts imply, or flatly state, that *qigong* practices are the 'essence' (*jinghua*) of traditional Chinese culture and therefore a national 'treasure' (*zhenbao*) to be put in the service of the nation and the world at large, where it will catalyse the revival of Chinese 'spiritual civilisation' and the return of the Chinese nation to its rightful place in history. Detailed technical discussions of individual practices are woven into a shared cultural-nationalist subtext which presents the vast array of *qigong* practices as a living embodiment of the greatness of the Chinese historical legacy.

Following the conventions of a certain genre of Chinese historiography, this literature tends to consist of lengthy compilations of annotated excerpts drawn from the classical religious and medical canon, which are reinterpreted in the light of contemporary practices. The *History of*

Chinese Qigong, the first comprehensive history of *qigong* practices published in the PRC, for instance, provides a description often repeated as a standard definition of sorts. It defines *qigong* as follows:

Taking the strengthening of the harmony [*xietiao xing*] of humanity's organism as its primary goal, using the adjustment of mind [*tiaoxin*], breath [*tiaoxi*] and posture [*tiaoxing*] to cultivate heart and mind [*shenxin*], that is *qigong.* (Li 1988: 2)

Accordingly, *qigong* is a process of self-consciously cultivating one's 'life activities', including breath, thought (*siwei*), and physical body, of which thought is the most important. These activities should be goal oriented, conscious (*yishi*), and planned (*jihua*) and therefore completely different from the instincts of animals. They should first and foremost benefit the health of people, for example, by promoting physical vigour (*yuanqi*), fighting disease, and promoting self-healing abilities, intelligence, and developing the human potential. Any such techniques that allow the practitioner to enter a '*qigong* state' (*qigong tai*) where 'body and mind are one' (*shenxin ru yi*) and one 'forgets both oneself and everything else' (*wu wo liang wang*) can be called *qigong.*

Li noted that the term '*qigong*' is a recent invention (see the following discussion) but argued that such practices have existed outside China for a long time under different names. Within China, they could be divided into a few main schools: 'guiding and stretching' (*daoyin*), 'circulating qi' (*xingqi*), 'preserving thought' (*cunsi*), and cultivating the 'internal cinnabar field' (*neidan*) (Li 1988: 1–5). Throughout history, these were created by imitating nature (*fangsheng*), leading to practices with names like 'Five Animals' (*wu qin xi*) or 'Turtle Breathing' (*gui xi*). This was not merely based on mimicking the appearance of nature but on the observation of the laws governing the macrocosm, which through introspection (*neixing*) were applied to the microcosmic laws governing the organs and *qi* channels (*jingluo*) in the body (Li 1988: II–IV, 28–31).

Where the *Complete Book* begins with Pengzu, the *History* traces *qigong* practices back to labour and agricultural activities of the Lower Palaeolithic, when they were transmitted independently as a part of medicine, religion, education, and warfare. Today's *qigong*, argued Li, therefore encapsulates the sum of 5000 years of Chinese people's collective experience. Having acknowledged that such practices never formed an independent subject until the invention of the term *qigong* in the twentieth century, the remaining 450-odd pages of the *History* confidently excavates *qigong* from the many faces it assumed throughout Chinese imperial history. The same approach, of confidently excavating *qigong*, is taken in the *Great Encyclopaedia of Chinese Qigong* (1995), a 1700-page tome edited by Zhang Zhenhuan, a powerful patron of the Chinese *qigong* milieu and first director of the Chinese Qigong Research Association, as well as in the four-volume strong *Collection of Qigong Therapeutic Methods* (Tao and Yang 1981, 1982, 1984, 1989) and the 14-volume *Chinese Classical Qigong Library* (1991).

The notion of an internally consistent set of *qigong* exercises at the core of China's mythical, 1000-year-old culture also continues to inform the official textbook used to teach *qigong* in traditional Chinese medical colleges in the PRC. Compiled by 30 professors from Chinese medical colleges and universities in every major province (Liu 2012), it argues that *qigong* has a history of 2000–3000 years and was developed in Buddhist, Daoist, medical, martial art, 'folk' (*minjian*), and Confucian traditions. Its English translation, published in 2010, argues in the introduction that 'if you ask 100 *qigong* practitioners what *qigong* is, you may get 101 different answers' (ibid.: 3). Accordingly, *tuna*,[3] *daoyin*, and so on were all 'ancient cultivation and refinement methods' (*xiulian famen*), and '*qigong*' is an 'all-inclusive contemporary term that applies to all traditional mind-body-breathing integration exercises and techniques' and refers to 'the skill of body-mind exercise that integrates body, breath and mind adjustments into one' (ibid.: 4). In this social world, exercises and techniques developing that skill are believed to be found littered across the classical literature, where they symbolise the historical continuity and transcendent greatness of an immeasurably profound but obscure culture which harbours the potential to revitalise the Chinese nation and humanity at large.

Qigong as Social Signifier

The Chinese *qigong* literature stands in stark contrast with the deconstructive methodology of the social scientific literature. Accordingly, the creation of the term *qigong* was a 'political act' intimately tied to the takeover of the Communist Party in 1949, when the state reversed its earlier policy of opposing traditional Chinese medicine and began to use local healers to mitigate a severe shortage in modern medical doctors (Palmer 2007: 29). The term was invented when a local Communist Party leader heard of a young Party member named Liu Guizhen (1920–1983), who had been miraculously healed from his numerous illnesses by an exercise practised by a paternal uncle in his village. Impressed with Liu's sudden return to health, the leader sent him to return to the village and learn the practice in its entirety.

Upon his return, Liu was assigned to teach it in a local sanatorium for Party members and to work with local hospital officials in order to cleanse it from its 'superstitious' background and turn it into a modern medical method. The reformulated practice replaced the original names of the exercises (e.g. 'The Claw of the Golden Dragon Sitting in Meditation in the Chan Chamber') with more scientific-sounding terms (e.g. 'I practise Sitting Meditation for a Better Health'). The group discussed a general name for these newly created practices, and after considering 'spiritual therapy' (*jingshen liaofa*), 'psychological therapy' (*xinli liaofa*), and 'incantation therapy' (*zhuyou liaofa*) they settled on 'qigong therapy' (*qigong liaofa*). As Liu explained, 'the character "*qi*" here means breath, and "*gong*" means a constant exercise to regulate breath and posture, that is to say, what popular parlance calls to practise until one has mastery [*you gongfu*]; to use medical perspectives to organise and research this *qigong* method; and to use it for therapy and hygiene, while removing the superstitious dross of old [...]' (Palmer 2007: 30–32).[4]

A similar account is presented by Otehode (2009) and Penny and Otehode (2016). They state that the name '*qigong*' was chosen for such practices because the character '*qi*' may be interpreted to refer both to oxygen (*yangqi*)—a biomedically endorsed concept—and to the Chinese medical notion of 'primordial *qi*' (*yuanqi*). According to Penny and Otehode (2016: 73), contrary to the attempt to prove the ancient pedigree of *qigong* with the use of the term in classical Chinese literature, the Tangshan Qigong Sanitorium founded by Liu at first used the term *qigong* (气工) with the character *gong* (工), referring to 'work', 'labour', 'skill', 'trade', 'profession', and so on, rather than *gong* (功) in the sense of 'meritorious deed' or 'achievement'.[5]

One of the practices created by Liu, named 'health maintenance training method' (*baojiangong*), illustrates the reinvention of *qigong* in the early 1950s: it consisted of 18 selected movements taken from *neigong*, a generic term referring to 'soft' or 'internal' (*nei*) practices focussing on the circulation of *qi* (as opposed to the 'hard' or 'external' [*wai*] type of physical practices found in martial arts); *daoyin*, a loosely defined category of bending and stretching exercises found in early Han-dynasty medical manuscripts, medieval Daoist scriptures, and Tang-dynasty immortality practices (Kohn 2008); as well as *shi er duan jin,* a seated exercise related to the Eight Pieces of Brocade (*ba duan jin*) commonly attributed to the Ming dynasty. The newly created practice was judged to '[accord] with the structure of the human body' by a Soviet professor at the Beijing Medical University, who added 3 more movements himself, bringing the total movements to 21. *Baojiangong* was later included in the 'Outline of Chinese Traditional Medicine' (1959), where it was described as a '*qigong* therapy with "a long history"' (Otehode 2009: 245).[6]

During the Cultural Revolution, all official *qigong*-related activities came to a halt and Liu Guizhen was removed from his position. But with the beginning of the Opening and Reform period from the late 1970s, a 'cultural fever' (*wenhua re*) began to spread in the PRC, and interest surged in *qigong*, martial arts, the *yijing*, the study of the classics, and other facets of traditional culture violently opposed during the Cultural Revolution. It is in this context that the myth of *chu shan le* imbued the medicalised '*qigong* therapy' of the 1950s with new significance, and *qigong* grew into a sweeping social movement, involving at its peak during the 1980s and 1990s up to one-fifth of the PRC's urban population (Palmer 2007: 6). By the time of the ban of *qigong*-related activities in the PRC following the crack-down on the Falun Gong group in 1999, the

Chinese *qigong* fever had become the 'largest mass cultural, social, and religious movement in urban post-Mao China' (Palmer 2008: 80). Individual groups such as Falun Gong or Zhong Gong had gained more followers than the Chinese Communist Party (Palmer 2008, 2011) and enjoyed considerable institutional support at the highest echelons of the Party bureaucracy, the medical establishment, and the military-industrial complex (Palmer 2007).

While some *qigong* groups were motivated by more commercial motives (Palmer 2011) and Falun Gong by the mid-1990s had turned into a salvationist movement in opposition to the Communist Party (Ownby 2008; Penny 2012), more ideologically inclined groups such as Zhineng Qigong explicitly premised their beliefs and practices on the mythical return of Chinese spiritual civilisation and dedicated much of their effort to cultivating an intimate ideological symbiosis with post-Mao ideology (Winiger forthcoming). Much of the non-Chinese academic literature on the Chinese *qigong* movement, however, has focussed on the cathartic and far more visible performance of 'spontaneous *qigong*' (*zifa gong*) in public parks (Chen 1995; Micollier 1999; Ots 1991, 1994).

Echoing the anthropological turn towards the body emerging in the early 1990s, this literature understood the various, often bizarre beliefs and practices circulating in the *qigong* fever as embodied expressions of emotions and behaviour not sanctioned during the highly repressive social environment of the Mao era. As Chen wrote, 'practitioners believe that trees have special powers of *qi* that can revive the force of *qi* in their own bodies. Many individuals can be seen hugging trees, rubbing their bodies around the trunk of trees, dancing in circles around trees, or sitting quietly before a tree' (Chen 1995: 354). 'At once a healing art, a daily regimen of exercise, and a spiritual revival', such practices created a 'social arena where trance, possession, and existence within otherworldly times and spaces were common practices of daily life' (ibid.: 347–348). Paradoxically, considering the term *qigong* was invented by a Party cadre, and *qigong* practices were promoted by the state during the 1950s and early 1960s and again throughout the 1980s and 1990s, these studies demonstrate how *qigong* enabled a withdrawal from the totalitarian grip of the state and the renegotiation of the self in relation to it in a safe space exempted from the normative pressures of urban life.

Reading this account against the emic understanding of *qigong* found in the Chinese literature, the practices themselves seem to play a negligible role—they appear as supporting actors in a larger, socio-political drama and figure as 'signifiers of other, broader societal shifts' as opposed to 'being understood in their own right' (Brosnan, Vuolanto and Danell, this volume, p. 2). Thus far, this literature has described the emergence of the Chinese *qigong* movement in the 1950s as an 'invented tradition' (Hsu 2008; Otehode 2009; Palmer 2007; Penny and Otehode 2016); in terms of its revival after the Cultural Revolution (Heise 1999; Miura 1989; Otehode 2009; Palmer 2007); the transmission of *qigong* in the PRC as a form of ritualised embodied knowledge vis-à-vis the institutionalisation of traditional Chinese medicine (Hsu 1999) and as a form of contested medical knowledge in China's transition to a market-economy (Chen 2003); the construction of *qigong* and *qi*-related paranormal abilities within religious, nationalist, and scientific discourses (Despeux 1997; Karchmer 2002; Jianhui Li and Fu 2015; Palmer 2007; Penny 1993; Van der Veer 2010; Xu 1999); and the highly visible cathartic exercises (*zifa gong*) with their possibilities of escape from the purview of an oppressive state (Chen 1995; Micollier 1999; Ots 1991, 1994; Lim 2009). Studies of *qigong* outside China have tended to focus on the question of authenticity and commodification in the context of the contemporary Western spiritual market place (Komjathy 2006; Siegler 2011).

Indeed, its portrayal in the social scientific literature seems to suggest that *qigong* proliferated due to little or no instrumental utility of its own, and few attempts have been made to understand what Hsu and Lim (2016), following Latour (2000), term the 'thing'—that is, *qigong* practices—in its own right. Other than a general discussion of the phenomenology of *qigong* (Murakawa 2002), no alternative model has been proposed to put the experiential reality produced by such practices into dialogue with the Cartesian conception of the body-mind. Instead, according to Brosnan, Vuolanto and Danell, 'the focus is on how [*qigong*] is perceived by, experienced by or mediates relationships between people' (p. 2).

This problem is well exemplified by Xu (1999: 961), who compared anthropological studies on *qigong* with studies of bodily practices whose practical value does not enter the picture and are apparently unrelated to each other if not for their shared fate in providing a canvas for an intense, embodied political struggle. As Xu argues:

> Joseph Alter's study of Indian wrestling (1993), for example, tracks the wrestlers' self-conscious reappropriation of their bodies from the power of the state through a regimented discipline aimed at resisting docility. John Donohue's study of the Japanese martial art karate (1993) explores how, in the West, karate's symbolic and ritual functions create a psychological dynamic that counters the prevalent fragmentation of urban life. Douglas Wile's research on Chinese *taijiquan* (1996) similarly reconstructs the cultural/historical context in which this martial art was created. He shows that what motivated nineteenth-century literati to create *taijiquan* was its representational function rather than its practical utility.

A notable exception seems to be found in Sagli's (2008) study of Norwegian practitioners of the 'Biyun' style of *qigong*. However, although Sagli describes the phenomenology of Biyun in some detail, her theoretical framework draws heavily on Despret (2004) and suggests that 'learning to affect' and 'be affected' by *qigong* is closely tied to a relationship of 'trust', 'interest', 'authority', and 'expectation' between the affected, that is, the Biyin-*qigong* teacher and his or her students. Like Despret, Sagli uses Gregory Bateson's understanding of 'authority' as 'when anyone who is under the influence of that authority does everything possible to make whatever this person says to be true' (Sagli 2008: 549; Despret 2004: 118). Students who learnt 'to be a nose' (that can perceive *qi*) were thus 'able to obtain results that confirmed their expectations because it mattered to them that what the teacher took to be true was true' (Sagli 2008: 549). Biyun practitioners, located in a context of trust, interest, expectation, and authority, exhibited what Despret refers to as a 'preference for agreement' towards their fellow practitioners and the Biyun teacher. Sagli thus eschews fundamentally engaging with the phenomenology of practice and reproduces the Cartesian assumption that the body is 'duped' by the mind. *Qigong* practice, therefore, fundamentally revolves around charismatic leadership and social relations of power.

Though a valid argument within the discursive logic of its own social world, if biomedical epistemology has sustained a prolonged critique of biological reductionism, this line of argument may seem to perpetuate its own epistemic blindness—that is, it passes over what appears to be the most basic ontological claim made by practitioners of any type of *qigong*: that their practice is not a matter of 'body politics' (Chen 1999) but principally revolves around the experiential apprehension of *qi*, believed to create material improvements to their physical or spiritual well-being. Instead of exploring the phenomenon in its own right—to 'represent them as they would represent themselves' (Good 1994: 25)—this circumvents the ontological question of *qi* and produces yet another, internally undifferentiated site in which to discover embodied resistance, complicity, and renegotiation vis-a-vis state power. Much like the 'metaphor of construction', it could be argued, this 'once had excellent shock value, but now it has become tired' (Hacking 1999: 35).

This 'sociological reductionism' of the body to an artefact of broader social or political processes is particularly striking for two reasons. Firstly, the body, once treated by Enlightenment thinkers as an 'object to be distrusted, if not reviled' for its potential to muddle rational thought and distract from the pursuit of objectivity (Stoller 1997: xii), has since increasingly moved to the centre of social analysis. Owing to a sustained critique by phenomenologists in the tradition of Maurice Merleau-Ponty, the turn to the body in British sociology since the mid-1980s (Ozawa-De Silva 2002), the Foucauldian and feminist conception of the body as a product and locus of power, and a long 'career' of the body among anthropologists (Csordas 1999), the body has become recognised not only as a mirror or 'canvas' of social life but as a productive process of both grasping and generating embodied meaning.

Secondly, the absence of the 'thing in itself' is striking in view of the number of authors on the topic who have had prior first-hand experience with the beliefs and practices of their informants, only to gradually marginalise the ontological question posed by their own experience. The obstacles in the social world of the academic study of *qigong* are well illustrated by Frank (2000: 13): 'social construction', he argued, 'is, of course, an inadequate term for getting at the subjective *experience* of *qi*'. According to Frank, '[a]nthropology has always maintained its dirty little secret of ethnographers who crossed into territory where their own bodily experiences made traditional ethnographic modes of representation and interpretation obsolete'. Frank discusses three such anthropologists who have been professionally ostracised as a result (Frank Hamilton Cushing, Carlos Castañeda, and Paul Stoller) and proceeds to the experience of *qi* as described by Ots and several well-known Western *qigong* and *taiji quan* practitioners. Frank concludes that *qi* may be best understood as a verb rather than a noun: '[u]sing *qi* as a noun form somehow confines us to the expectation that we will be able to touch *it*, taste *it*, or shoot *it* through our fingers. When we use *qi* as a verb, [...] we have to accept our bodies as potentially solvable *physical* mysteries. We need to look at how muscles, bones, lymphatic nodes, etc., work together as a conduit for "doing *qi*," [...]' (ibid.: 26, emph. in orig.). Although Frank argues for a greater regard for the phenomenology of *qi* in discussions of *qigong* and martial arts, his conclusion by his own admission '[moves] around the edge of the concept in very much the same way that a boxer might move around the edge of an opponent in a sparring situation' (ibid.: 25, 26). In this way, Frank, too, sidesteps the basic ontological claim made in the social world of the Chinese *qigong* fever: that *qi* indeed can be touched and even emitted or 'shot' through the palms or fingers (*faqi*) to injure opponents or disperse tumours, that it can be tasted (or at least smelt), as in the 'fragrant *qigong*' (*xiang gong*) wildly popular in the PRC during the 1980s and 1990s, and that the discovery of the materiality of *qi* will spark a scientific revolution which will prove the equivalence, if not superiority, of a distinctly Chinese modernity.

The social world surrounding the academic literature of *qigong* thus reproduces a 'Cartesian-Kantian epistemology that considers religious worlds to be either "objective" realities that are cognitively inaccessible or "subjective" cultural-linguistic fabrications' (Gleig: 100)—something that is 'performed', 'enacted', 'done', or 'experienced' but never truly real. Not unlike the 'conceptual uplifting' which retrospectively discovered a transcendent category of internally consistent *qigong* practices in Chinese history, or the transformation of 'Golden Dragon Sitting in Meditation' into the 'I practise Sitting Meditation' congruent with the modernist imaginary of Chinese socialism, this effectively marginalises the rich technical, practical, and phenomenological dimensions of *qigong*. Following Zhan (2014), this may be understood as a process of 'bifurcation' by which *qigong* practices are disarticulated into an empirical dimension, in need of bioscientific validation, and a conceptual dimension that inevitably revolves around what such practices can disclose about the anonymous socio-political processes of which *qigong* practices are but one expression.

Qigong as Breathing Exercise

Considering the widely diverging understandings of *qigong*—how is the term operationalised in the biomedical literature? Surprisingly, a large literature has been produced in the past 20 years evaluating the biomedical efficacy of *qigong* as though it were an internally coherent set of practices. New studies are published on a monthly basis and with increasing frequency.[7]

Typically, meta-analyses of *qigong* appear as aggregates of internally undifferentiated analytical categories such as 'mind-body', 'Chinese nursing', 'relaxation', or most often 'breathing' exercises. Where such studies are narrowed to *qigong*, various types, intensities, and styles of *qigong* practice are routinely collapsed into a single category and their efficacy generalised to *qigong* on the basis of an aggregate of its clinical efficacy. Calls to improve the design of clinical trials, made in nearly every systematic review of *qigong*, have focussed on rehearsing methodological challenges shared by non-pharmacological interventions in general, rather than interrogating the manner of approaching the subject.

This problem is exemplified in a study by Oh et al. (2008), who described their intervention as follows:

> 30 min of gentle stretching and body movement in standing postures to stimulate the body along the energy channels (stimulate the body along the energy channels, flying bird, monkey shaking the arm and leg, shaking the body to cleanse and detoxify body,[...]); 15 min movement in seated posture [Dao Yin exercise for face, head, neck, shoulders, waist, lower back, legs, feet]; and 30 min of breathing exercise, meditation and visualization based on Chinese medicine principles of energy channel and channeling human energy with nature including natural breathing, chest breathing, abdominal breathing, breathing for energy regulation, circulation, and

relaxation; 'Five gates' breathing; feeling the Qi (nature's/cosmic energy) and visualization.

What precisely is understood by 'monkey shaking the arm and leg' and what 'Chinese medicine principles' this practice is based on is left to the imagination of the reader. As specificity and type of *qigong* intervention is not considered in the inclusion criteria of systematic reviews or meta-analyses, unnamed and loosely described practices are lumped in with highly formalised practices such as *baduanjin* ('Eight Pieces of Brocade') (Li et al. 2014) first recorded in the Song dynasty (960–1279). Thus, a systematic review of studies on the effectiveness of *qigong* in cardiac rehabilitation (Chan et al. 2012) included, among well-known practices such as *baduanjin*, Guolin Qigong and *wuqinxi* ('Five Animals Exercise'), a study on a 'newly developed intervention [...] established on a Chinese Chan tradition' named 'Chanwuyi (i.e., Zen, martial art and healing), from the Shaolin Temple'. In addition to dieting and 'listening to the body', this required subjects to '[f]oster self-awareness and self-control: keep calm and relaxed when feeling distressed and angry by practicing self-guided massages (i.e., qigong), e.g., rolling their hands slowly up and down between the chest and the abdomen; resting their hands on their abdomen while quietly observing their breathing in and out; and massaging their nasal bridge' and to 'practice Shaolin Mind–Body exercises', which are explained as 'somewhat like Tai Chi and meditation, [...] sets of breathing exercises and slow movements that emphasize smooth, gentle and calm movements' (Chan et al. 2012: 285, 286). Similarly, a Cochrane review of *qigong* for the primary prevention of cardiovascular disease (Hartley et al. 2015) included both a study of *baduanjin* and a protocol based on '[...] basic movements to affect body awareness, balance and coordination, breathing and muscular tension; and [...] relaxation and mindfulness meditation with self-performed body massage at the end' (Stenlund et al. 2009: 763).

A more nuanced approach is taken by a systematic overview of RCTs, published in the *Journal of the Royal Society of Medicine* (Lee et al. 2011). The study acknowledges that '[t]here are numerous distinct forms of qigong' and distinguished between two 'main groups': 'internal' *qigong* ('a physical and mental training method for the cultivation of oneself to achieve optimal health in both mind and body') and 'external' *qigong* ('where *qigong* practitioners direct or emit their *qi*-energy to the patient with the intention to clear *qi*-blockages or balance the flow of *qi* within that patient') (ibid.: 1, 2). This distinction was also used in an earlier review of pain conditions (Lee et al. 2007, 2009). The differentiation between biomedically plausible 'internal' *qigong* practices and those based on the 'external' emission of *qi,* however, produced the paradoxical result of making the evidence for 'external' *qigong* appear more convincing ('The evidence [...] is encouraging') than 'internal' *qigong* ('the existing trial evidence is not convincing enough to suggest that internal *qigong* is an effective modality [...]'). As noted by Lee et al. (2009: 6), the studies under review were further limited by the 'expertise of *qigong* practitioners, the pluralism of *qigong*, frequency and duration of treatment, [...] and heterogeneous comparison groups'. Although the distinction made between internal and external *qigong* provides a basic typology, what is taken to constitute 'internal qigong' varies widely.

In a mixed-methods study of *qigong* in cancer care, Klein et al. (2016) attempted to address the 'pluralism of *qigong*' by expanding on the internal-external distinction with an analysis of the effectiveness of individual intervention protocols. The authors included 'Medical Qigong', 'Gou Lin [sic] Qigong', 'Qigong/Tai Chi Easy™', 'Kuala Lumpur Qigong', and several types of *taijiquan*, which the authors classify with one or more of the following categories: 'Gentle/integrated/repetitious/flowing/weight-bearing exercises', 'Stylised exercises', 'Meditation/mindfulness', 'Breath regulation', 'Energy cultivation', 'Relaxation', and 'Self-massage' (Klein et al. 2016: 3212, 3216). No further distinctions are made for 'breath regulation' or 'energy cultivation', of which in the world of Chinese *qigong* practitioners several hundred techniques, practice styles, variations, and intensities were circulated. The authors report that '[n]o conclusions can be suggested regarding superiority of one Qigong style or form over another' but nonetheless make a number of suggestions for health professionals recommending *qigong* practice (Klein et al. 2016: 3216, 3219).

Klein et al.'s approach takes a critical step in a rapprochement between the social worlds of Chinese *qigong*, social science, and biomedical understandings by developing a typology to more accurately capture the variety of *qigong* practices and per-protocol evaluation of treatment efficacy. Nonetheless, Klein's analysis remains problematic. The case of the effect of 'Kuala Lumpur Qigong' on reported quality of life of Malaysian breast cancer survivors included in Klein is instructive. Curiously, the only mentions of 'Kuala Lumpur Qigong' indexed by popular search engines refer back to the study cited by Klein et al. (2016). The original study (Loh et al. 2014) named the intervention as '*Zhi Neng* Qigong' (*zhineng qigong*), one of the most popular *qigong* groups active in the PRC during the 1980s and 1990s, when it reached between 3.57 and 10 million practitioners. Zhineng Qigong is best known for having operated a 'medicine-less hospital', a large rehabilitation and training centre on former military premises in northern China which treated chronically ill patients using Zhineng Qigong only. Most patients attended the centre as a last resort and were unable to afford biomedical care or were given little hope by it. Between 1989 and 1999, the centre trained and treated over 310,000 patients and practitioners using Zhineng Qigong, conducted research with several major universities in the PRC, and published a five-volume collection of research results, including a 365-page volume on medical research (Winiger forthcoming).[8]

The Zhineng Qigong intervention described by Loh, Lee, and Murray ('a low-moderate intensity internal Qigong […] programme') involved weekly, 90-minute face-to-face meetings with an instructor, repeated for eight weeks. The exercises included '*Peng Qi Guan Ding Fa*' ('Lift Qi Up Pour Qi Down'), a slow-moving practice performed while standing, and '*San Xin Bing Zhan Zhuang*' ('Three Centres Merge Standing Form'), whereby the practitioner stands quietly holding a fixed posture. Supplementary exercises named '*Kai He La Qi*' ('Open-Close Pulling Qi'), '*Dun Qiang*' ('Wall Squats'), and '*Chen Qi*' ('Stretching Qi') were also taught, and the intervention group was 'encouraged' to practise twice a week for 30 minutes.

Although Loh et al. clearly specify a relatively standardised *qigong* practice with a long record of use with cancer patients and found an improvement in Quality of Life scores over a control group of line dancers, the study remains problematic for two reasons. Firstly, both *Peng Qi Guan Ding Fa* and *Kai He La Qi* are not 'internal' *qigong* practices but are rather based on gathering 'external *qi*' of nature—in Zhineng Qigong terminology referred to as '*hunyuan qi*'—and guiding it through the body using slow hand movements (Winiger forthcoming). Insofar as *hunyuan qi* is gathered into the practitioner's own body and not that of a second person these two practices may be understood as 'internal' in the sense of Lee et al. (2011). However, this classification appears at odds with the belief of Zhineng Qigong practitioners that the efficacy of *Peng Qi Guan Ding Fa* and *Kai He La Qi*—unlike more advanced stages in the Zhineng Qigong practice system, such as *Xing Shen Zhuang* ('Body Mind Form') or *Wu Yuan Zhuang* ('Five-One Form')—lies in increasing the quality and quantity of *qi* in the body by transferring external *hunyuan qi* into the body, and the physical movements are deliberately minimised and merely serve to facilitate this process. Indeed, experienced practitioners may perform the practice with little or no physical movement.

Secondly, the intervention, described by the authors as 'low-moderate intensity', is significantly less demanding than the practice regime common among Chinese Zhineng Qigong practitioners in the PRC during the 1980s and 1990s, particularly those suffering from cancer. At the Zhineng Qigong rehabilitation centre, the practice routine consisted of at least eight hours of practice per day for a period of either 24 or 50 days, conducted in a highly disciplined, live-in residential setting. Success stories of cancer patients published in the group's internal magazine regularly reported intensive regimes exceeding this routine, suggesting that highly committed or desperate patients practised for even longer. An analysis of 4501 cases of cancer patients treated at the rehabilitation centre between March 1993 and November 1996 reported an average duration of stay of 2–4 months (shortest 24 days, longest 3 years 7 months) (Winiger forthcoming). The sample included 972 patients admitted to the centre after relapsing from surgery. Of 378 patients with breast cancer, 19 were discharged as 'cured'. For all types of cancer, 95.33% of patients reported some degree of efficacy (ibid.). Putting aside the shaky methodology of uncontrolled retrospective studies conducted by *qigong* enthusiasts in the PRC during the 1990s—and the larger question of whether cancer can be cured with *qigong*, a point where the social worlds of *qigong* inevitably collide—this illustrates how even a highly formalised *qigong* practice such as Zhineng Qigong is construed rather differently in the social world of the Chinese *qigong* movement and that of contemporary biomedical studies.

Discussion

As suggested by the stark divergence of the *qigong* across these three social worlds, rather than using the term as a normative category of internally consistent practices, it may be more usefully understood as a 'nominal repository' (Star and Griesemer 1989: 410) cutting across the social worlds of the Chinese *qigong* movement, social scientists, and bio-medical researchers. Unlike a formalised normative category, this has afforded sufficient ambiguity to create the appearance of coherence between each social world: as a convenient collection of 'things that might be individually removed without collapsing or changing the structure of a whole', the term maintains a sense of heterogeneity with-out confronting internal contradictions (Star 2010: 603). The interpre-tive flexibility or 'affordance' (Gibson 1979; Hutchby 2001) of *qigong* has allowed it to travel from the urban public parks, cathartic mass gath-erings, and government-sponsored research associations of the Chinese *qigong* fever to the pages of social scientists who conducted fieldwork in the PRC during the 1980s and 1990s and to the sample groups, sham interventions, and statistical aggregates of the RCT without running up against the apparently incommensurable understandings projected into such practices by each social world.

The suggestion that social constructivist arguments about the Chinese *qigong* movement have come at the expense of the 'thing in itself', how-ever, should not be taken as an endorsement of an essentialist under-standing of such practices. Neither does the radical constructivist position—that *qigong*, like other (bio)medical treatment modalities, enacts a segmented and potentially self-contradictory ontology of its sub-ject (Mol 2002)—point a way towards a rapprochement between Chinese practitioners, social science, and biomedicine. Retreating into a 'prag-matic ethos of healing' ('doing whatever works', Quah 2003) may inter-mediately accommodate such practices in the context of patient-centred healthcare and private health insurance. In the long run, however, if the cultural-nationalist subtext of the practice is unquestionably accepted by practitioners, if the deconstructionist methodology of social science decentres the 'thing in itself' to the point of irrelevance, and if the biomedical evaluation of efficacy remains based on an arbitrary catch-all term for various oriental self-cultivation practices, using *qigong* as a normative category becomes a liability rather than a starting point for the exploration and application of alternative health modalities.

Notes

1. Search string: (qigong[Title] OR "qi gong"[Title]) AND (Review[ptyp] AND "2007/03/19"[PDAT]: "2017/03/17"[PDAT]).
2. As Palmer (2007: 194) notes, '[i]t was common in qigong circles to speak of over 3000 denominations', ranging from a 'handful of disciples' to 'tens of millions of followers'. Ji, Wu ,and, Liang here limit themselves to relatively well-established groups with a considerable number of followers.
3. Exhaling turbid *qi* and inhaling pure *qi*, not to be confused with *tuina*, the massage technique.
4. Translated literally, *qigong* refers to the 'mastery' or 'skill' (*gong* 功) of vital energy or 'breath' (*qi* 气). Usage of the term *qi* varies between 'cosmological, health-related, martial, literary, sexual, and environmental contexts' (Frank 1997, in Frank 2000: 13; see also Kubny 1995).
5. Penny and Otehode (2016: 74) and Otehode (2009: 244) also suggest geographical variation in the choice of the term before *qigong* became widely accepted, including 'deep breath therapy' (*shen huxifa*), 'light breath therapy' (*qian huxifa*), 'movements for breathing and massage' (*huxi anmo yundong*), 'breathing therapy for nourishing life' (*huxi yangshengfa*), and 'quiet sitting therapy' (*jingzuo liaofa*) which in medical journals were presented as 'medical exercises' (*yiliao tiyu*) and 'preventive therapies' (*yufang liaofa*).
6. According to Otehode (2009: 249), Soviet science, in particular Pavlovian physiology, also played a significant role during the 1950s in providing *qigong* with a theoretical basis acceptable with its status as a 'national medical heritage'.
7. A PubMed search for 'qigong' (search string: "qigong"[MeSH Terms] OR "qigong"[All Fields]) shows that the number of publications referring to *qigong* has increased from 3 in 1990 to 6 in 2000, 15 in 2005, 23 in 2010, and 45 in 2016.
8. An overview of this material translated to English may be found in the appendix of Winiger (forthcoming).

References

Adams, V. (2002). Randomized controlled crime: Postcolonial sciences in alternative medicine research. *Social Studies of Science, 32*(5/6), 659–690.

Chan, C. L.-W., Wang, C.-W., Ho, R. T.-H., Ho, A. H.-Y., Ziea, E. T.-C., Taam Wong, V. C.-W., et al. (2012). A systematic review of the effectiveness of qigong exercise in cardiac rehabilitation. *The American Journal of Chinese Medicine, 40*(02), 255–267.

Chau, A. Y. (Ed.). (2010). *Religion in contemporary China: Revitalization and innovation*. London and New York: Routledge.

Chen, N. (1995). Urban spaces and experiences of qigong. In D. Davis, R. Kraus, B. Naughton, & E. Perry (Eds.), *Urban spaces in contemporary China: The potential for autonomy and community in post-Mao China* (pp. 347–361). Cambridge and Washington, DC: Woodrow Wilson Center Press.

Chen, N. (1999). Cultivating qi and body politic. *Harvard Asia Pacific Review, 4*, 45–49.

Chen, N. (2003). *Breathing spaces: Qigong, psychiatry, and healing in China*. New York: Columbia University Press.

Csordas, T. J. (1999). The body's career in anthropology. In H. L. Moore (Ed.), *Anthropological theory today* (pp. 172–205). Cambridge: Polity Press.

Despeux, C. (1997). Le qigong, une expression de la modernité Chinoise. In J. Gernet & M. Kalinowski (Eds.), *En suivant la Voie Royale. Mélanges en homage à Léon Vandermeersch* (pp. 267–281). Paris: École Francaise d'Extrême-Orient.

Despret, V. (2004). The body we care for: Figures of anthropo-zoo-genesis. *Body & Society, 10*(2/3), 111–134.

Edwards, D., Ashmore, M., & Potter, J. (1995). Death and furniture: The rhetoric, politics and theology of bottom line arguments against relativism. *History of the Human Sciences, 8*(2), 25–49.

Farquhar, J., & Zhang, Q. (2012). *Ten thousand things: Nurturing life in contemporary Beijing*. Cambridge, MA and London, England: MIT Press.

Feng, H., & Zhou, X. (1990). *Daojiao qigong baodian*. Taiyuan: Shanxi kexue jiaoyu chubanshe.

Frank, A. (2000). Experiencing qi. *Text, Practice, Performance, 2*, 13–31.

Fujimura, J. H. (1987). Constructing 'do-able' problems in cancer research: Articulating alignment. *Social Studies of Science, 17*(2), 257–293.

Gao, H., Hu, N., & Cheng, L. (1991). *Zhonghua gudian qigong wenku*. Beijing: Beijing chu ban she: Xin hua shu dian Beijing fa xing suo fa xing.

Gibson, J. J. (1979). *The ecological approach to visual perception*. Boston: Houghton Mifflin.

Gleig, A. (2012). Researching new religious movements from the inside out and the outside in. *Nova Religio, 16*(1), 88–103.

Good, B. (1994). *Medicine, rationality and experience: An anthropological perspective.* Cambridge; New York: Cambridge University Press.

Hacking, I. (1999). *The social construction of what?* Cambridge, MA and London, England: Harvard University Press.

Hartley, L., Lee, M. S., Kwong, J. S., Flowers, N., Todkill, D., Ernst, E., et al. (2015). Qigong for the primary prevention of cardiovascular disease. In The Cochrane Collaboration (ed.), *Cochrane database of systematic reviews.* Chichester, UK: John Wiley & Sons.

Heise, T. (1999). *Qigong in der VR China: Entwicklung, Theorie und Praxis.* Berlin: VWB.

Hsu, E. (1999). *The transmission of Chinese medicine.* Cambridge, UK and New York, NY: Cambridge University Press.

Hsu, E. (2008). The history of Chinese medicine in the People's Republic of China and its globalization. *East Asian Science, Technology and Society, 2*(4), 465–484.

Hsu, E., & Lim, C. H. (2016). *Enskilment into the environment: The Yijin Jing Worlds of Jin and Qi.* Preprint: Max-Planck-Institut für Wissenschaftsgeschichte.

Huang, H.-Y. (2013). *Psycho-boom: The rise of psychotherapy in contemporary urban China.* Doctoral dissertation, Harvard University.

Hutchby, I. (2001). Technologies, texts and affordances. *Sociology, 35*(2), 441–456.

Iskra, A. (forthcoming). *Strengthening the nation through self-discovery: The body-heart-soul movement in the PRC.* Doctoral dissertation, The University of Hong Kong.

Ji, Y., Wu, H., & Liang, K. (Eds.). (1993). *Zhongguo Dangdai Qigong Quanshu.* Beijing: Renmin Renti Chubanshe.

Karchmer, E. (2002). Magic, science and qigong in contemporary China. In S. D. Blum & L. M. Jensen (Eds.), *China off center: Mapping the margins of the middle kingdom* (pp. 311–322). Honolulu: University of Hawai'i Press.

Keshet, Y. (2011). Energy medicine and hybrid knowledge construction: The formation of new cultural-epistemological rules of discourse. *Cultural Sociology, 5*(4), 501–518.

Klein, P. J., Schneider, R., & Rhoads, C. J. (2016). Qigong in cancer care: A systematic review and construct analysis of effective qigong therapy. *Supportive Care in Cancer, 24*(7), 3209–3222.

Kleinman, A. (1988). *The illness narratives: Suffering, healing, and the human condition.* New York: Basic Books.

Kohn, L. (2008). *Chinese healing exercises: The tradition of Daoyin.* Honolulu: University of Hawai'i Press.

Komjathy, L. (2006). Qigong in America. In *Daoist body cultivation: Traditional models and contemporary practices* (pp. 203–235). Magdalena, NM: Three Pines Press.

Kubny, M. (1995). *Qi – Lebenskraftkonzepte in China: Definitionen, Theorien Und Grundlagen.* München: LMU München.

Latour, B. (2000). When things strike back: A possible contribution of "science studies" to the social sciences. *The British Journal of Sociology, 51*(1), 107–123.

Lee, M. S., Oh, B., & Ernst, E. (2011). Qigong for healthcare: An overview of systematic reviews. *JRSM Short Reports, 2*(2), 7.

Lee, M. S., Pittler, M. H., & Ernst, E. (2007). External qigong for pain conditions: A systematic review of randomized clinical trials. *The Journal of Pain, 8*(11), 827–831.

Lee, M. S., Pittler, M. H., & Ernst, E. (2009). Internal qigong for pain conditions: A systematic review. *The Journal of Pain, 10*(11), 1121–1127.e14.

Li, Jianhui, & Fu, Z. (2015). The craziness for extra-sensory perception: Qigong fever and the science–pseudoscience debate in China. *Zygon®, 50*(2), 534–547.

Li, Junpeng. (2014). The religion of the nonreligious and the politics of the apolitical: The transformation of Falun Gong from healing practice to political movement. *Politics and Religion, 7*(01), 177–208.

Li, R., Jin, L., Hong, P., He, Z.-H., Huang, C.-Y., Zhao, J.-X., et al. (2014). The effect of baduanjin on promoting the physical fitness and health of adults. *Evidence-Based Complementary and Alternative Medicine, 2014,* 1–8.

Li, Z. (1988). *Zhongguo Qigong Shi.* Zhengzhou: Henan Kexue Jishu Chubanshe.

Lim, Chee Han. (2009). *Purging the ghost of Descartes: Conducting zhineng qigong in Singapore.* Doctoral dissertation, Australian National University.

Liu, T. (Ed.). (2012). *Zhongyi Qigong Xue.* Beijing: Zhongguo Zhongyiyao Chubanshe.

Loh, S. Y., Lee, S. Y., & Murray, L. (2014). The Kuala Lumpur qigong trial for women in the cancer survivorship phase-efficacy of a three-arm act to improve QOL. *Asian Pacific Journal of Cancer Prevention, 15*(19), 8127–8134.

Micollier, E. (1999). Control and release of emotions in qigong practice. *China Perspectives, 24,* 22–30.

Miura, K. (1989). The revival of Qi: Qigong in contemporary China. In L. Kohn (Ed.), *Taoist meditation and longevity techniques* (pp. 331–358). Ann Arbor, MI: Center for Chinese Studies, The University of Michigan.

Mol, A. (2002). *The body multiple: Ontology in medical practice.* Durham: Duke University Press.

Murakawa, H. (2002). *Phenomenology of the experience of qigong: A preliminary research design for the intentional bodily practices.* Doctoral dissertation, California Institute of Integral Studies, San Francisco, California.

Ning, A. M. (2013). How "alternative" is CAM? Rethinking conventional dichotomies between biomedicine and complementary/alternative medicine. *Health: An Interdisciplinary Journal for the Social Study of Health, Illness and Medicine, 17*(2), 135–158.

Oh, B., Butow, P., Mullan, B., & Clarke, S. (2008). Medical qigong for cancer patients: Pilot study of impact on quality of life, side effects of treatment and inflammation. *The American Journal of Chinese Medicine, 36*(03), 459–472.

Otehode, U. (2009). The creation and re-emergence of qigong in China. In Y. Ashiwa & D. L. Wank (Eds.), *Making religion, making the state: The politics of religion in modern China* (pp. 241–266). Stanford: Stanford University Press.

Ots, T. (1991). *Stiller Körper, lauter Leib: Aufstieg und Untergang der jungen chinesischen Heilbewegung Kranich-qigong.* Doctoral dissertation, Universität Hamburg, Hamburg.

Ots, T. (1994). The silenced body—The expressive Leib: On the dialectic of mind and life in Chinese cathartic healing. In T. J. Csordas (Ed.), *Embodiment and experience—The existential ground of culture and self* (pp. 116–139). Cambridge: Cambridge University Press.

Ownby, D. (2008). *Falun Gong and the future of China.* Oxford and New York: Oxford University Press.

Ozawa-De Silva, C. (2002). Beyond the body/mind? Japanese contemporary thinkers on alternative sociologies of the body. *Body & Society, 8*(2), 21–38.

Palmer, D. (2007). *Qigong fever: Body, science, and utopia in China.* New York: Columbia University Press.

Palmer, D. (2008). Embodying Utopia charisma in the post-Mao Qigong craze. *Nova Religio, 12*(2), 69–89.

Palmer, D. (2011). Chinese religious innovation in the Qigong movement: The case of Zhonggong. In *Religion in contemporary China: Revitalization and innovation* (pp. 182–202). London: Routledge.

Penny, B. (1993). Qigong, Daoism and science: Some contexts for the qigong boom. In M. Lee & A. D. Stefanowska (Eds.), *Modernization of the Chinese past* (pp. 166–179). Sydney: Wild Peony.

Penny, B. (2012). *The religion of Falun Gong.* Chicago and London: The University of Chicago Press.

Penny, B., & Otehode, U. (2016). Qigong therapy in 1950s China. *East Asian History, 40,* 69–84.

Quah, S. R. (2003). Traditional healing systems and the ethos of science. *Social Science & Medicine, 57*(10), 1997–2012.

Sagli, G. (2008). Learning and experiencing Chinese qigong in Norway. *East Asian Science, Technology and Society, 2*(4), 545–566.

Siegler, E. (2011). Daoism beyond Modernity: The "Healing Tao" as postmodern movement. In D. A. Palmer & X. Liu (Eds.), *Daoism in the twentieth century: Between eternity and modernity* (pp. 274–293). Los Angeles: University of California Press.

Star, S. L. (2010). This is not a boundary object: Reflections on the origin of a concept. *Science, Technology, & Human Values, 35*(5), 601–617.

Star, S. L., & Griesemer, J. R. (1989). Institutional ecology, "translations" and boundary objects: Amateurs and professionals in Berkeley's Museum of Vertebrate Zoology, 1907–39. *Social Studies of Science, 19*(3), 387–420.

Stenlund, T., Birgander, L. S., Lindahl, B., Nilsson, L., & Ahlgren, C. (2009). Effects of qigong in patients with burnout: A randomized controlled trial. *Journal of Rehabilitation Medicine, 41*(9), 761–767.

Stoller, P. (1997). *Sensuous scholarship*. Philadelphia: University of Pennsylvania Press.

Tao, B., & Yang, W. (1981). *Qigong liaofa jijin (di yi ce)*. Beijing: Renmin weisheng chubanshe.

Tao, B., & Yang, W. (1982). *Qigong liaofa jijin (di er ce)*. Beijing: Renmin weisheng chubanshe.

Tao, B., & Yang, W. (1984). *Qigong liaofa jijin (di san ce)*. Beijing: Renmin weisheng chubanshe.

Tao, B., & Yang, W. (1989). *Qigong liaofa ji jin (di si ce)*. Beijing: Renmin weisheng chubanshe.

Van der Veer, P. (2010). Body and mind in qi gong and yoga: A comparative perspective on India and China. *Eranos Yearbook, 69*, 128–141.

Winiger, F. (forthcoming). Doctoral thesis, The University of Hong Kong, Hong Kong.

Winiger, F. (forthcoming). *Curing capitalism: "Zhineng qigong", Datong and the globalisation of Chinese socialist spiritual civilization*. Doctoral dissertation, The University of Hong Kong.

Xu, J. (1999). Body, discourse, and the cultural politics of contemporary Chinese Qigong. *The Journal of Asian Studies, 58*(4), 961.

Zhan, M. (2014). The empirical as conceptual: Transdisciplinary engagements with an "experiential medicine". *Science, Technology & Human Values, 39*(2), 236–263.

Zhang, Z. (Ed.). (1995). *Zhonghua qigong dadian*. Beijing: Tuanjie chubanshe.

Part II

Doing CAM in Different Contexts: Politics, Regulation and Materiality

5

Towards the Glocalisation of Complementary and Alternative Medicine: Homeopathy, Acupuncture and Traditional Chinese Medicine Practice and Regulation in Brazil and Portugal

Joana Almeida, Pâmela Siegel,
and Nelson Filice De Barros

Introduction

Much has been written about complementary and alternative medicine (CAM) in Western societies in the last decades. Early sociological research on CAM (Baer et al. 1998; Cant and Sharma 1999; Saks 1995; Siahpush 1999; Wardwell 1994) showed how CAM practice and regulation have become globalised since the 1960s and 1970s in these societies. Western populations have seen increasing use of CAM for health and well-being (Sointu 2006; WHO 2013). CAM practitioners have gradually gained professional status and been regulated across a variety

J. Almeida (✉)
University of Bedfordshire, Luton, Bedfordshire, UK

P. Siegel • N. F. De Barros
State University of Campinas, Campinas, São Paulo, Brazil

© The Author(s) 2018
C. Brosnan et al. (eds.), *Complementary and Alternative Medicine*, Health, Technology and Society, https://doi.org/10.1007/978-3-319-73939-7_5

113

of Western countries, such as the United Kingdom (Saks 2015), Australia (Baer 2006), the United States (Baer et al. 1998; Saks 2015) and Canada (Kelner et al. 2006; Welsh and Boon 2015). Mainstream healthcare professionals have increasingly embraced some form of CAM in their practice—such is the case in the United States (Winnick 2006), France (Ramsey 1999), Australia (Eastwood 2000) and New Zealand (Dew 2000).

In addition, supra-state organisations, such as the World Health Organisation (WHO), the Pan-American Health Organisation (PAHO) and the European Union (EU), have proposed 'global', 'Pan-American' and 'Pan-European' governances of CAM, respectively. The WHO's Traditional Medicine Strategy for 2014–2023 (2013), the PAHO's Health of the Indigenous Peoples of the Americas 2005–2007 Action Plan (2004) and the EU's aspirations to set up a European health policy on CAM (EUROCAM 2014) are three good examples of this transnational governance. Indeed, there has been a global institutionalisation of CAM yet simultaneously a construction and promotion of CAM as a local particularism.

Forces of global homogenisation therefore have interpenetrated, and been shaped by, the local. Wiesener et al. (2012), for example, have concluded that although many European countries have moved towards some form of CAM regulation, it has been difficult to identify a pattern in terms of which CAM therapies have been legally practised and regulated and by whom they have been practised. Furthermore, the PAHO has addressed the cultural diversity of the Americas and the multiethnic and multilingual character of this continent. This suggests that the globalisation of CAM has intersected with local contexts and growing particularisations.

The intersection of global and local forces in CAM practice and regulation, however, has remained blurred in sociological analysis, in part due to the significant lack of qualitative comparative studies on CAM to date. Therefore, this chapter introduces CAM in the sociological literature as a 'glocal' (Robertson 1995) phenomenon, that is, as a universalism-particularism issue (Robertson 2000). To bring this 'glocalised' dimension into focus, we analyse the differences in CAM practice and regulation in two countries with a long-standing economic, political and cultural relationship—and therefore with significant levels of intercultural hybridism: Brazil and Portugal. Homeopathy, acupuncture and traditional Chinese medicine (TCM) present three cases in point in terms of their distinctive status in these two countries.

We use a wide range of documentary sources: mainly, official documents, such as bills and reports; virtual documents, such as schools' and organisations' websites and blogs; and mass-media outputs, such as newspapers. We also use research papers from the sociology and history fields to complement our analysis of CAM practice and regulation over time in both countries. All of these are sources of data in their own right, significant in terms of content and, for some, in the part they play in CAM's practice and regulation (Bryman 2016).

We start by presenting some theoretical considerations on CAM as a glocal and culture-dependent phenomenon. We then present the practice and regulation of homeopathy, acupuncture and TCM over time, in Brazil and then in Portugal. Finally, we put these 'practices' and 'regulations' into comparative perspective.

CAM as a Glocal Phenomenon

The terms 'glocal' and 'glocalisation', although popularised in the 1990s in several fields, can be traced back to the Japanese capitalist business and marketing world in the 1980s to express 'global thinking and local acting' strategies (Jain et al. 2012). In other words, being glocal meant tailoring and advertising goods and services on a global scale to differentiated local markets (Robertson 1995). According to Pitta and Franzak (2008), this integration of the global and the local has become the axiom for contemporary marketing managers.

One of the best examples of glocalisation in the contemporary business world has been that of fast-food chains. McDonald's, although being a paradigmatic example of rationalisation and globalisation of marketing strategies (Ritzer 1993), has become sensitive to cultural characteristics and customs and has implemented glocal strategies adapted to different countries. Authors like Barber (1992) see the global and the local, or the universal and the particular, as being inevitably in tension: a McWorld of homogenisation versus a Jihad (meaning struggle-oriented) world of particularisation and 'retribalisation'; in other words, a tension between cultural homogenisation and cultural heterogenisation (Appadurai 1990). Robertson (2012), however, disagrees with the existence of such tension and claims that localisation is a manifestation of globalisation. He posits that the term globalisation should be replaced by the term glocalisation, which has the advantage of highlighting the concern with local needs and preferences.

Since the 1990s, the dynamics of the glocal have become increasingly salient in other fields such as culture and health, where practices have become locally territorialised but globally connected. For example, Robertson (2012) has argued that the concern with a spatio-cultural dimension and the promotion of locality have spread throughout many fields and have been a main characteristic of postmodern societies. He goes on to say that the WHO's attempt to promote 'glocal health' by reactivating indigenous medical traditions is an example of the importance of space and particularism in recent supra-state policies (the Regional Strategy for Traditional Medicine in the Western Pacific from 2012 being a good example—(WHO 2012)).

In the case of CAM, we have seen how challenges to nation-states by supra-state agencies with regard to its governance have been handled in differing ways that suggest differences in the spatio-cultural dimensions of each country; or, following Jasanoff (2005), in ways that suggest different 'civic epistemologies'—that is, culturally specific knowledges and social orders. For example, while in the United Kingdom, CAM therapies have mostly achieved a self-regulatory status and homeopathy has received the support of the royal family, in Australia, homeopathy has been marginalised and largely discredited (Brosnan et al., this volume), and in France, CAM practice is only legitimised for medical doctors (Ramsey 1999). Furthermore, some countries have regulated some forms of CAM as therapies and others as medication, and still others as professions (Wiesener et al. 2012). The variety of nation-states' responses to CAM regulation clearly suggests that there is little prospect of a one-dimensional globalisation process of CAM but rather many modes of CAM globalisation.

Furthermore, as Brosnan et al. (this volume) have stated, CAM has been transformed by national cultures while also intervening in the formation of these cultures, and in their relationships with other cultures through 'intercultural hybridity' and 'intercontinental crossover culture' (Pieterse 1995). Using the globalisation-glocalisation debate and Jasanoff's concept of 'civic epistemologies', we want to capture: (1) the way the globalisation of homeopathy, acupuncture and TCM has been reinterpreted locally by Brazilian and Portuguese cultures and (2) how homeopathy, acupuncture and TCM in Brazil and Portugal have been involved in intercultural hybridism and knowledge networks over time and therefore been shaped by each other and by other cultures, influencing the relationship between these two countries.

Homeopathy, Acupuncture and TCM in Brazil

Brazil is the largest Latin American and Lusophone country and the fifth largest country in the world. The country was a Portuguese colony until the decolonisation of the Americas during the early nineteenth century, leading to its independence. Brazil has been a republic since the end of the nineteenth century, when the monarchy collapsed. Nowadays, it is a federative republic with 26 states and one federal district. Each state is divided into administrative regions called municipalities. The National Congress (*Congresso Nacional*) is the Brazilian legislative body. The Federal Medical Council (*Conselho Federal de Medicina*) oversees the medical practice within the country.

Brazilian society was under populist dictatorships and military regimes during a great part of the twentieth century, ending with the restoration of democracy and the amendment of the constitution in 1988. The new constitution regulated the Unified Health System (*Sistema Único de Saúde*—SUS), allowing for universal healthcare access (Viana 2000). Additionally, the SUS foundation was based on the Brazilian experience taken from international organisations such as the WHO, the PAHO and the World Bank, which emphasised decentralisation of basic health services and the expansion of the role of the state in the assistance to society, reaching out to a larger share of the population (Viana 2000).

Brazil was inhabited by indigenous people when the Portuguese first arrived. This local, indigenous culture—which emphasises the natural environment as a source of medicine and a place for cure—has been in danger for many centuries but still remains today. The indigenous population has generally been a little under 0.5% of the population of the country, although it has increased in recent years (Maggi 2014). A specific healthcare model for indigenous people is laid out in the 1988 Brazilian federal constitution. Brazil thus has a long-lasting history of traditional healing systems as practised by native Indians and has been very disposed to holistic health—which is a main tenet of CAM, yet a marginal perspective in mainstream health.

A brief overview of the history and status of homeopathy in Brazil reveals the intersection of global and local forces over time. Liévano (2013) argues that Brazil and India have been the most prominent countries in the development of homeopathy, in that they have integrated this therapy into their national healthcare systems. Furthermore, both countries had been colonised by European countries, a fact that influenced homeopathy's development as they received many European immigrants who functioned as globalising agents of this therapy (whose codified terminology and principles are of German nature).

Homeopathy in Brazil has had seven main historical phases: its implementation (1840–1859), its expansion (1860–1882), the resistance to it (1882–1900), its golden period (1900–1930), its academic decline (1930–1970), its revival (1970–1990) (Luz 1996) and its current contradictory phase. Homeopathy's implementation period started with the arrival of Benoît Mure—a French homeopath with socialist aspirations—in Brazil (although there has been earlier evidence of contact with this therapy, marked by various Brazilian figures' correspondence with the founder of homeopathy, Samuel Hahnemann (1755–1843), and the introduction of homeopathic literature and doctoral theses on homeopathy) (Liévano 2013). During this phase, intense disputes occurred in the press between homeopaths and members of the Imperial Academy of Medicine (later renamed the National Academy of Medicine), mainly due to an epistemic opposition. The homeopaths defended a modern therapeutic rationality which contradicted the mechanistic tenets of conventional medicine, considering them old-fashioned and ineffective;

meanwhile, conventional medical bodies tried to block the attempts of legitimising homeopathy in Brazil (Luz 1996).

In the transition to homeopathy's expansion phase, in 1859, the Hahnemann Institute of Rio de Janeiro was founded. During this expansion period, homeopathy was disseminated among the lower classes, and various laboratories, pharmacies, health centres and clinics for free treatment of the needy population were established (Luz 1996). This was quite the opposite of what happened in Europe, where homeopathy was mostly used by members of the nobility or royalty and was known as the 'therapy of the rich' (as the case study of Portugal shows).

Homeopathy's period of resistance expressed the battles of traditional homeopaths against several attempts—by the Imperial Academy of Medicine, the Faculty of Medicine of Rio de Janeiro and the Public Hygiene League—to block the practice. Nevertheless, the homeopaths continued publishing their findings in national and international conventions, in a context dominated by the Pasteurian revolution and the expansion of public hygiene (Luz 1996). The homeopathic practice also expanded socially through the support of philanthropic and religious institutions and indigenous spiritual centres.

During homeopathy's golden period, two homeopathic faculties were established, one in Rio de Janeiro and another in Rio Grande do Sul, as well as a homeopathic hospital. Another landmark was the First Brazilian Convention of Homeopathy held in 1926. During this same period, however, sanitary medicine advocates such as the Brazilian medical doctors Oswaldo Cruz and Carlos Chagas tried to discredit homeopathy within the nation (Luz 1996).

The academic decline of homeopathy occurred between 1930 and 1970 and was strongly influenced by the intense development of medical specialties, the pharmaceutical industry and the use of antibiotics. In other words, the downfall was due to the growth of medical technologies that gained worldwide acceptance, despite the ongoing support of the Brazilian military who sympathised with the homeopathic philosophy.

The revival of homeopathy after 1970 reflects the beginning of a new societal movement towards the use of less invasive therapies. A main reason for this was the great urban development, which caused a wave of concerns among the middle class about their healthcare (Luz 2005). This phase saw an expansion of healthcare centres, homeopathic pharmacies and organic health food stores in the largest municipalities. Furthermore, opportunities to practise homeopathy became available to medical doctors. In 1979, homeopathy was recognised by the Brazilian Medical Association as a medical specialty, and in 1980, it was also accepted by the Federal Medical Council (Luz 1996). In 1981, the Brazilian Homeopathic Medical Association was created and charged with establishing directives for courses in the training of the 'homeopathic physician' (Galhardi and Barros 2008). The therapy started to be offered in several states and municipalities until 1985, when the first bill for its integration into the public health services was published. Yet homeopathic practice was still being established through individual, isolated and sometimes discontinued initiatives—revealing the need for specific guidelines to regulate its practice within the SUS (Barros et al. 2007; Salles and Schraiber 2009; Loch-Neckel et al. 2010).

In 2006, the Health Ministry published the National Policy for Integrative and Complementary Practices (PNPIC) within the SUS under Act 971, promoting the implementation of different integrative practices: homeopathy, acupuncture/TCM, phytotherapy, social thermalism/chrenotherapy and anthroposophical medicine (Ministry of Health of Brazil 2006). Nevertheless, homeopathy is currently stuck in a contradictory phase, which is supportive of its development as a therapy within the public healthcare system, yet hinders it as a profession because of political and historical difficulties outside the SUS. Homeopathy has been statutorily regulated as a therapy which may be practised by different healthcare professionals (doctors, nurses, pharmacists and dentists) within the SUS, but it remains unregulated as a profession outside the public system, and traditional homeopaths have been able to survive only through self-regulation.

Similar to that of homeopathy, the development of acupuncture and TCM in Brazil arose from transnational cultural networks and intercultural communication. In the late 1950s, Frederico J. Spaeth, an immigrant Luxembourgish physiotherapist, arrived in Brazil and started the first courses on acupuncture in São Paulo and later in Rio de Janeiro. Together with physician Evaldo Martins Leite, Spaeth dedicated decades of effort to expanding and disseminating multi-professional acupuncture in Brazil, despite legal resistance that put both in prison in the 1970s. As a medical doctor, Martins Leite was acquitted of the charges quickly, but Spaeth remained jailed for a longer period as he did not have a medical degree and was accused of charlatanism (Rocha and Gallian 2016). Spaeth imported the so-called French School of acupuncture, mainly based on the works of George Soulié de Morant (1878–1955). Nevertheless, it was not until 1970 that courses on traditional Chinese acupuncture were taught in Brazil by the Chinese themselves—most notably by Wu Chao-Hsiang, in Rio de Janeiro; and Liu Pai Lin and Wu Tou Kwang, in São Paulo (Tesser 2010).

In the following decades, acupuncture gradually attained recognition as a medical therapy in Brazil. In 1995, the Federal Medical Council recognised acupuncture as a medical speciality (Conselho Federal de Medicina 2001); yet it was only in 2002 that the Ministry of Education regulated courses on the therapy, which were organised and taught by medical doctors (Colégio Médico Brasileiro de Acupuntura 2012). Following globalising trends, acupuncture's practice has been detached from TCM within the SUS.

Although the integration of homeopathy, acupuncture and TCM to the public health system has been occurring progressively since the 1980s, it was boosted by the creation of the SUS in 1988 and the already-mentioned PNPIC in 2006. To date, there is no statutory regulation of homeopathy, acupuncture and TCM as health professions in Brazil, although since 1986 several bills have been sent to the National Congress aimed at such. Several allied healthcare professions—such as physiotherapy, nursing, psychology and speech therapy—have at some point regulated the use of acupuncture and TCM, mostly as specialties. However, the Federal Medical Council has legally questioned the right of other healthcare professionals to use these therapies. After the implementation of the PNPIC within the SUS, there was an attempt to allocate the practice of acupuncture as a private medical act. Nevertheless, all the arguments presented along this line were rejected by former President Dilma Rousseff in the final text approved in July 2013 by the National Congress, a decision that is still being upheld at the time of writing (Presidência da República 2013).

To conclude, homeopathy, acupuncture and TCM have been integrated as therapies in Brazil within the SUS since 2006, although their practice there goes further back in time than that. Furthermore, homeopathy became a medical specialty earlier than acupuncture, and acupuncture's practice became detached from TCM. These therapies have been medicalised within the SUS, and although they are regulated as multi-professional practices, they have not been legitimised as professions outside the public healthcare system. Medical doctors and other allied healthcare professionals have functioned as mediators between global CAM and local Brazilian culture. Furthermore, the importation and hybridisation of homeopathy, acupuncture and TCM by European and Asian immigrants who functioned as globalising agents of CAM and intercultural brokers in Brazil is also an aspect of note. We look now at the case of homeopathy, acupuncture and TCM in Portugal.

Homeopathy, Acupuncture and TCM in Portugal

Portugal is a Southern European country, which has been a republic since October of 1910, when the monarchy ended. Portugal performed a key role during colonial times, with Brazil being one of its most valuable colonies. From 1926 to 1933, the country lived under a military dictatorship, and in 1933, the *Estado Novo* (New State) and its fascist right-wing dictatorship was installed. The authoritarian *Estado Novo* lasted for four decades, until 1974, when the Carnation Revolution (*Revolução dos Cravos*) put an end to the regime, and the Prime Minister Marcello Caetano, the successor of the long serving dictator António de Oliveira Salazar, was exiled to Brazil (Saraiva 1999).

The democratic republic was restored in Portugal in 1974, and in 1976, a new constitution was adopted. In 1979, the national health system (*Sistema Nacional de Saúde*—SNS) was created, stressing the democratic principles of universality, generality and gratuity. However, since the early 1990s, the SNS has undergone major changes including financial ones, such as the creation of public-private partnerships. This has put its earlier principles into question (Barros et al. 2011). The Central Administration of the Health System (*Administração Central do Sistema de Saúde*—ACSS) is the governmental institute in charge of the management of the SNS.

Following the global and European trends towards regulating CAM in Western countries, the statuses of some CAM therapies in Portugal have recently changed. It is estimated that there are 20,000 CAM practitioners in the country (Margato 2016). In July 2013, the government approved Act 71/2013 (*Lei do Enquadramento Base das Terapêuticas Não Convencionais*), which extended regulation to seven CAM therapies: homeopathy, acupuncture, TCM, osteopathy, chiropractic therapies, naturopathy and phytotherapy. Amongst these, homeopathy, acupuncture and TCM are very interesting case studies because, although all are included in Act 71/2013, they have each gained different statuses within Portuguese society and the medical profession over time. When compared to their Brazilian counterparts, they make the universalism-particularism debate a pertinent one.

In the same way as they did in Brazil, knowledge networks and interculturalism played a major role in the introduction of homeopathy to the country. Authors like Mira (1947), Araújo (2005) and Pereira et al. (2005) have documented that medical and pharmaceutical interest in homeopathy in Portugal goes back to the early nineteenth century. According to Pereira et al. (2005), homeopathy was introduced in Portugal during the 1830s, via the influence of Parisian culture. Hahnemann lived in Paris, and so the city became a centre of homeopathy's dissemination—not only for Portugal but also for most Western countries, including Brazil (Pereira et al. 2005). Pereira et al. (2005) also state that the introduction of homeopathy in Brazil by French homeopath Benoît Mure in the 1830s and 1840s contributed to its popularity in Portugal, due to the strong cultural, political and economic ties between these two countries. Finally, Spain—where homeopathy was more integrated, supported by the Royal Family and already being practised by medical doctors and pharmacists—was also a vehicle for the dissemination of homeopathy in Portugal due to its geographical proximity (Pereira et al. 2005).

Amongst the first medical doctors to practise homeopathy in Portugal were Henrique de Burnay—who, although Belgian, lived in Portugal—and Florêncio Peres Furtado Galvão, Professor in the Faculty of Medicine at the University of Coimbra, who obtained his PhD in 1835 and referred in his thesis to homeopathy. Interestingly, homeopathy was taught in some medical courses by academics, such as Furtado Galvão himself. By 1859, Furtado Galvão, Professor of 'Materia Medica' and Pharmaceutical Studies, was teaching Hahnemann's doctrines in his courses, which were attended by medical students but also by future pharmacists at the School of Pharmacy from the University of Coimbra (Pereira et al. 2005; Araújo 2005). Therefore, conclude Pereira et al. (2005), the University of Coimbra performed a crucial role in the dissemination of homeopathy among medical doctors and pharmacists in Portugal during the nineteenth century.

In parallel with the enthusiasm for homeopathy from medical doctors and pharmacists in the nineteenth century, there was another type of enthusiast—mainly autodidacts—who argued for the institutionalisation of homeopathy and were very critical of allopathic medicine. Consequently, and in the same way as in Brazil, Portuguese society has seen the development of two groups of homeopathic practitioners since the eighteenth century: the healers and the 'charlatans' who usually lack a biomedical background, and the medical doctors who complement their conventional medical knowledge with homeopathy or even convert their practice to homeopathy (Pereira et al. 2005).

Homeopathy also obtained the support of personalities from the Portuguese aristocracy and from the political and artistic spheres over the centuries. In the nineteenth century, the left-wing liberal MP Manuel da Silva Passos and the Duke of Saldanha were major advocates for Hahnemann's theory—both in their private lives, through their successful personal use of homeopathy, and in public, through attempts to institutionalise homeopathy into the mainstream healthcare system and within medical education (Pereira et al. 2005). The Duke of Saldanha was the director of a CAM journal, the *Gazeta Homeopática de Lisboa*.

Another event which contributed to the increasing acceptance of homeopathy within Portuguese medical circles was the nomination of Samuel Hahnemann as honorary member of the Medical Science Society of Lisbon (*Sociedade de Ciências Médicas de Lisboa*) in 1839 by Lima Leitão, the Society's president and a medical doctor supportive of homeopathy. Leitão was friends with Silvestre Pinheiro Ferreira, a Portuguese bourgeois advocate of homeopathy exiled in Paris who was a friend of Hahnemann. The nomination of Hahnemann and the recognition of his contribution to humanity and medicine by the Medical Science Society of Lisbon, therefore, is an important achievement in the history of the institutionalisation of homeopathy in Portugal (Pereira et al. 2005). Nevertheless, it also gave rise to several protests from within the medical profession and among doctors themselves who did not believe in homeopathy and protested its institutional acceptance (Pereira et al. 2005). Since then, the divisions within the medical profession between those who support or embrace homeopathy and those who do not believe in its scientific validity have endured. Indeed, Martins e Silva (1990) suggested in 1990, more than one century after Hahnemann's nomination, that the increasing practice of CAM among the population and among the medical doctors themselves was a sociocultural anomaly which should be tackled in three ways: (1) by increasing the educational level of the population, (2) by disseminating conventional medicine through the media and (3) by developing critical thinking in medical professionals in relation to CAM.

The difficulties encountered in homeopathy's struggle to gain legitimacy in Portugal over time can be attributed to the medical resistance towards the homeopathic ideology, which has persisted there. At the end of the 1990s, when CAM practitioners were able to lobby the government to pay attention to their situation, two CAM Bill projects were presented to the Portuguese parliament requesting the regulation of six CAM therapies: homeopathy, acupuncture, osteopathy, chiropractic, naturopathy and phytotherapy (Almeida and Gabe, 2016). These projects marked the beginning of a long-standing political battle, which involved representatives of these therapies, the medical profession and the state. The result was the creation of Act 45/2003, which regulated the aforementioned CAM therapies and which was later replaced by Act 71/2013, which added TCM to the list.

Today, homeopathy is regulated as a profession through Act 71/2013 but has yet to wait for the government to issue its educational standards.

Moreover, homeopathy remains unregulated for medical doctors. The latter are not permitted to call themselves homeopaths, as according to the Portuguese Medical Council's Code of Ethics (Assembleia da República Portuguesa 2009), titles other than doctor are prohibited from membership. Despite this, medical doctors' practice of CAM in Portugal has persisted. At present, there are at least two medical associations for homeopathy within the country: the Homeopathic Society of Portugal (*Sociedade Homeopática de Portugal*—SHP), founded in 2003 by a small group of medical doctors and pharmacists, and the Portuguese Society of Homeopathy (*Sociedade Portuguesa de Homeopatia*–SPH) (Almeida 2012). As Almeida (2012) has shown, the extent to which these associations have set up courses in homeopathy—for medical doctors and other healthcare professionals or for people without previous formal healthcare training—remains ambiguous, as very little information has been disclosed on the topic.

The history of acupuncture and TCM in Portugal is more recent than that of homeopathy. Again, intercultural engagement played a main role in the introduction of these therapies to the country. The first traces of Western, medicalised acupuncture go back to the Portuguese soldier and missionary Fernão Mendez Pinto, who mentioned this therapy as a medical treatment in Japan in a book entitled *Pilgrimage of Fernão Mendez Pinto* from 1614—which was then translated into Spanish in 1620, French in 1628 and English in 1663 (Lu and Lu 2013). Although the medical practice of acupuncture goes back to the 1970s, it was only at the turn of the twenty-first century, in 2001, that medical doctors acquired the legal right to practise this therapy as a 'medical competency' (Almeida 2012). Until then, many medical doctors used to travel to France, where acupuncture was already implemented in medical courses, to acquire training and education in the practice (SPMA 2016). Interestingly, at the same time as the political battle over CAM regulation in the country, in 2001, the Portuguese Medical Society of Acupuncture (*Sociedade Portuguesa Médica de Acupunctura*—SPMA) was founded and tasked with establishing criteria to determine competency in 'medical acupuncture'. In 2002, the Portuguese Medical Council approved and applied these criteria to medical doctors (Almeida 2012). The SPMA represents the interests of medical doctors who practise 'medical acupuncture' and aims to contribute to the promotion and scientific research of this therapy.

The SPMA is a member of international medical federations such as the International Council of Medical Acupuncture and Related Techniques (ICMART) and the Iberic-American Federation of Medical Societies of Acupuncture (Filasma).

This move towards the institutional medical acceptance of acupuncture led to the creation of a postgraduate course in 'medical acupuncture', accredited by the Medical Council and held at universities approved by the Ministry of Education and in partnership with the SPMA. The first institution to welcome this course was the Abel Salazar Biomedical Science Institute (ICBAS) in Porto in 2003, followed by the Faculty of Medicine at the University of Coimbra in 2007, the Faculty of Medical Sciences at the New University of Lisbon in 2010 and the School of Medical Sciences at the University of Minho in 2012. According to the SPMA (2016), there are more than 180 medical doctors with training in 'medical acupuncture' in the country, at least 63 of whom have acquired the SPMA's accreditation in medical acupuncture (Gomes 2009). Many medical doctors have started offering acupuncture treatments within the SNS, in hospitals and health centres, and around 150 medical doctors have enrolled in one of the four postgraduate courses offered in the country (SPMA 2016).

Some aspects of this postgraduate course in 'medical acupuncture' are worth mentioning in more detail. The course is designed solely for medical doctors and delivered by medical doctors, and the content of the course covers such aspects as 'neuro-anatomical and neuro-physiological notions of acupuncture', 'evidence-based research and medicine', 'theoretical notions of TCM', study of the meridians and pressure points and clinical indications and side effects of acupuncture. After completion of the course, candidates still must demonstrate continuing practice over 12 months under the supervision of an accredited 'medical acupuncturist', submit a report with ten case studies where medical acupuncture treatment has been applied, contribute to the training and education in acupuncture of other medical doctors, publish articles on medical acupuncture, attend refresher courses and promote medical acupuncture (SPMA 2016).

Acupuncture, therefore, has been medicalised in the country, restricted to medical doctors within the SNS and detached from TCM. Acupuncture and TCM, however, have also been practised outside the SNS by traditional practitioners who have acquired training and education through non-medical professional schools or associations. Both therapies are covered by Act 71/2013, although only acupuncture has seen its educational standards approved by the state to design and propose appropriate BSc courses. Since Act 71/2013, the Central Administration of the Health System has received 3500 applications to acquire the professional credentials in one of the five CAM therapies (excluding homeopathy and TCM) (Margato 2016).

It can thus be stated that significant changes have been made concerning the status of homeopathy, acupuncture and TCM in Portuguese society, Act 71/2013 being the best evidence of it. However, they do not share the same status within the Portuguese medical establishment. While acupuncture has been medicalised and can legally be practised as a speciality by medical doctors within the SNS, homeopathy and TCM are banned from medical practice, even though homeopathy has a longer traditional history in Portuguese medical circles than acupuncture. A main reason for this ban has been their perceived poor scientific plausibility when compared to acupuncture.

The operation of global dynamics of CAM thus has gone hand in hand with local loyalties, particularly in relation to the power of the medical profession and scientific knowledge in state development of CAM policies within and outside the public health system. Furthermore, in the same way as in Brazil, Portuguese society has been the recipient of cultural influences from other European cultures and the Brazilian culture itself, as well as from many intellectuals and cognitive agents, leading to a boundary-crossing mixture of CAM regulations and practices.

Discussion

Brazil and Portugal have clearly participated in the globalising trend of CAM governance over the last decades, in that both countries have been concerned with the integration of homeopathy, acupuncture and TCM into their healthcare systems. Yet this global, homogenised trend has also involved the incorporation of locality, in that both countries have differed in the way they have conducted such governance. Therefore, Brazil and Portugal have presented different modes of globalisation of CAM. Table 5.1 summarises the main differences and similarities in homeopathy, acupuncture and TCM practice and regulation in both countries over time.

Brazil regulated homeopathy in 1979 and acupuncture in 1995, as medical specialities, and in 2006, these therapies were incorporated into the SUS together with TCM, phytotherapy, social thermalism/chrenotherapy and anthroposophical medicine through Act 971, which sanctions the PNPIC. These therapies have been regulated to be practised by different healthcare professionals within the public health system, although they

Table 5.1 Practice and regulation of homeopathy, acupuncture and TCM in Brazil and Portugal

	Homeopathy	Acupuncture	TCM
Brazil	• Introduced in the nineteenth century • Regulated as a medical speciality in 1979 • Self-regulated as a profession • Statutorily regulated as a therapy within the SUS in 2006 • Practised by medical doctors and allied health professionals within the SUS	• Introduced in the twentieth century • Regulated as a medical speciality in 1995 • Self-regulated as a profession • Statutorily regulated as a therapy within the SUS in 2006 • Practised by medical doctors and allied health professionals within the SUS	• Introduced in the twentieth century • Unregulated as a medical speciality • Self-regulated as a profession • Statutorily regulated as a therapy within the SUS in 2006 • Practised by medical doctors and allied health professionals within the SUS
Portugal	• Introduced in the nineteenth century • Unregulated as a medical speciality • Statutorily regulated as a profession in 2013 • Not included in the SNS	• Introduced in the twentieth century • Regulated as a medical speciality in 2001 • Statutorily regulated as a profession in 2013 • Practised by medical doctors within the SNS	• Introduced in the twentieth century • Unregulated as a medical speciality • Statutorily regulated as a profession in 2013 • Not included in the SNS

remain marginalised as professions and statutorily unregulated outside the SUS. Given the long-standing tradition of indigenous health beliefs, practices and knowledge-making in Brazil and the role of international organisations such as the PAHO in stimulating indigenous health, it is relatively surprising that the Brazilian state is resistant to protecting traditional medical knowledge and to extending regulation to homeopathy, acupuncture and TCM outside the SUS. On the contrary, the biomedical epistemic framework has prevailed.

In Portugal, in turn, acupuncture has remained the only CAM therapy regulated for medical doctors and has been clearly detached from TCM within medical circles. Homeopathy is still discredited and marginalised by the Portuguese Medical Council, although there are medical doctors practising it privately in the country. Medical doctors are the only health professionals practising acupuncture within the SNS, although this SNS practice is still rare and not much advocated. In 2013, however, homeopathy, acupuncture and TCM, together with osteopathy, chiropractic, naturopathy and phytotherapy, were statutorily regulated through Act 71/2013 and became professions to be practised by traditional CAM practitioners yet outside the SNS. The country, therefore, has recently turned into a political culture in which diverse health knowledges have been legitimised outside the SNS, yet they have often been in tension and in conflict inside a healing culture where biomedical expertise has tended to prevail.

These different directions and divergent policy framings that homeopathy, acupuncture and TCM have taken within Brazilian and Portuguese healthcare systems, although having been developed as part of a global governance of CAM, have pointed to a degree of glocalisation (Robertson 1995), as global policies and decision-making on these therapies have become locally territorialised, that is, reinterpreted locally, leading to a myriad of practices and regulations. Homeopathy, acupuncture and TCM practice and regulation in these two countries have been influenced by different 'civic epistemologies' (Jasanoff 2005), that is, different national cultures around the status of professionals, knowledge and expertise. These national cultures have been inextricably bound up with 'power', 'resistance' or 'liberation' (Robertson 2000). In Portugal, the practice and regulation of homeopathy, acupuncture and TCM within the public healthcare system have been conducted with strong involvement of the state and the hegemonic medical power, as acupuncture's practice limitation to medical doctors within the SNS has shown. In Brazil, in turn, the practice and regulation of these therapies, although also controlled by the state, have been more pluralistic and open to different health professionals within the SUS. Looking across the two countries, Portuguese medical expertise remains tied to the medical profession, which has emerged as an authoritative presence in the CAM policy arena within the SNS. In Brazil, despite the diverse attempts of the medical profession to retain full medical expertise over CAM practice over time, the latter has been liberated to other health professionals within the SUS.

This heterogenisation of CAM governance, however, has been interpenetrated by homogenisation trends. Brazil has clearly medicalised homeopathy, acupuncture and TCM through their integration into the SUS, and Portugal has clearly medicalised acupuncture through its exclusive practice by medical doctors within the SNS and therefore transformed their practice. In both countries, the contrast between those intellectuals, usually from the medical field, who have attempted to discard, reject, omit or redefine the global flow of these therapies and those who have been less tied to a scientific episteme and sought a more flexible and inclusive healthcare has been worthy of noting. As shown, both countries have witnessed epistemic tensions within the medical profession, between those who have disbelieved in these therapies' effectiveness and those who have embraced them. Furthermore, both countries have also witnessed the epistemic division between two types of homeopathic, acupuncture and TCM practitioners over time: those without a biomedical background and those with a biomedical background who have embraced these therapies as complements to their practice or even as alternatives.

Another important issue arising from the comparison of these two countries has to do with the selective incorporation, cultural hybridisation and re-embedding of national cultures (Pieterse 1995). In other words, 'the tendency for nation-states to "copy" ideas and practices from other societies' (Robertson 1995: 41). Homeopathy has been present within Brazilian and Portuguese medical circles since the nineteenth century. Acupuncture and TCM, in turn, have also been present in both countries since the early twentieth century. In both countries, there were many attempts by European and Asian agents to import and incorporate the knowledge and practice of these therapies over time. In Brazil, the dissemination of homeopathy saw the influence of the Portuguese and French, while the importation of acupuncture saw the influence of the Luxembourgish and Asian nationals. In Portugal, the Parisian culture, Brazilian agents and the status of homeopathy in Spain were the main vehicles of dissemination of homeopathy. Furthermore, Portuguese medical doctors used to travel to France to acquire training in acupuncture prior to its regulation as a medical competency in 2001. Unavoidably, Brazil and Portugal have engaged in crossover culture, by learning and copying practices from other societies and being influenced by such interdependencies and 'hybridised national cultures' (Robertson 1995). Consequently, due to their long-standing economic, cultural and political relationship, it has been clear that these two countries have exchanged homeopathic, acupuncture and TCM knowledge over time, which, in turn, shaped and reinforced that same relationship.

To conclude, the sameness and the difference present in the current status of homeopathy, acupuncture and TCM in Brazil and Portugal have allowed us to emphasise the concern with the local issues and the significance of the concept of glocalisation for the sociology of CAM. In other words, by comparing homeopathy, acupuncture and TCM status in these two countries, we have shown the misleading conception of the globalisation of these practices as a one-dimensional process. Instead, we should see the global flow of these, and potentially other CAM practices, as being increasingly expressed in terms of locality and particularity. Furthermore, this comparative analysis has also allowed us to present the nation-state as a local expression of globalisation and a major agent of diversity and localisation. As Featherstone (1990) has stated, CAM's global culture by no means entails a weakening of the sovereignty of nation-states; rather, it operates within diverse local discourses, preferences and intergroup struggles, which have given rise to various brands of CAM. Other future country comparisons should be put forward in order to de-ethnocentrise this subfield of sociology.

References

Almeida, J. (2012). The differential incorporation of CAM into the medical establishment: The case of acupuncture and homeopathy in Portugal. *Health Sociology Review, 21*(1), 5–22.

Almeida, J., & Gabe, J. (2016). CAM within a field force of countervailing powers: The case of Portugal. *Social Science and Medicine, 155*, 73–81.

Appadurai, A. (1990). Disjuncture and difference in the global cultural economy. *Theory, Culture & Society, 7*, 295–310.

Araújo, Y. L. M. M. (2005). Heterodoxias da arte de curar portuguesa de oitocentos—o caso da homeopatia. *Revista da Faculdade de Letras*, Porto. III Série. 6: 153–167.

Assembleia da República Portuguesa. (2009). Ordem dos Médicos. Regulamento no 14/2009. In Diário da Assembleia da República, 2.ª série – No. 8 – 13/1/2009, 1355–1369.

Baer, H. A. (2006). The drive for legitimation in Australian naturopathy: Successes and dilemmas. *Social Science & Medicine, 63*, 1771–1783.

Baer, H. A., Jen, C., Tanassi, L. M., Tsia, C., & Wahbeh, H. (1998). The drive for professionalization in acupuncture: A preliminary view from the San Francisco bay area. *Social Science & Medicine, 46*(4–5), 533–537.

Barber, B. R. (1992). Jihad vs. McWorld. *The Atlantic, 269*(3), 53–65.

Barros, N. F., Siegel, P., & Simoni, C. (2007). Política nacional de práticas integrativas e complementares no SUS: passos para o pluralismo na saúde. *Cadernos de Saúde Pública, 23*(12), 3066–3069.

Barros, P. P., Machado, S. R., & de Almeida Simões, J. (2011). *Portugal health system review*. European observatory on health systems and policies. Denmark: WHO Regional Office for Europe.

Bryman, A. (2016). *Social research methods*. Oxford: Oxford University Press.

Cant, S., & Sharma, U. (1999). *A new medical pluralism? Alternative medicine, doctors, patients and the state*. London: UCL Press.

Colégio Médico Brasileiro de Acupuntura. (2012). No Brasil, a residência médica em acupuntura tem carga horária de 5.760 horas, durante dois anos, em nove universidades do país. *Colégio Médico Brasileiro de Acupuntura Webpage* 25 July. Retrieved November 9, 2017, from http://www.maxpress-net.com.br/Conteudo/1,516155,No_Brasil_a_residencia_medica_em_Acupuntura_tem_carga_horaria_de_5760_horas_durante_dois_anos_em_nove_universidades_do_p,516155,9.htm

Conselho Federal de Medicina. (2001). *Ementa: fundamento para o conselho federal de medicina editar resoluções reconhecendo especialidades médicas.* Brasília, 18 April. Retrieved November 9, 2017, from http://www.portalmedico.org.br/notasdespachos/CFM/2001/85_2001.pdf.

Dew, K. (2000). Deviant insiders: Medical acupuncturists in New Zealand. *Social Science & Medicine, 50*(12), 1785–1795.

Eastwood, H. (2000). Why are Australian GPs using alternative medicine? Postmodernisation, consumerism and the shift towards holistic health. *Journal of Sociology, 36*(2), 133–156.

EUROCAM. (2014). *CAM 2020: The contribution of complementary and alternative medicine to sustainable healthcare in Europe.* Brussels: EUROCAM.

Featherstone, M. (1990). Global culture: An introduction. In M. Featherstone (Ed.), *Global culture: Nationalism, globalization and modernity* (pp. 1–14). London: Sage Publications.

Galhardi, W. M. P., & Barros, N. F. (2008). The teaching of homeopathy and its practice in the Brazilian public health system. *Interface, 12*(25), 247–266.

Gomes, C. (2009). Alguns hospitais públicos já têm consultas de acupuntura. *Jornal Público Webpage.* Caderno Principal, Portugal, 11 April. Retrieved November 9, 2017, from http://www.mynetpress.pt/pdf/2009/abril/2009041119b0f4.pdf.

Jain, M., Khalil, S., Le, A. N., & Cheng, J. M. (2012). The glocalisation of channels of distribution: A case study. *Management Decision, 50*(3), 521–538.

Jasanoff, S. (2005). *Designs on nature: Science and democracy in Europe and the United States.* Princeton, NJ: Princeton University Press.

Kelner, M., Wellman, B., Welsh, S., & Boon, H. (2006). How far can complementary and alternative medicine go? The case of chiropractic and homeopathy. *Social Science & Medicine, 63*, 2617–2627.

Liévano, C. L. S. (2013). Breve mirada al desarrollo de la historia de la homeopatía en el mundo durante los dos últimos siglos. *Universidad Nacional de Colombia. Facultad de Medicina.* Maestría en Medicina Alternativa (unpublished).

Loch-Neckel, G., Carmignan, F., & Crepaldi, M. A. (2010). A homeopatia no SUS na perspectiva de estudantes da área da saúde. *Revista Brasileira de Educação Médica, 34*(1), 82–90.

Lu, D. P., & Lu, G. P. (2013). An historical review and perspective on the impact of acupuncture on U.S. medicine and society. *Medical Acupuncture, 25*(5), 311–316.

Luz, M. T. (1996). *A Arte de curar versus a ciência dasdoenças: história social da homeopatia no Brasil*. São Paulo: Dynamis.

Luz, M. T. (2005). Cultura contemporânea e medicinas alternativas: Novos paradigmas em saúde no fim do século XX. *PHYSIS: Revista Saúde Coletiva, 15*, 145–176.

Maggi, R. S. (2014). Indigenous health in Brazil. *Revista Brasileira de Saúde Materno Infantil, 14*(1), 13–16.

Margato, D. (2016). Medicinas alternativas com licenças bloqueadas. *Jornal de Notícias Webpage*, 1 November. Retrieved November 9, 2017, from http://www.jn.pt/nacional/interior/apenas-105-cedulas-definitivas-para-terapias-5473840.html.

Martins e Silva, J. (1990). Medicinas alternativas, homeopatia e ciência médica. *Acta Médica Portuguesa, 3*, 301–304.

Ministry of Health of Brazil. (2006). *Política nacional de práticas integrativas e complementares no SUS—PNPIC-SUS*. Secretaria de Atenção à Saúde. Departamento de Atenção Básica. Brasília: Ministério da Saúde. (Série B. Textos Básicos de Saúde).

Mira, M. F. (1947). *História da medicina Portuguesa*. Lisboa: Edição da Empresa Nacional de Publicidade.

Pan-American Health Organisation. (2004). *Health of the indigenous peoples initiative. Strategic direction and plan of action 2003–2007*. Regional Office of the World Health Organisation.

Pereira, A. L., Pita, J. R., & Araújo, Y. L. (2005). L'influence sur la réception de l'homéopathie au Portugal. *Revue D'Histoire de la Pharmacie, 93*(348), 569–578.

Pieterse, J. N. (1995). Glocalisation as hybridization. In M. Featherstone, S. Lash, & R. Robertson (Eds.), *Global modernities* (pp. 45–68). London: Sage Publications.

Pitta, D. A., & Franzak, F. F. (2008). Foundations for building share of heart in global brands. *Journal of Product & Brand Management., 17*(2), 64–72.

Presidência da República. (2013). *Mensagem° 287, de 10 de Julho de 2013*. Retrieved November 9, 2017, from http://www.planalto.gov.br/ccivil_03/_Ato2011-2014/2013/Msg/VEP-287.htm.

Ramsey, M. (1999). Alternative medicine in modern France. *Medical History, 43*, 286–322.

Ritzer, G. (1993). *The McDonaldization of society: An investigation into the changing character of contemporary social life*. London: Sage Publications.

Robertson, R. (1995). Glocalisation: Time-space and homogeneity-heterogeneity. In M. Featherstone, S. Lash, & R. Robertson (Eds.), *Global modernities* (pp. 25–44). London: Sage Publications.

Robertson, R. (2000). *Globalization: Social theory and global culture* (6th ed.). London: Sage Publications.

Robertson, R. (2012). Globalisation or glocalisation? *The Journal of International Communication, 18*(2), 33–52.

Rocha, S. P., & Gallian, D. M. C. (2016). A acupuntura no Brasil: uma concepção de desafios e lutas omitidos ou esquecidos pela história—Entrevista com dr. Evaldo Martins Leite. *Interface: Comunicação, Saúde e Educação, 20*(56), 239–247.

Saks, M. (1995). *Professions and the public interest. Medical power, altruism and alternative medicine*. London, New York: Routledge.

Saks, M. (2015). Health policy and complementary and alternative medicine. In E. Kuhlmann, R. Blank, I. Bourgeault, & C. Wendt (Eds.), *The Palgrave international handbook of healthcare policy and governance* (pp. 494–509). London: Palgrave Macmillan.

Salles, S. A. C., & Schraiber, L. B. (2009). Gestores do SUS: apoio e resistências à homeopatia. *Cadernos de Saúde Pública, 25*(1), 195–202.

Saraiva, J. H. (1999). *História concisa de Portugal*. Mem Martins: Publicações Europa-América.

Siahpush, M. (1999). A critical review of the sociology of alternative medicine: Research on users, practitioners and the orthodoxy. *Health: An Interdisciplinary Journal for the Social Study of Health, Illness and Medicine, 4*(2), 159–178.

Sociedade Portuguesa Médica de Acupunctura. (2016). Competência; acupunctura. *SPMA Webpage*. Retrieved November 9, 2017, from http://www.spma.pt/competencias/criterios/.

Sointu, E. (2006). The search for wellbeing in alternative and complementary health practices. *Sociology of Health & Illness, 28*(3), 330–349.

Tesser, C. D. (org). (2010). *Medicinas complementares: o que é necessário saber* (Homeopatia e Medicina Tradicional Chinesa/Acupuntura). São Paulo: Editora UNESP.

Viana, A. L. D. (2000). As políticas de saúde nas décadas de 80 e 90: o (longo) período de reformas. In A. M. Canesqui (org). *Ciências sociais e saúde para ensino médico* (pp. 113–133). São Paulo: Hucitec.

Wardwell, W. I. (1994). Alternative medicine in the United States. *Social Science & Medicine, 38*(8), 1061–1068.

Welsh, S., & Boon, H. (2015). Traditional Chinese medicine and acupuncture practitioners and the Canadian health care system: The role of the state in creating the necessary vacancies. In N. K. Gale & J. V. McHale (Eds.), *Handbook of complementary and alternative medicine—Perspectives from social science and law*. London: Routledge.

Wiesener, S., Falkenberg, T., Hegyi, G., Hök, J., Di Sarsina, P. R., & Fønnebø, V. (2012). Legal status and regulation of complementary and alternative medicine in Europe. *Forsch Komplementmed, 19*(2), 29–36.

Winnick, T. A. (2006). Medical doctors and complementary and alternative medicine: The context of holistic practice. *Health: An Interdisciplinary Journal for the Social Study of Health, Illness and Medicine, 10*(2), 149–173.

World Health Organisation. (2012). *The regional strategy for traditional medicine in the western pacific*. Western Pacific Region. Manila: WHO.

World Health Organisation. (2013). *WHO traditional medicine strategy: 2014–2023*. Geneva: WHO.

6

A 'Miracle Bed' and a 'Second Heart': Technology and Users of Complementary and Alternative Medicine in the Context of Medical Diversity in Post-Soviet Kyrgyzstan

Danuta Penkala-Gawęcka

Introduction

It was in 2011, just at the beginning of my ethnographic fieldwork in Bishkek, the capital of Kyrgyzstan, when I heard about a 'miracle bed' for the first time. My new acquaintance Sayra,[1] a friend of my friend, told me with palpable excitement about this bed, provided by a company from South Korea—Nuga Medical—which, in Sayra's words, proved to be an excellent therapeutic device. She maintained that using the 'Korean bed' had greatly helped her in numerous ailments, including sore throat, ear ache, kidney troubles and aching legs. This story sparked my interest, so the next day I accompanied Sayra to the 'Nuga Best' centre and then visited it alone several times. As I found out, that facility was very popular in Bishkek.

D. Penkala-Gawęcka (✉)
Department of Ethnology and Cultural Anthropology, Adam Mickiewicz University, Poznań, Poland

© The Author(s) 2018
C. Brosnan et al. (eds.), *Complementary and Alternative Medicine*, Health, Technology and Society, https://doi.org/10.1007/978-3-319-73939-7_6

Therapies using the Nuga Best (NB) bed-massager and other devices offered at the centre illustrate the wide array of non-biomedical services available to the inhabitants of Bishkek. Post-Soviet Kyrgyzstan and particularly its urban centres are sites of great medical diversity. Alongside biomedical care, a broad range of complementary and alternative medicine (CAM)[2] therapies are at people's disposal. While previous governmental support for folk medicine, connected with an overall revaluation of Kyrgyz culture in the newly independent Kyrgyz Republic, has weakened in recent years, an official tolerant attitude towards such non-biomedical therapies that are practised mainly by medical doctors has remained relatively stable.

In this chapter, I discuss the dynamics of CAM in Kyrgyzstan—the role and place of its particular segments. However, if we are to understand the transformations it has undergone, we should also consider broader contexts. Among other factors, political economy, the politics of nationalism, the state's 'modernising' efforts and the impact of globalisation contribute to the changing status of CAM. A contextual approach is widely promoted by medical anthropologists, although it is admitted that we have to take into account 'increasingly complex contexts in order to understand the researched phenomenon adequately', while (…) never being able to consider *enough* contexts' (Dilger and Hadolt 2015: 143; cf. Andersen and Risør 2014). In my view, contextual research in Kyrgyzstan is necessary in studying the local medical diversity and CAM's place within it. This can help capture changes in its position within the post-Soviet period, which, in turn, may be useful when we research such specific entanglements as, for example, the NB network in Bishkek, discussed in this chapter.

In addition to examining these broader contextual factors, the chapter provides an analysis of how context shapes local CAM technologies. Many CAM therapies are based on specific technologies, some more or less complicated. It is noticeable that much anthropological research has been conducted on globalised biomedical technologies and their appropriation in different settings (Hardon and Moyer 2014; Lock 2004: 87) whereas less attention has been devoted to the role of CAM technologies. As Lock (2007: 274) points out, what is worth examining is not only 'the importation of technologies associated with the biosciences, but also (…) the global movement of indigenous medicinals and local technologies in multiple directions'. In addition, she rightly stresses that such studies can reveal 'the metamedical context in which technologies of all kinds are mobilized and applied in practice' (Lock 2007: 275).

In this chapter, the focus is on CAM technologies offered by Nuga Medical, specifically the NB bed-massager and some other devices. Their introduction and popularisation can be interpreted as the result of globalisation and glocalisation processes; such new therapies are often, in many ways, adapted to the local socio-economic conditions. I will discuss the process of marketing these products and accompanying knowledge and, in particular, attitudes and practices of patients who use these technologies. Relations between various actors engaged in NB activities in Bishkek will also be examined. I consider, in particular, the role of non-human actors in the NB network and how they are associated with human actors, especially patients—and how aspirations, hopes and capabilities of the latter influence the network. These sections, which form the main body of the chapter, are preceded by a presentation of the adopted analytic approach and a section on methods. In the conclusion, I will sum up my findings on Bishkek's NB network and comment on the reasons for its popularity and durability.

Analytic Approach

The perspective applied in this chapter draws from the concept of medical pluralism, which—although criticised for several reasons—has been continuously applied in medical anthropology research since Charles Leslie's contribution of the 1970s (Leslie 1976). This concept remains a useful analytical tool for studies of CAM and biomedicine in different contexts, and its newer variants such as 'medicoscapes' embrace effects of transnational flows and globalisation processes (see Hörbst and Wolf 2014; Hsu 2008; Johannessen 2006; Parkin 2013; Penkala-Gawęcka and Rajtar 2016). Another term, 'medical diversity', according to Parkin,

> refers to more than medical pluralism, if by the latter is meant a number of medical traditions coexisting relatively insulated from each other within a region. Diversification is more than this and implies mutual borrowing of

ideas, practices and styles between them, and by implication more differentiated strategies adopted by patients in search of cure. (2013: 125)

Such a situation is observed in Kyrgyzstan; therefore, the notion of medical diversity underpins my analysis of people's perceptions of health and illness and related health-seeking strategies that were at the centre of my research conducted in Bishkek (cf Penkala-Gawęcka 2016).

I have found inspirations from Latour's Actor-Network Theory (ANT) useful in the analysis of Nuga Medical technologies in Bishkek. In fact, it is not a 'theory' but rather a method which enables the tracing of processes of networking, establishing and destabilising relations between actors. In Cressman's (2009: 2) words, ANT contains concepts that make it a valuable tool within the social study of technology. As Latour (2005: 12) points out in his famous phrase, the researcher has 'to follow the actors', not impose some order but 'try to catch up with their often wild innovations' and trace new associations that have not already been assembled. Importantly, this approach 'extends the word actor—or actant—to *non-human, non-individual* entities' (Latour 1996: 369), '*any thing* that does modify a state of affairs by making a difference is an actor' (Latour 2005: 71). ANT puts stress on materiality and relationality, and it is non-human agency, namely this of the NB bed, together with its materiality, which seems crucial in the studied case. The bed definitely is an actor, since—as will be shown—it acts, makes a difference, influences and changes other actors' activities.

In ANT's approach, new, heterogeneous and fluid associations are traced, in which both humans and non-humans act, and the latter are, as Latour puts it, 'full-blown actors' rendering network interactions more durable (2005: 68–70). The network described here, involving complex relations between fluctuating patients, therapeutic devices, personnel and managers of the centre, with changing locations and constant innovations, is characterised by heterogeneity, openness and fluidity. It may be presented and analysed with the use of the ANT perspective, since this is a situation 'where innovations proliferate, where group boundaries are uncertain, when the range of entities to be taken into account fluctuates' (Latour 2005: 11).

Additionally, I have found Johannessen's remarks considering medical pluralism to be 'ordered into networks that are fluid and flexible' (2006: 14) substantiated, as well as her claim that 'the starting point for any analysis of networks in medical pluralism is (…) to observe what people do and say' (2006: 9). Similarly, Law (2007: 2) notes that ANT is firmly grounded in empirical case studies, and they are typical of the anthropological approach. In the same vein as Johannessen, I argue that in the analysis carried out here, combining the use of the concept of medical diversity with an actor-network approach is a useful perspective. According to this approach, overlapping networks which consist of diverse practitioners of biomedicine and CAM, patients and their relatives, managers, knowledge bases and ethical principles, therapeutic methods and techniques, medicines and other objects used in treatment/ healing, medical infrastructure, organisation and so on constitute a local form of medical diversity. Although I concentrate in my analysis on a specific network—the NB—I do not lose sight of other important features of medical diversity in Bishkek, especially the changing role and place of various CAM disciplines.

Methods

The research that I carried out in Kyrgyzstan, on people's health-seeking strategies, resulted from my long-standing interests in medical anthropology and the Central Asian region—including the status of CAM in different locations—and was funded by a grant from the National Centre of Science in Poland.[3] This chapter is based on materials gathered during three seasons of ethnographic fieldwork in Bishkek between 2011 and 2013 (about four months altogether). My general aim was to study people's health-related choices, strategies and practices in the urban environment where a wide range of therapeutic options, both biomedical and non-biomedical, were available. My interlocutors were of diverse ethnic backgrounds but mainly the Kyrgyz (who constitute the majority of Kyrgyzstan's population—72.6%) and Russians. Among them were women and men (but predominantly women), people of different ages and professions, incumbent residents of the city and newcomers from other regions. I approached them in many ways: through my previous contacts or rather accidentally; in biomedical institutions (e.g., hospitals, clinics), physicians' and CAM practitioners' offices, pharmacies and healers' consultation rooms; in the streets, parks and bazaars. They were mostly 'ordinary' people but also several biomedical and non-biomedical professionals and healthcare officials.

I used qualitative research methods typical of the anthropological approach: unstructured or partly structured interviews and loose talks, sometimes during brief encounters and sometimes in the course of several longer meetings with the same people. I talked to a total of nearly 80 people and the majority of interviews were recorded. An important part of my fieldwork was observation, including participant observation during therapeutic sessions of various practitioners, in pharmacies, bazaars or shops selling locally produced healthy beverages.

During my visits at the NB centre in Bishkek, I attended the so-called presentation (which I discuss further later) combined with the patients' use of the NB bed and other devices, made observations and had short talks with the personnel. But first and foremost, I carried on many conversations with people who came there to get treatment, often waiting in long queues. So, I followed the actors of the NB network, visitors in particular, not only during presentations and the bed trials but also directly before and after that, as well as in other circumstances—for example, while talking with Sayra about her experiences with the bed and many other kinds of CAM treatments. Presentations in the NB centre were held in Russian and in my conversations with people I used Russian, as a kind of lingua franca in Kyrgyzstan, especially in big cities. I also followed the most important non-human actor, the bed, mainly through visitors' and personnel's descriptions of its particular abilities and strengths, through manifestations of the users' feelings and experiences and while observing the 'miracle bed' in action. At the same time, I traced the bed's and other devices' history—their invention, development, and global and local expansion—primarily using the website information of the Nuga Medical Company, its products and NB facilities in Russia and Central Asia.

Additionally, local newspapers and magazines as well as TV programmes served as sources of valuable information about the situation of the healthcare system and its reform and, to some extent, the position of CAM in Kyrgyzstan. The latter topic was presented on TV and in the newspapers, mostly as advertisements of particular therapies and/or practitioners. Some special magazines with healers' advertisements and advertising articles were also available.

Medical Diversity in Bishkek and the Status of CAM in the Kyrgyz Republic

Complementary and alternative treatments of diverse origins and shapes occupy an important place in the 'medical landscape' of Bishkek. Among them are the medical traditions of the Kyrgyz and other ethnic groups of this multinational country, therapies offered by practitioners of Chinese, Korean or Tibetan medicines and various new or relatively new methods and techniques which have been arriving since the 1980s and especially since the beginning of the 1990s from Russia and other parts of the former Soviet Union, as well as from the West. Therapies of foreign origins often undergo significant local adaptations and modifications in the process of glocalisation. It should be noted that despite the long-lasting persecution and spread of atheistic propaganda during the Soviet times, many local, traditional methods of treatment, including spiritual healing, survived and are currently popular among the people, even in urban centres (Penkala-Gawęcka 2017b). Therefore, although medical diversity is nowadays particularly rich, it is not a new phenomenon in Kyrgyzstan, similar to other countries of the Central Asian region. Lindquist (2006: 30–37) describes how in the Soviet Union 'alternative medicine' developed semi-underground and then more openly, especially during the period of 'late socialism' and perestroika. Among those methods were folk medicine, treatment with 'bio-energy' (by the so-called *ekstrasensy*) and other para-scientific techniques, as well as acupuncture and Tibetan medicine. Despite the official ideology, some kinds of non-biomedical therapies gained acceptance and were allowed to move to the margins of biomedicine. Thus, there was no sharp boundary between biomedicine and certain CAM modalities.

Dramatic political, economic and social changes which followed the dissolution of the Soviet Union near the end of 1991 also impacted the situation of healthcare in Central Asia, including the newly independent Republic of Kyrgyzstan. Shortcomings of the Soviet state medical system (Field 2002) became clearly visible and intensified by the economic crisis. Transformation to the market economy induced the decline of the centralised healthcare system, and although state medical institutions still play the most important role, private healthcare facilities have been opened. Diverse CAM therapies began to flourish and underwent commercialisation, especially in urban contexts. A relatively new phenomenon in Kyrgyzstan is the presence of some globally spread CAM technologies, enabled thanks to the opening up of the country to the influences of globally operating corporations such as Nuga Medical.

At the same time, different CAM modalities are strongly based on local medical traditions. After the collapse of the USSR, the Kyrgyz Republic and the other newly independent Central Asian states strove to legitimise their sovereignty by references to the cultural heritage of their titular nations. Such nationalist tendencies favoured 'medical revivalism' (cf. Lock and Nichter 2002: 7–8; Ferzacca 2002)—the process of revalidating folk medicine (for Central Asia see Penkala-Gawecka 2002; Hohmann 2010). In Kyrgyzstan, this trend saw the establishment, under the auspices of the Ministry of Health, of the Republican Centre of Folk Medicine in Bishkek (known as 'Beyish'—'Paradise') at the beginning of the 1990s. The Centre was an educational institution which carried out courses for healers and granted them licences and at the same time offered medical services. So, there were attempts at registration and some standardisation of healers' practices. It is worth mentioning that 'Beyish' employed both biomedical doctors and healers, and its 'integrative' efforts comprised production of medicines based on folk remedies. The other reason for such a supportive attitude of the authorities to local medical traditions, as well as other CAM treatments, was obviously a dramatic deterioration of the healthcare system after the breakup of the Soviet Union. There is no space to discuss this here, but it should be noted that the situation of healthcare in Kyrgyzstan, despite wide-ranging reforms since the mid-1990s, still leaves a lot to be desired. Among the most serious problems are underfunding of healthcare, corruption and poor quality of medical education, the mass economic migration of physicians and other health workers to Kazakhstan and Russia and uneven distribution of medical facilities within the country. Additionally, people are faced with economic barriers in access to healthcare, although there has been an increase in public financing, and even officially free basic services involve costs because of the persistence of informal payments (Johnson 2009: 231–298; Ibraimova et al. 2011; Penkala-Gawęcka 2016).

However, the process of professionalisation of folk healers has been stopped during the last decade; they can work freely in the market but without official backing. 'Beyish', which had given them substantial support, was closed down in 2011, following the directive issued by the Prime Minister of the Kyrgyz Republic regarding its transformation into the International Academy of Traditional and Experimental Medicine. According to the statement given during an opening ceremony by the Deputy Minister of Health, 'Beyish' had not fulfilled its mission: 'quacks, *ekstrasensy* and often common charlatans, i.e. people distant from medicine had worked [at the Centre] before'. He pointed out that the newly founded institution should take a 'scientific direction' and work in close collaboration with the Ministry of Health (Nichiporova 2011). In my view, such a turn has mainly been caused by governmental modernising efforts. As a result, shamans and other 'traditional' healers are no longer treated as carriers of national traditions but, in the official discourse, more and more often presented as charlatans. Nevertheless, these changes in the official policy towards folk healing do not affect the great popularity of healers among the people, which is largely connected with patients' dissatisfaction with the healthcare system and common distrust of doctors (Penkala-Gawęcka 2016).

The other segments of CAM in Kyrgyzstan, especially treatments practised by biomedical doctors, have a much more stable position. For example, acupuncture, hirudotherapy (treatment with leeches) and some other branches of CAM are taught at special post-graduate courses for physicians at the Department of Physiotherapy and Traditional Medicine of the Kyrgyz National Medical University in Bishkek. In fact, these CAM disciplines are usually treated as part of biomedicine, and practitioners of such therapies who have professional training may be employed in clinics or hospitals. Thus, the blurring of 'therapeutic boundaries' (cf. Naraindas et al. 2014), already observed in the decline stage of the Soviet Union, is characteristic of relations between biomedicine and these CAM practices, but at the same time the boundary between them (together with bio-medicine) and folk healing seems to be strengthened as the result of the changes in the policy towards healers mentioned earlier. This may be seen as an example of 'boundary work' which is grounded in different knowl-edge claims: in the case of segments of CAM described earlier, claims to scientific knowledge as the base of these practices (see Brosnan, Vuolanto and Danell, in Chapter 1).

Legitimacy and authority of such CAM practitioners, who are bio-medical doctors, are largely based on their biomedical competence, and this 'bureaucratic legitimacy'[4] is obviously most important for their work in healthcare institutions. However, they often refer also to 'tradition' as the source of legitimacy, which in this case may be traditional Chinese or Korean medicine, or 'ancient Oriental massage' or some kind of Kyrgyz folk medicine. Such 'mixed' legitimisation may help them attract a diver-sified urban clientele—people of different ethnic and social backgrounds, having different ideas of health and illness and varied expectations (Penkala-Gawęcka 2017a).

I argue here, in line with an ANT approach, that authority and agency should not be restricted to human actors. Medical devices and instru-ments, among other things, gain their legitimisation mostly through 'the reference to the scientific establishment' (Lindquist 2006: 37–38). I have found it striking that, in the Soviet times, the authority of science, per-sonalised in esteemed medical professionals (especially 'academics'— members of the Academy of Sciences of the USSR), enabled the introduction of various medical inventions without standard clinical tri-als, and this kind of legitimacy is still valid in today's Kyrgyzstan. Numerous CAM technologies appeal to patients through their claims to science, although they are usually not grounded in evidence-based medi-cine. Most of them are imported from Russia or Ukraine, some from other places and some are locally invented.

In the following sections I will examine the case of South Korean Nuga Medical Company products—in particular, the NB bed, which arrived in Bishkek in 2006 and gained popularity there. After a brief description of the company, its products and their introduction to Kyrgyzstan, I will show how Nuga Medical operates in Bishkek and focus on the attitudes and practices of patients who use the bed and other devices in search of good and inexpensive treatment.

Nuga Medical Company and Its Products

The company, which can be found on the Internet under the names NB and Nuga Medical Company, was founded in South Korea in 2002, with its head office in Seoul. It is an ambitious, successfully developing enterprise that has been quickly expanding its network all over the world. According to the information provided by the personnel of NB in Bishkek in 2011, this firm operated in 75 countries and, as they claimed, had 6500 establishments (showrooms connected with treatment facilities) similar to the one that I visited. However, the data found in 2017 on the NB Korean site indicates sales networks 'reaching over 3500 places [perhaps, centres] in about 105 countries', with plans of further globalisation and the goal 'to propagate Nuga Medical's health culture throughout every country in the whole world'. In the words of Nuga Global Chairman, Cho Syung Hyun, their 'corporate mission' is 'to contribute to the human health by providing the best service with our best technology and love'.[5]

In parallel to the expansion of the sales network, through 'distributors' in many countries, the company improves its products and introduces new ones. Generally, it advertises them as special medical instruments—thermal acupressure massagers that combine 'the ancient Eastern healing arts of acupressure, massage, modern chiropractic theory, far infrared light therapy, and modern technology'[6]—but there are also on sale, for example, various newer 'beauty care products' such as anti-wrinkle emulsions and creams. However, the stress is put on the unique therapeutic properties of the patented material invented by NB, called tourmanium, which contains tourmaline, germanium, volcanic rocks and 'elvan rocks' (a variety of quartz-porphyry). It is processed in high temperatures to get 'tourmanium ceramic', in the shape of small discs, that are said to produce far infrared rays and emit negative ions beneficial to the body. There is a wide range of recommended therapeutic uses of NB products and the listed benefits include, among others, relief of pains, especially back and neck pains, as well as headaches, stress relief and strengthening the nervous system, enhancement of blood circulation and oxygenation, regulation of the digestive system, blood sugar control and improvement of the activities of internal organs.

Among advertised technological inventions, the main actor is undoubtedly the NB bed, a flagship product of NB—a thermal bed-massager combining heating and acupressure with the use of spinal rolling massagers ('internal heating projectors'). It is presented as a unique invention which successfully integrates principles of Oriental and Western medicines. The bed has been available in several successive, improved versions. The original jade roller-massagers were substituted with tourmanium ones, which were promoted as producing better results due to the increased emission of negative ions (presumably, the issue of cost may also have been a consideration). The newest bed variety, N5—ergonomic, with some innovations and a folder-type design—is advertised as the number one world-class product of Korea.[7] There are numerous other NB products with tourmanium discs, such as mattresses and heat mats of various sizes, a cushion, a neck pillow, waist belts and small five—or nine—ball external projectors designed to be used by the patient on various parts of the body. Another product is a low-frequency wave pad meant to reduce fat and increase metabolism. Among the popular devices there is also the so-called second heart, a kind of foot massager based on acupressure principles which, it is claimed, brings many health benefits including positive cardiovascular effects. In addition, tourmanium jewellery (necklaces and bracelets) have been produced for a number of years, and the newer products include wristwatches (with watch straps made of NB ceramic) and a range of cosmetics.

NB Network in Bishkek

If we approach medical diversity in Bishkek as 'ordered into fluid and flexible networks', in line with Johannessen's proposal quoted earlier, the NB network may be considered one of them. It comprises distributors, managers, consultants/sale assistants, patients, 'miracle beds', 'second hearts' and other devices, teaching aids, promotion materials, presentation schemes, the NB anthem, people's public testimonials, the company's rules and requirements, changing venues and so on. It overlaps with other 'therapeutic networks' which form the local medical diversity since patients move between them. At the same time Bishkek's NB network can be recognised as a node within the NB Company global network.

In connection with the process of globalisation of NB, we can observe some particular features of its advertising in Russia and Central Asia. They shed light on the specificities of glocalisation of these products in different markets. I noticed that marketing efforts in Russia include comparisons of NB therapies to the 'forgotten Russian traditions', namely the use of the upper surface of bread ovens as the place where old people used to lie and 'heat their bones'. In Volgograd's NB centre, such a pseudo-oven was built and patients could lie on the NB mattress placed on top of this structure.[8] On the websites of the NB centres in Kyrgyzstan and Uzbekistan, we can find some brief mentions of Eastern medical traditions connected with NB products; however, it seems that references to family values and kin obligations are much more important. They are revealed in the story of Cho Syung Hyun whose invention of the 'miracle bed' is depicted as an act of love and deep gratitude of the son towards his widowed mother whose health had suffered due to her efforts to provide a livelihood for the family.[9] It should be stressed that this picture of modern technology embedded in traditional values can successfully appeal to people in Central Asia, where family and kinship ties which entail mutual support and obligations remain crucial. I did not find this kind of information, for example, on the NB United Kingdom and Ireland website.[10]

The process of the NB networking started in Bishkek in 2006. The venue has not been stable; NB had changed it perhaps twice before renting rooms at the Drama Theatre where it was located during the period of my research, and then it moved again. However, together with expanding this network, other NB networks in Bishkek have emerged, probably overlapping with the original one, and there are presently three centres in the city.[11] I do not know how the NB activities were introduced and organised in the first years in Kyrgyzstan. The NB websites state that an entrepreneur, Evgeniy Kim, became the exclusive distributor of Nuga

Medical's products in Kyrgyzstan in 2014, which can be seen as an attempt to regulate and stabilise the NB network. During the procedure of signing the agreement on distribution in Seoul, the aim of promoting people's health in Kyrgyzstan was strongly stressed.[12] The new NB facilities have been established not only in Bishkek but also in other cities and towns, such as Osh and Kara Balta.

The NB centres are commercial institutions, with the aim to sell Nuga Medical products, especially the most expensive NB beds. Their activities in Kyrgyzstan, similar to other NB facilities in different countries, were organised in such a way that free trials of the bed should act as an incentive for ultimate purchase, although its cost—for the local population—was very high. The number of visits and 'trials' of the bed was not limited, but participants were obliged to listen to the 'presentations' and were strongly encouraged to bring new persons who might be interested in buying the bed. The main task of the personnel was to convince the visitors about the enormous health benefits of using the bed on a daily basis, at home. They tried to achieve this goal in many ways, described later; however, bodily contact with the NB bed was treated as the most important means to make people believe that this device was necessary to ensure them health. In addition, the staff (not necessarily with medical training) were locally recruited; as I observed, they were of various ethnic backgrounds (Kyrgyz, Russian and others), supposedly with good interpersonal skills.

The range of devices offered by Kyrgyzstan's first NB centre has not been unchanging. During my later research seasons in Bishkek, the bed model which had been used there in 2011 (NM-5000) was replaced by a newer one, which was said to provide a more gentle treatment. And recently the model N4, a slightly older 'brother' of the newest innovation, N5, has been introduced to Kyrgyzstan's facilities.[13] Besides the bed, a fairly wide array of NB products, including many of those described earlier, were offered during presentations in 2011.

As my interlocutors maintained, the enterprise, with its prime product—the bed—quickly gained popularity after its introduction. In the course of my visits to the NB centre in 2011, I observed surroundings of the Drama Theatre crowded with people. I was astonished to see so many visitors waiting for their turn, often for a long time. The NB network was fluid and changing—there were regular patients and many newcomers, some of them from nearby towns and villages. The company's policy of attracting more and more people through existing participants' contacts fostered further extension of the network. According to this policy, those regular patients who brought newcomers were given precedence; therefore, it was a strong incentive to attract new patients, usually recruited from the circle of relatives, friends and fellow workers. Thus, Sayra, whom I accompanied during my initial visit, was happy that we could enter together and jump the queue.

Most people knew the centre's rules and requirements and brought a sheet, slippers or a pair of socks and a cotton sock for placing over a handheld device—an 'external projector'—while using it. Others were offered those accessories for a small fee at the entrance. There were about 25 people of different ethnic backgrounds (mainly Kyrgyz and Russian), with the majority being older women, allowed at one time. All of us were invited to take seats in front of a woman in a blue gown (like the rest of the personnel) who would give a 'presentation' (in Russian), as this event was called. It was easily noticeable that the presentation proceeded in accordance with a provided, repeatable scheme. It bore many traits of corporate meetings or psychotherapeutic sessions, such as public testimonials by regular and new visitors, common singing of the NB anthem and other songs, choral recitation of NB advertising slogans, common exercises to the rhythm of music and other behaviours demonstrating participants' shared values and community spirit. The presenter continually asked the public for applause to encourage those who made testimonials. It should be noted that the personnel avoided using such words as 'treatment' or 'medical instrument', and the place itself was called a 'demonstration-exhibition room', most likely because of the lack of licence for providing medical services.

The extensive presentation of NB principles and therapeutic values of its products was divided in two parts and took about 40 minutes altogether, with pauses for visitors' testimonials. The whole event lasted more than one-and-a-half hours, including the time for trials of the bed and other appliances by the participants, which took about half an hour. The presentation focused on detailed descriptions of the NB technology—the production of tourmanium ceramic, technical details of this 'unique invention' and health benefits of the particular NB products, especially when used regularly at home. However, it was also replete with characteristic rhetorical figures and marketing hooks. For example, the presenter used phrases such as 'With Nuga Best comes health' and encouraged the participants to repeat them. She employed various 'teaching aids' such as a spine model to show how the NB bed rollers worked on it, or small glass containers with samples of 'bad' and 'good' (oxygenated) blood (presumably fake blood), and also presented NB products: a pillow, a belt, mats and jewellery. Short films explaining the company's mission, showing tourmanium's beneficial qualities and therapeutic procedures using NB products were an important part of the presentation. Promotional materials in Russian were also available and the walls of the room were full of advertising posters.

The woman who led the meeting sounded very convincing, was energetic and well prepared. Other personnel—four younger women—listened to her presentation and then, during the trials, helped the patients properly use NB beds and other devices. The session was arranged in such a way that, after the first part of the presentation, one-half of the participants could use the beds while the others did some exercises and listened to the second part, waiting for their turn. Although I had revealed my research aims to the personnel at the entrance, I was later encouraged to try the bed but decided to confine myself to the 'second heart' since some people told me that they had felt bad after first NB bed uses. When we were about to leave, another group was already waiting in the lobby.

During my further research seasons, I observed that the arrangements at the NB centre in Bishkek had somewhat changed and in 2013 people waited in smaller groups outside the building, since there was a possibility to book a visit in advance. However, financial conditions were not changed and patients could use the bed at the centre for free.

Relations Between the Main Actors: Patients, NB Bed, Personnel

In this section, I will analyse relations between the main actors of Bishkek's NB network, namely the patients, the personnel and the NB bed. I argue that the central actor is the 'miracle bed', since diverse strategies of the patients and the personnel are focused on it. In the analysis, I will pay most attention to the patients, their expectations, hopes and dreams, centred on the bed, but my intention is also to show how patients' attitudes and practices are connected with the personnel's aims and strategies.

As can be seen from the patients' comments, the most powerful incentive for visiting the NB centre was the 'Korean bed'. This was manifested in the manner of speaking about the NB centre and how people find their way there—I was usually told that they had somehow, in most cases through family or friends' advice, learned about 'the bed' and wanted to try it. They expanded then on their experiences and feelings connected with the bed's use, and this object was definitely at the centre of their attention. It was often described as a miraculous object of desire, much more than a 'thing', something highly valued, epitomising health and well-being. However, the process of recovering from various illnesses is not quick and easy. Patients spoke about unpleasant sensations and even worsening symptoms after first trying the bed but were convinced that those experiences were normal, indicating the start of cleansing the organism. They maintained: 'all people say that there should be cleansing at the beginning of the treatment'. People also claimed that the use of the bed should be continual, so they tried to come to the NB unit as often as possible. It was a commonly held view that if the therapy was interrupted, health problems would come back. Such experiences were often described during visitors' testimonials at the centre and the personnel's statements reinforced that view. For example, an older woman explained that when she was regularly using the bed for four days, her heart troubles stopped, but after a three-day break she felt weak again and the heartache returned. The presenter asked her why it was like that and the woman answered: 'Oh, I think I should buy it [the bed] or come here [regularly] if I want to feel good', which was rewarded with loud applause.

When I talked with a Dungan woman in her early 40s, Zamira, who suffered from serious heart problems, she expressed her astonishment at the fact that the bed, which was so expensive, was available to use for free. To take advantage of that opportunity, she had regularly attended the centre for two months, despite the long distance from the village where her family lived. In her words, the bed was her rescue; thanks to using it she felt much better and that condition was confirmed by medical tests.

Nevertheless, Zamira's unattainable dream was to have the bed at home. She said: 'Once a day is not enough. If it could be used three times a day, or at least two … But this is for us a lot of money'. Similarly, many other people told about their great desire to get the bed for continuous home use. I heard statements of this kind: 'then we would not need doctors anymore!', which confirmed my observations about common negative assessments of medical personnel in Kyrgyzstan. As my research revealed, opinions of doctors' poor professional and moral standards were widely shared and in many cases resulted in 'doctor-avoiding strategies', since therapeutic encounters with them were perceived as risky (for more on this, see Penkala-Gawęcka 2016).

While expressing their desire to purchase the bed, people complained that it was something out of reach (its cost ranged between 2500 and 3000 USD at the time of my research). Only one man, who came to the NB facilities for the first time, told me that he would check the bed and buy it if it turned out to be effective. When I mentioned the high price of this device, he answered: 'When it comes to health, money does not matter'. For most people that dream could not be fulfilled.

The ideas about the bed and its special position in patients' views may be considered, in part, the result of the specificity of advertising and marketing of this product. Nevertheless, I argue that the bed's agency could be greatly enhanced by people's own bodily experiences and sensations during therapeutic sessions and consequent feelings about the bed's efficacy, which was often stressed by my interlocutors. In addition, other users' opinions played an important role—mostly those of close and trusted persons but also those expressed by co-participants in the course of presentations. Such interactions have been important for granting the NB bed agency, the quality of being an actor. The materiality of the bed and other products seems crucial in this respect. This can be seen while observing people's use of these devices and listening to their stories. Bodily contact with the bed is an intense experience, since it emits heat and a person can feel rolling massagers moving along her/his spine. Although these feelings can be unpleasant or even painful, convictions about the bed's healing powers are often very strong and, as mentioned earlier, such experiences are considered to be signs that prove the start of the process of treatment. So, in a way, the bed's activity alone may be the proof of its strength and efficacy. Similarly, foot sensations during the use of the 'second heart' are treated as indications of the device's action. Notably, its name also suggests capability to help in heart troubles.

A story told by a middle-aged woman, Ainura, is a good example of the relations between a patient and a NB appliance. She could only afford a pillow, but this pillow became so close, so intimate to her that she felt it necessary to have it always with her. Ainura took that pillow everywhere and applied it when she felt any pain. She concluded: 'Such a doctor came to my home!' Nonetheless, she dreamed about buying the bed and declared that would do her best to achieve this goal.

The personnel of the NB centre in Bishkek, in line with the global promotion of Nuga Medical Company products, very clearly placed the bed at the central position, constantly pointing out that one can regain or maintain his/her health thanks to using the bed. The woman who gave the presentation started her description of the products with this invention, introducing it as 'the bed-massager beautifully named Nuga Best NM-5000, multifunctional and universal'. Later, after showing various other devices and describing their therapeutic effects she summed up: 'these things serve to make us healthy from head to toe'. However, she clearly explained then that the other products are only 'additions' to the main hero of her story, namely the bed. Its extraordinary functions, combining infrared rays with acupressure and massage, 'would not only restore one's well-being, but also provide hundred-percent health'. Of course, the workers were interested in selling the product, which was not easy because very few people could afford it. During the meeting described earlier, the presenter pointed out that the bed would be excellent for the household, since all family members could use it in turn. Besides, she explained that the best results could be obtained if the bed was used early in the morning and late in the evening. And the punchline was: 'So we ought to have this thing at home!' Thus, since both the patients and the NB centre personnel focus their attention, feelings and interests on the bed-massager, it may be recognised as the prime actor in the NB network, endowed with agency and strongly influencing people's ideas, strategies and practices.

What were the patients' and personnel's particular strategies in the aforementioned context? Although the former were very eager to get the bed and the latter to sell it, the cost was an enormous barrier to the desired purchase. The patients' main strategy was, therefore, to take advantage of the free use of the bed and continue therapy on site as long as possible. This was enabled according to the company's rules, but—as I explained earlier—access to the bed was obstructed for those who could not bring a newcomer. Such patients not only had to wait for a long time but also could not use some of the other devices. For example, during the presentation, a woman interested in the successive use of the belt for 'muscle stimulation' was told that it would only be possible if she came with somebody new. Additionally, the rules and limitations might be changed, as my interlocutors' stories revealed. The use of the 'second heart' was charged at a small amount of money on occasions, but the access to it and some other NB devices was temporarily facilitated during special promotion arrangements. Supposedly, such arrangements depended on the personnel's observations and suggestions put forward to their managers.

Since the purchase of the bed was out of reach for the majority of patients, many of them were confined to buying another, less expensive device or a few devices in turn, which often required them to save money for several months. The most popular among the women and the least expensive things were tourmanium jewellery items, such as necklaces and bracelets. Some people also bought mats, pillows or belts. The often expressed desire to 'get more' (and, ultimately, the bed) was enhanced by the personnel who encouraged potential customers in various ways, such as describing somebody's determination and efforts to buy a dreamed-of thing. For instance, the presenter introduced a Kyrgyz woman in her 70s and praised her as a very special person who had saved money from her small pension for 9 months to buy tourmanium jewellery, which helped her feel better. The woman explained then that her ultimate aim was to purchase the bed. She said that she was already very close to achieving her goal, since she had fed a bullock during summer and sold it but did not get enough money. Despite this, she still desperately wanted the bed and claimed that she would save the missing amount of money from her pension.

During the presentation, although the bed was always at the forefront, other products were also recommended. In line with the personnel's

message: 'even if we have only a few such devices at home, we can econo-
mise on medicines', the patients strove to make the most of the products
that they had managed to buy. For example, mats could be used by all
family members and even friends and neighbours. Importantly, people
were often creative about the ways of using purchased things. Some scope
for creativity was given by the personnel who described different methods
of NB products' usage, such as removing bad smells from the refrigerator
by placing the bead necklace inside. The same item, however, was used by
one of my interlocutors, a middle-aged Russian woman, in yet another
way. She inserted the beads into her vagina for some 'female trouble', following the advice passed on by her friend.

As the analysis reveals, associations and interactions between the NB
network's actors are complex and fluctuating. Various human and non-
human actors in this network depend on each other, while at the centre
is, definitely, the NB bed as an object of hopes and desire, endowed with
its own agency and capability to 'change things'.

Discussion and Closing Remarks

My intention in this chapter was to examine Bishkek's NB network by
demonstrating relations between heterogeneous actors. In this analysis, I
focused on people who come with hope to improve their health through
the use of the 'miracle bed'; on the bed itself, which epitomises health and
well-being; and on personnel who act as mediators and facilitators (or
'limiters') providing, in a specific way, access to this desired object. The
associations and interactions between these actors were changing, subject
to negotiations, and the network was fluent and fluctuating. Following
the actors during my research I could observe that they changed each
other and that the main non-human actor, the bed, strongly influenced
the attitudes and practices of other actors. In fact, it acted (Latour 1996)
as the human actors did.

In their search for better health, the patients tried to comply with the
rules and requirements imposed by the personnel. As I noticed, they
patiently participated in long presentations and agreed to give testimonials about the effects of the bed and other devices on their health, although

it must have been tiring for the regular users. It seemed to me that they rather tended to treat it as a barrier they had to climb over before they could lie down on the bed. Strikingly, it was the materiality of the NB products which was at the centre of people's interests, since the bodily contact with them was recognised as crucial for the therapy. The strategies of the NB products' users in Bishkek were designed to make the most of these devices. If the patients managed to buy such a thing, they used it extensively and sometimes in ways unanticipated by the inventors. These findings are in line with the results of ethnographic studies which show how patients creatively appropriate medical technologies for their own ends (Hardon and Moyer 2014).

The NB networks in Bishkek are important parts of the local CAM landscape. It was evident during my research that the 'Korean bed' was well known among the city dwellers. Many research participants who were not actual users said that they had used it before and wanted to repeat this experience or at least had heard about the NB bed. The further development and durability of the NB networks prove its continuous popularity. Medical diversity in the city offers various therapeutic options, but many of them, both biomedical and provided by CAM institutions, are beyond the means of the majority of people. Among the reasons for the popularity of the NB medical services, people's economic conditions definitely play a significant role. However, a special appeal of the 'miracle bed' to people should also be taken into account. This lies in its extraordinary qualities demonstrated by skilful advertisement and spread by word of mouth and accounts of personal experience. Its vision as a 'family doctor' solving all health problems seems particularly attractive. Nevertheless, from an ANT perspective, it is primarily the connections between numerous heterogeneous actors that can provide the stability of the network. In Law's (2007: 9) words, it is the configuration of the network that produces durability. In this case, this involves the interplay between patients' and personnel's attitudes, interests and expectations, focused—for both kinds of actors—on the main actor, the NB bed. Fundamentally, the profound agency of the bed itself makes this network enduring and stable, albeit at the same time fluent and changing.

Notes

1. Pseudonyms are used throughout the chapter to preserve the anonymity of the interlocutors.
2. An exhaustive discussion on complementary and alternative medicine (CAM) has been provided by Brosnan, Vuolanto and Danell (in Chapter 1). The authors point out the controversy over terminology and the inevitable relationship of CAM to biomedicine. In this chapter, I do not discuss these issues and use the term CAM for convenience.
3. National Centre of Science (Narodowe Centrum Nauki), grant number N N109 186440.
4. I differentiate between 'bureaucratic' (or 'rational') and 'traditional' legitimacy referring to Max Weber's classical typology of political legitimacy adapted to the medical field (Lindquist 2001, 2006). However, they are rather mixed modes of legitimisation that are characteristic of not only CAM practitioners who are biomedical doctors but also of healers whose methods, although based on tradition, are usually hybridised.
5. http://www.nugamedical.com/new_eng/introduce/vision.php, http://www.nugamedical.com/new_eng/introduce/ceo.php (accessed 25.04.2017).
6. http://www.nugabest.tv/global/bbs/board.php?bo_table=001&wr_id=1 (accessed 23.04.2017).
7. http://www.nugamedical.com/new_eng/ (accessed 02.05.2017).
8. https://www.youtube.com/watch?v=zO4zJgTsKe0&t=29s (accessed 6.05.2017).
9. https://ok.ru/nugabest9l, http://nuga-best.uz/5-2/ (accessed 5.05.2017).
10. http://www.nuga-best.co.uk/ (accessed 6.05.2017).
11. https://ok.ru/nugabest9l (accessed 6.05.2017).
12. http://nugamedical.com/new_eng/news/news_view.php?no=1881, https://ok.ru/nugabest9l (accessed 6.05.2017).
13. https://ok.ru/nugabest9l (accessed 02.05.2017).

References

Andersen, R. S., & Risør, M. B. (2014). The importance of contextualization. Anthropological reflections on descriptive analysis, its limitations and implications. *Anthropology & Medicine, 21*(3), 345–356.

Cressman, D. (2009). *A brief overview of Actor-Network Theory: Punctualization, heterogeneous engineering & translation*. Paper for Simon Frasier University ACT Lab/Centre for Policy Research on Science & Technology (CPROST), pp. 1–17. Retrieved November 11, 2017, from https://www.sfu.ca/communication/research/centres/cprost/recent-papers/2009/a-brief-overview-of-actor-network-theory--punctualization--heter.html.

Dilger, H., & Hadolt, B. (2015). 'Medicine in context'. An epistemological trajectory. *Medicine Anthropology Theory, 2*(3), 128–153.

Ferzacca, S. (2002). Governing bodies in new order Indonesia. In M. Lock & M. Nichter (Eds.), *Horizons in medical anthropology: Essays in honour of Charles Leslie* (pp. 35–57). London and New York: Routledge.

Field, M. G. (2002). The Soviet legacy: The past as a prologue. In M. McKee, J. Healy, & J. Falkingham (Eds.), *Health care in Central Asia* (pp. 67–75). Buckingham: WHO, Open University Press.

Hardon, A., & Moyer, E. (2014). Medical technologies: Flows, frictions and new socialities. *Anthropology & Medicine, 21*(2), 107–112.

Hohmann, S. (2010). National identity and invented tradition: The rehabilitation of traditional medicine in post-Soviet Uzbekistan. *The China and Eurasia Quarterly Forum, 8*(3), 129–148.

Hörbst, V., & Wolf, A. (2014). ARVs and ARTs: Medicoscapes and the unequal place-making for biomedical treatments in sub-Saharan Africa. *Medical Anthropology Quarterly, 28*(2), 182–202.

Hsu, E. (2008). Medical pluralism. In K. Heggenhougen & S. Quah (Eds.), *International encyclopedia of public health* (Vol. 4, pp. 316–321). Amsterdam: Elsevier.

Ibraimova, A., Akkazieva, B., Ibraimov, A., Manzhieva, E., & Rechel, B. (2011). Kyrgyzstan: Health system review. *Health Systems in Transition, 13*(3), 1–152.

Johannessen, H. (2006). Introduction: Body and self in medical pluralism. In H. Johannessen & I. Lázár (Eds.), *Multiple medical realities: Patients and healers in biomedical, alternative and traditional medicine* (pp. 1–17). New York and Oxford: Berghahn Books.

Johnson, E. J. (2009) *Authoritarian regimes and non-governmental organizations: Transitions in health care provision in Central Asia*. PhD diss. Ann Arbor: ProQuest.

Latour, B. (1996). On actor-network theory: A few clarifications. *Soziale Welt, 47*(4), 369–381.

Latour, B. (2005). *Reassembling the social: An introduction to actor-network-theory*. Oxford: Oxford University Press.

Law, J. (2007). Actor network theory and material semiotics (version of 25th April 2007). Retrieved March 6, 2016, from http://www.heterogeneities.net/publications/Law2007ANTandMaterialSemiotics.pdf.

Leslie, C. M. (Ed.). (1976). *Asian medical systems. A comparative study.* Berkeley: University of California Press.

Lindquist, G. (2001). The culture of charisma: Wielding legitimacy in contemporary Russian healing. *Anthropology Today, 17*(2), 3–8.

Lindquist, G. (2006). *Conjuring hope: Magic and healing in contemporary Russia.* New York: Berghahn Books.

Lock, M. (2004). Biomedical technologies: Anthropological approaches. In C. R. Ember & M. Ember (Eds.), *Encyclopedia of medical anthropology: Health and illness in the world's cultures topics* (Vol. 1, pp. 109–116). New York: Kluwer Academic/Plenum Publishers.

Lock, M. (2007). Medical anthropology: Intimations for the future. In F. Saillant & S. Genest (Eds.), *Medical anthropology: Regional perspectives and shared concerns* (pp. 267–288). Oxford: Blackwell Publishing.

Lock, M., & Nichter, M. (2002). From documenting medical pluralism to critical interpretations of globalized health knowledge, policies, and practices. In M. Lock & M. Nichter (Eds.), *Horizons in medical anthropology: Essays in honour of Charles Leslie* (pp. 1–34). London and New York: Routledge.

Naraindas, H., Quack, J., & Sax, W. S. (Eds.). (2014). *Asymmetrical conversations: Contestations, circumventions, and the blurring of therapeutic boundaries.* New York: Berghahn Books.

Nichiporova, N. (2011). Traditsii v eksperimente. *Vecherniy Bishkek*, December 20. Retrieved April 24, 2017, from http://members.vb.kg/2011/12/20/panorama/7.html.

Parkin, D. (2013). Medical crises and therapeutic talk. *Anthropology & Medicine, 20*(2), 124–141.

Penkala-Gawęcka, D. (2002). Korean medicine in Kazakhstan: Ideas, practices and patients. *Anthropology & Medicine, 9*(3), 315–336.

Penkala-Gawęcka, D. (2016). Risky encounters with doctors? Medical diversity and health-related strategies of the inhabitants of Bishkek, Kyrgyzstan. *Anthropology & Medicine, 23*(2), 135–154.

Penkala-Gawęcka, D. (2017a). Legitimacy and authority of complementary medicine practitioners in post-Soviet Kyrgyzstan. The role and use of tradition. *Rocznik Orientalistyczny, 70*(1), 20–32.

Penkala-Gawęcka, D. (2017b). Perceptions of health and illness, and the role of healers in Kyrgyzstan. *Public Health Panorama, 3*(1), 80–87.

Penkala-Gawęcka, D., & Rajtar, M. (2016). Introduction to the special issue "medical pluralism and beyond". *Anthropology & Medicine, 23*(2), 129–134.

7

Translation of Complementary and Alternative Medicine in Swedish Politics

Jenny-Ann Brodin Danell

Introduction

Some of the most important boundaries to complementary and alternative medicine (CAM) are set up by national legislations and regulations. Among other things, regulations define professional boundaries in terms of which professions are allowed to diagnose and treat patients, what qualifies as medical training, and what modalities are included in public and/or conventional healthcare. Regulations also set up boundaries of what is economically subsidised and supported by general health insurances. However, such regulations vary substantially in different national contexts (CAMDOC Alliance 2010; Fisher and Ward 1994; Wiesener et al. 2012). Many countries, such as those in Southern Europe, have relatively strict regulations and limit the performance of CAM modalities to trained medical professionals. Other actors are more or less banned from treating patients. In Northern Europe, CAM treatments can be performed by almost anyone, although there are restrictions on

J.-A. B. Danell (✉)
Department of Sociology, Umeå University, Umeå, Sweden

© The Author(s) 2018
C. Brosnan et al. (eds.), *Complementary and Alternative Medicine*, Health,
Technology and Society, https://doi.org/10.1007/978-3-319-73939-7_7

specific patient groups and medical acts, such as treatment of pregnant women and small children and the performance of surgery and use of X-rays. In other countries, such as Hungary and Slovenia, some CAM modalities are limited to medical doctors, while other CAM modalities are open to other professions (CAMDOC Alliance 2010). There are also substantial differences in how CAM is regulated, from direct government-administrated regulations of healthcare professionals to government-sanctioned systems (where control of titles, certificates, and education is delegated to national medical associations) and self-regulation (where CAM professionals develop and maintain their own standards). In some countries, there are also official registers of 'approved' CAM profession-als. It is worth noting that the last system might overlap with the other two (CAMDOC Alliance 2010). A number of studies indicate an increase in professionalisation and self-regulation of CAM, for example, by establishing educational standards, ethical guidelines, and uniform titles (Clarke et al. 2004; Saks 1999; Welsh et al. 2004).

Because CAM is often questioned and contested, especially in scien-tific and medical contexts (e.g., Angell and Kassirer 1998; Singh and Ernst 2008; Werneke et al. 2004), an intriguing question is how the political understanding of this phenomenon is established and expressed. This chapter will analyse the political debate on CAM in one national context, Sweden. In particular, the focus is on how CAM is 'translated' in the Swedish parliament. What are defined as political problems, and what goals and solutions are offered? What actors are involved in these processes? The focus is also on how issues related to CAM are interlinked with broader political agendas.

The main analysis was inspired by actor network theory (e.g., Latour 1996; Latour 2005). The basic idea was to analyse how the political understanding of CAM is established—or translated—in terms of how a heterogeneous network on this topic has stabilised in the Swedish parlia-ment. In the analysis, I borrowed some key ideas from Michel Callon (1986). In general, translation refers to processes that allow a network to be formed. According to Callon, this involves four steps. In the first step, problematisation, problems and main actors are defined. In the second step, interessement or interposition, various kinds of negotiations take place (e.g., on goals). In this step, the main actors also try to recruit other actors into the networks. In the last two steps, enrolment and mobilisation, the involvement of other actors is accepted and confirmed. Other actors, or allies, are also made into legitimate speakers of the network.

Data and Method

Empirically, this chapter draws upon 99 motions in the Swedish parliament during the time period 1980–2015. The choice of Swedish material is a pragmatic one, motivated by my own knowledge about the political and healthcare context. As I will discuss later in the section, Sweden is not unique, either concerning the position of CAM or the healthcare sector in general. Rather the contrary, Sweden has many similarities with other Scandinavian and Northern European countries, where one could expect similar political debates. The time period is also selected for pragmatic reasons because parliamentary documents in Sweden are available in electronic versions starting from 1980.

The documents were retrieved from the parliamentary database (www. riksdagen.se) using the general key words 'complementary medicine', 'alternative medicine', and 'integrative medicine' and hopefully including all motions on CAM during the time period. Potentially, there could be documents on single CAM traditions, such as acupuncture or homeopathy, that are not covered by the keywords, but these should be exceptions because general terms are usually used along with more specific terms. There are also other document types available in the database, such as committee reports, public investigations, protocols from debates, and written questions to the ministers. However, the motions are the most argumentative type of document, and this motivated the choice of such documents for this study. Compared to public investigations, which usually are written by researchers or other experts, the motions are a type of document where the politicians express themselves with their own words and formulate ideological standpoints. All members in the parliament have the opportunity to submit motions, but the vast majority are from the political opposition. Motions are prepared by single members or by a group of parliamentarians, representing one or several political parties.

Normally they consist of a proposal for parliamentary decision and of a motivation of the proposal. Motions are considered by one of the parliamentary committees. The committees are responsible for preparing parliamentary decisions (i.e., to decide what proposals they support) and the result of their work is presented in committee reports and statements. These documents normally include summaries of the motions and also serve as the basis for debate in the chamber. In this particular debate, the Committee of Social Affairs has considered most of the motions.

The analysis was performed in different steps with help from MAXQDA 11 software. Because the documents are of varying length, and because some of them are concerned with several topics, the first phase consisted of lexical searching and automatic coding of key words (such as 'complementary medicine') in which the main goal was to identify what parts of the documents were dealing with CAM. In the second step, qualitative content analysis (Graneheim and Lundman 2004) was performed on the identified sections in order to capture what issues the politicians wrote about. In this phase, the main focus was on the manifest and outspoken dimensions of the motions. The motions were also coded in terms of background information (concerning what political party is represented, in what political committees it is presented, and year of publication). This resulted in a large number of codes that were later sorted in broader themes (so-called parent codes) and sub-codes. In the third step, the focus was on how CAM is translated by different actors by following the links and associations in the documents. In practice, this was an iterative process of exploring the material from various starting points, for example, from single codes, co-variation of codes (which is possible to detect by a co-variation matrix in the software), and striking meaning units. All quotations were translated from Swedish to English in the last step of the analysis. The goal has been to keep the translations close to the linguistic characteristics of the original documents. However, some adjustments to make the quotations comprehensible have been necessary.

The Swedish Healthcare System and Its Relation to CAM

To grasp the political debate over CAM in Sweden, it is helpful to have a brief background of the Swedish healthcare system and its relation to CAM. First of all, Sweden is characterised by a strong relationship between the state and the healthcare sector. As early as the seventeenth century, doctors were paid by some municipalities to deliver healthcare for the poor population. Later, when hospitals were established in the late 1800s, the vast majority were funded by public means. As a consequence, most healthcare professionals, such as doctors, nurses, and midwives, were (and still are) employed in the public healthcare system (Palier 2006). Since the 1920s, the organisation and funding of healthcare has primarily been arranged at the municipality level. In a comparative perspective, Sweden has one of the most decentralised healthcare sectors in Europe. In the 1990s, the healthcare sector was reformatted along with the ideal on new public management. This opened it up to private enterprises, which, if they fulfil specific requirements, can offer healthcare that is funded by public means. One of the most important changes was the introduction of *vårdval* (choice of care), which means that the patient has the right to choose the deliverer of care. This choice is usually made at the level of the healthcare centre and not of single healthcare professionals (Magnussen et al. 2009).

There are many ways of defining healthcare systems, for example, by focusing on welfare regimes, institutional settings, or expenditures (Bergqvist et al. 2013). In focusing on welfare regimes, which are assumed to capture similar political ideologies, the Swedish healthcare system is often defined as social democratic or Scandinavian, along with countries such as Austria, Belgium, Denmark, Finland, the Netherlands, and Norway (Esping-Andersen 1990; Ferrera 1996). At the core of healthcare policies in Sweden lie universalistic and egalitarian ideals, that all inhabitants should have equal access to health regardless of income, gender, ethnicity, and so on (Magnussen et al. 2009). This type of healthcare system tends to be characterised by generous subsidies and interventionist states (Esping-Andersen 1990).

As in many other Western societies, medical doctors have developed strong professional autonomy and strong professional associations in Sweden. In 1663, the *Collegium Medicorum* was established, and this medical association was in control of medical practice. However, in the late 1800s, this professional autonomy was lost to the public authorities, and since 1960 healthcare has been under surveillance by the National Board of Health and Welfare (Palier 2006). In 1960, the so-called *Quackery Law* (*Lag om förbud i vissa fall mot verksamhet på hälso- och sjukvårdens område [Law on prohibition in some cases on activities in the area of healthcare]*, 1960: 409) was established, which, among other things, stated that only approved medical professionals were allowed to treat diseases. From 1999 the main parts of this law have been incorporated within the general law for patient security (*Patientsäkerhetslagen*, 2010: 659). There is no special regulation for CAM in Sweden. Instead the general regulations for the healthcare sector are applied (Wiesener et al. 2012). The most important is *Hälso-och sjukvårdslagen [Healthcare Act]* (1982: 763), which, among other things, states that healthcare professionals should conduct care in compliance with established scientific knowledge and proven clinical practices.

The Main Actors and the Overall Pattern of the Debate

As expected from the choice of empirical material, the main actors in this particular debate are the politicians who have written the motions. They are the ones that define political problems, negotiate on goals and solutions, enrol other actors into the debate, and mobilise various values and ideas to support their claims. These politicians, in turn, represent political parties in the Swedish parliament. Twenty-five per cent of the motions were written by representatives of *Centerpartiet*, followed by representatives of *Moderaterna* (22 per cent), *Miljöpartiet* (19 per cent), *Socialdemokraterna* (16 per cent), and *Folkpartiet*, *Vänsterpartiet*, and *Kristdemokraterna* (5–6 per cent each).[1]

Centerpartiet has a background of representing farmers and regional interests in Sweden. Today they are usually defined as a liberal and market-oriented party along with *Folkpartiet*. Although *Centerpartiet* and *Folkpartiet* are relatively small parties, they have been involved in several governmental coalitions with liberal and conservative parties during this debate (1979–1981, 1981–1982, 1991–1994, 2006–2010, and 2010–2014). *Moderaterna* is a liberal conservative party and is also characterised by its market orientation. During this time period, they have been the largest right-wing party, leading most liberal and conservative coalitions. In 1991, a Christian social conservative party, *Kristdemokraterna*, entered parliament. Since then, they have been part of all liberal and conservative governmental coalitions, although as the smallest party in the parliament. Another party who has entered the parliament during this debate is the environmental or green party, *Miljöpartiet*. They were established in 1980, entered parliament in 1988, lost their mandates during the right-wing coalition of 1991–1994, but returned to the parliament after that. Since 2010, they have collaborated with *Socialdemokraterna*, the social democrats. *Socialdemokraterna* has been the largest party in the Swedish parliament throughout the time period studied here. They have also been leading the government during several election periods, alone (1982–1986, 1986–1990, 1990–1991, 1994–1996, and 1996–2006) or in coalition with *Miljöpartiet* (2014–present). *Vänsterpartiet* is a relatively small left-wing socialist party. They have not been part of any Swedish government. Two parties, which have been represented in the parliament during parts of the time period, have not been active in this debate in terms of any written motions. Both of these parties, *Ny Demokrati* and *Sverigedemokraterna*, can be defined as nationalist or social conservative.

The debate on CAM has been active to different extents over the years. At the beginning of the time period, one or two motions were presented each year, with a small increase at the end of the 1980s. The most active period was during the years 2003–2008, with 7 or 8 motions per year, including a peak in 2005 with 12 motions.

When looking more carefully at the problematisation of CAM, two main types of political problems can be identified. In the first one, the problems are focused on public health issues. In the second one, which also is the most recurrent, the focus is on CAM itself and on more specific circumstances affecting CAM use or CAM practice. There are also a few examples in which issues involving CAM are parts of non-health-related debates, for example, concerning taxes, research politics, or environmental issues.

Political Problems: Public Health Issues

In the first type of political problem, a number of relatively broad public health issues can be identified, such as increasing costs for health insurance and long-term sick leaves, increasing medication, lack of preventive healthcare, long waits for doctor appointments, and negative changes in lifestyle. A recurrent argument is that public and/or conventional healthcare is poorly prepared to deal with such problems and that CAM might offer a contribution, in most cases along with other forms of healthcare. In some of the motions, limitations or failures of public healthcare are explicitly associated with basic characteristics of conventional medicine, such as a focus on diagnosis, the treatment of sickness/diseases, and the extensive use of medications. For example, two of the most active politicians in this debate, both representing *Moderaterna*, argued for economic interventions to promote CAM against the backdrop of public health issues:

> The rising sickness rate among the Swedish population is not only a large public health problem, but has become by far the largest economic strain on the Swedish economy by weighing the transfer systems with large expenditure on health insurance. Behind the sickness rate, there is widespread illness, which the health care [system] is poorly equipped to take care of. The Swedish health care system has been, and still is, organised to take care of diagnosed diseases and injuries. (MOT 2008/09: Sk324)

In contrast, CAM is often associated in the political debate with active patient choices, healthy lifestyles, and health promotion. Two representatives of *Centerpartiet*, also very active in the debate, took their point of departure in general problems of rising costs and increased medication:

The cost of drugs is rising faster in Sweden than in any other country. The cost of health insurance is increasing. This is very unsatisfactory, both for humans and finances, and all agree that something must be done. But what? Why are people sick and why do they need so much medication? (MOT 2001/02: So223)

Later on in the motion the politicians elaborated on their critique of conventional healthcare and suggested CAM as an important complement for people who seek options outside conventional healthcare but also as a contribution to the general healthcare system:

Doctors in the past have fought against diseases, but where has it brought us? The constant pursuit of miracle cures for various diseases is often reflected in a lack of knowledge about how lifestyle and environmental factors affect our health. An increasing number of patients are concerned about the side effects of medications, and many have chosen to seek alternative treatment to get a better quality of life [...] We don't argue that this is the solution, but we are convinced that it is one of several factors that can reverse the unfortunate trend we find ourselves in. We are confident that resource-saving alternative medicine can relieve [public] care in several areas. (MOT 2001/02: So223)

Problematisation of CAM as a public health issue, or more precisely of CAM as a contribution or solution to public health issues, is clearly connected to liberal and conservative politicians in the debate. Almost none of these motions were written by representatives of *Socialdemokraterna, Miljöpartiet*, or *Vänsterpartiet.*

Political Problems: CAM Issues

In the second type of political problem, the focus is on CAM itself and on more specific constraints and circumstances that might delimit CAM use or practice. Here it is possible to identify a number of broad themes, such as unequal conditions, professional practice, legal constraints, lack of knowledge and research, and various forms of risks. As we will see later, some of these themes overlap. In the first theme, the main actors highlight that CAM cannot compete with public or conventional healthcare on equal terms, for example, concerning costs, taxes, education, availability, and professional autonomy. Concerning costs, one recurrent argument is that CAM users 'pay double', with already taxed money, because CAM treatments are provided within the private sector and have no tax exemptions. For example, representatives of several liberal and conservative parties stated in a joint motion: 'Many of these [treatments] are not funded by public means, instead it is the individual who pays, with taxed money. This causes unfair conditions and makes it into a matter of class' (MOT 2004/05: So432). The same logic is applied for CAM education, which is organised privately and paid out of pocket by the students. In these problematisations of CAM, it is possible to identify links both to ideals on free markets and open competition and to matters of social justice and class. These aspects need to be understood in relation to the system of Swedish higher education, which to a large extent is publicly funded, with no student fees and relatively generous student allowances and loans. So, even if parties like *Centerpartiet* often are associated with ideals on free markets and private enterprises, a typical argument on this issue is presented as follows.

> In the traditional Swedish education system, there is no complementary/alternative training. That means that people who are interested in such education must search for private alternatives. This, in turn, means that there is no free education and that there are no student allowances or loans. If one wants an education in the area of complementary [medicine], one must make a huge economic commitment. This is an injustice that should receive more attention and be reconsidered. (MOT 2002/03: So225)

Another theme concerns professional practice and legal constraints—and the fact that CAM practice, to a large extent, is relatively unregulated in Sweden. The main argument is that there is too little control of education, titles, and practitioners. This, in turn, opens up risks and uncertainty for individual patients and users but also for practitioners and healthcare providers. Common arguments are that it is difficult to know what education practitioners have, what the titles refer to, what the differences are between various treatments, and what is considered 'reliable', 'serious', or 'trustworthy'. More or less explicitly, these aspects are also connected to legal aspects, as stated in various regulations (such as the general health act). Or as one representative of *Moderaterna* summarised the problem: 'Because it is possible to establish oneself as a practitioner, without declaring professional competence or results, and this has become a large market, it is difficult for the consumers to make informed choices' (MOT 2006/07: So319). Some of the politicians also highlighted the problem of limited protection concerning specific patient groups and their right to reliable and scientific treatments. For example, representatives of *Folkpartiet* argued: 'We believe that mental illness is as serious as cancer, diabetes, and other diseases covered by the so-called quackery law. Patients with mental illness must be guaranteed expert and diligent care in accordance with science and proven experience' (MOT 2007/08: So484). The general focus in this motion was on limitations in current regulations, which leave the field open to non-professional and potentially manipulative practitioners. Patients with mental illness were identified as an exposed and unprotected group and the comparison with cancer and diabetes patients needs to be understood as the backdrop of current regulation, which set up certain limitations for practitioners without official licenses (e.g., regarding what disorders they are allowed to treat).

In several of the motions, CAM is presented as practices that fall outside the responsibilities of established control agencies such as the National Board of Health and Welfare and the National Board of Higher Education. There are also a number of motions that draw upon the so-called quackery law (which, at the time of most of the motions, had been replaced by the law for patient security and the general healthcare act) to distinguish between serious and non-serious practices in terms of quackery or to highlight risks with more or less uncontrolled professions. For example, representatives of *Folkpartiet* and *Miljöpartiet* wrote about professional boundaries and problems with information and valuation in connection to quackery:

> The legislation on quackery has been critically questioned with regard to developments in the so-called alternative medicine. The flora of commercial enterprises and clinics that has emerged, and the range of therapies,

treatments and effects on people's psychological state that are not based on science or proven experience and are practiced by people without medical qualifications or equivalent, cause concern. (MOT 2006/07: So235)

It is also of great importance to get increased control and to distinguish serious activities from—which of course exist—pure quackery. Information to the public is basic. People must know how control is maintained and what is trustworthy. It should not be necessary to be well educated to navigate among the different services. (MOT 2003/04: So625)

As indicated earlier, legal boundaries are not only framed as problematic to patients and users but also for healthcare professionals and providers. For example, against the backdrop of public health issues, such as increasing societal costs, representatives of *Centerpartiet* focused on the fact that licensed healthcare professionals could not practice CAM as part of their profession. In the following motion, the politicians touched upon unequal economic conditions but also on professional limitations caused by regulations:

It is not uncommon that medically trained [staff] pay thousands of [Swedish] crowns on private training because they discover that conventional health care is not enough. Many incorporate their skills in alternative medicine in daily health care, in silence. However, today this is not allowed. ... Licensed staff must, in principle, delegitimise themselves in order to practise alternative medicine. (MOT 1999/2000: So486)

Concerning limitations of CAM practice, two aspects in particular have been in focus in the debate. The first one focuses on the law for professional activities in the healthcare sector and on restrictions on which patient groups' non-licensed practitioners are allowed to treat (especially pregnant women and children under the age of eight) and the fact that this did not change when the so-called quackery law was replaced in 1999. The second aspect concerns rights to prescribe certain drugs and remedies or as representatives of *Centerpartiet* summarised the problem: 'There is growing concern that the availability of supplements and vitamins is limited for Swedish citizens' (MOT 2002/03_So225). This way of problematising CAM has been recurrent in the political debate since

2001, when the regulation on various supplements was adjusted to meet the directives of the EU. From being relatively uncontrolled and sold freely, they came under supervision of the Medical Product Agency and were only sold at public drug stores. At higher doses than daily recommendations, a prescription from licensed healthcare professionals is needed. This problematisation, in turn, is linked to issues on freedom of choice, availability, and unequal conditions compared to conventional healthcare. For example, two of the most active representatives of *Centerpartiet* argued that authorised CAM practitioners should have the right to prescribe supplements:

> One of the tools of complementary and alternative medicine is the ability to recommend supplements such as glucosamine. Now, since Sweden is adjusted to the EU regulation, the Medical Product Agency [*Läkemedelsverket*] must consider that supplements, when they have documented curative effects, should be classified as drugs. From October 1 2001, these may only be sold in pharmacies with a prescription. This means that remedies, which have shown curative effects, will not be available for the individual patient. It requires a doctor's appointment in healthcare that already is difficult to access, and also to a doctor who is not familiar with this medication. Complementary and alternative practitioners with authorisation and quality assurance, who have knowledge in glucosamine, ought to prescribe this drug. (MOT 2001/02: So623)

Another theme is related to lack of knowledge and research. One argument is that patients and users—but also healthcare professionals—have limited knowledge about CAM. In many of the motions this is explicitly connected to problems for patients and users to make informed choices, which, in turn, is connected to various risks. Healthcare professionals are assumed to have limited competence on CAM in general, or on specific treatments and remedies (as in the example earlier), which limits their ability to provide information about CAM treatments or to handle parallel treatments. In some cases, these problematisations are also connected to basic patient rights, as formulated in the general health regulation. For example, representatives of *Centerpartiet* argued:

District nurses and doctors are some of the health professionals who, in their daily work, are key actors in informing patients. According to the general health regulation, 2a §, patients should be given information about available treatments. Today, it is not always the case that these professionals have good knowledge about opportunities offered by representatives of alternative medicine. That is, from the patient perspective, unsatisfactory. (MOT 1997/98: So308)

In other cases, the need for knowledge and research is argued for in more general terms, for example, by drawing on public health issues and pointing at the need for explanations. Some of these propositions are also examples of when the political context not only is related to health but also is expanded to education and research politics. For example, representatives of *Miljöpartiet* argued for more research on CAM in a motion to the Committee on Education:

> Today, many people use drugs and treatments from alternative and complementary therapies. In this area, there is a great need of research that can distinguish which treatments are efficient from a health economic point of view. However, health is more than a strictly medical concern, and interdisciplinary research is needed to get an overall perspective. (MOT 2008/09: Ub8)

Lack of knowledge and research is closely connected to shortage of funding, lack of competence among conventionally trained researchers, and limited integration and/or acceptance in scientific contexts. This, in turn, draws upon basic conflicts between CAM and conventional medicine, especially concerning scientific methods. Representatives of *Vänsterpartiet* summarised the problem: 'Traditionally, there has been, and still is, a mutual distrust between complementary medicine and traditional scientific medicine, so-called school medicine' (MOT 2001/02: So398). There are also notions of a 'catch 22' moment for CAM research in which funding for research requires certain levels of establishment, but such establishment is difficult to achieve without research funding. Representatives of *Miljöpartiet* argued: 'Today there is a catch 22. A method must be proven to be effective in trials before the research grants are awarded and established researchers become interested [in CAM research]' (MOT 2002/03: So365).

Several of the motions identify common characteristics of CAM, such as a holistic view, as important to understanding why established scientific methods, such as randomised controlled trials, are unsuitable to investigate how CAM works. New or adapted research designs are needed. For example, a representative of *Centerpartiet* argued:

> Complementary alternative medicine is a treatment that is based on a holistic approach, based upon the individual. Because of this, it is difficult to use randomised trials. In other words, it is difficult to use conventional medical research methods and it is necessary to adapt the research methods to the discipline that will be examined. A suggestion is to apply the so-called black-box approach on complementary and alternative medicine. That, in turn, requires that someone in the research team has practical experience on how the complementary alternative treatment is performed. (MOT 2012/13: So494)

This problematisation also raises a more general critique of evidence-based medicine and established scientific methods. The motion continued:

> But then the question is how to understand evidence. How to interpret 'science and proven clinical conduct'? Can we expand the view on evidence to include all existent and relevant information on a problem area without abandoning a scientific approach? (MOT 2012/13: So494)

In contrast to the first theme of political problems, the second one is more diverse, in terms of both what is focused on and which main actors are involved. Here, all political parties are represented.

Negotiations on Goals and Solutions

Following the links from what are defined as political problems, we find a number of goals and suggested solutions and how these are negotiated. To some extent, goals and solutions can be divided into the same types as explained earlier—into goals related to public health and into goals concerning CAM use, practice, and knowledge production—but they also overlap. In particular, relatively specific political problems (such as the availability of drugs and remedies) can be linked both to general public health goals (such as the general well-being of the population) and more specific CAM goals (such as the availability of homeopathy).

First of all, it is important to note that the politicians often formulate a number of goals in the same motion and that these goals vary from very general to relatively specific. The proposals also differ in how explicit they are in terms of the connection between political problems and suggested interventions. At the most general level, many of the politicians formulate goals concerning the whole healthcare sector. For example, representatives of *Socialdemokraterna* stated that the general goal for the healthcare sector is to 'decrease sickness, sick leaves, and the costs associated to these' (MOT 1993/94: Sk44). Representatives of *Centerpartiet* formulated a similar goal: 'The goal of all health care must be that more people should have a healthier life. Here, alternative medicine can contribute to people and economy in an advantageous manner' (MOT 2000/01: So223). Such public health goals are stated in many documents, no matter what political party is represented or what political ideology they are associated with. But there are also general goals concerning individual possibilities, circumstances, and constraints. In these cases, the links to political ideologies are more apparent. A recurrent goal in the proposals written by liberal and conservative parties (especially *Centerpartiet* and *Moderaterna*) is to stimulate individuals to take more responsibility for their health or to take active healthcare decisions. For example, representatives of *Moderaterna* wrote: 'We must learn to promote health, not only treat sickness. It is a political duty and a human right. [...] From an individual perspective, the individual must be regarded as a competent actor between care providers and care recipients' (MOT 2013/14: Ub403) and 'Therefore, we ask for a review on how it can be possible to stimulate people to take a more active role in taking care of their health' (MOT 2014/15: 2406).

Looking at specific CAM goals, one of the most recurrent goals is to achieve more integration and collaboration between CAM and public and/or conventional healthcare. This is often formulated in very general terms, for example: 'Complementary preventive care should be involved in the health care framework' (MOT 2004/05: So603). Integration is presented as the answer to meet public health issues as well as individual preferences and needs. For example, integration is assumed to make CAM more accessible, reduce unequal conditions, bridge professional/ legal constraints (especially for healthcare professionals), support research, and improve the general knowledge about CAM treatments. Again, these goals are closely connected to general ideas on individual freedom, autonomy, and respect. For example, representatives of *Miljöpartiet* framed the goal of integration as follows: 'The goal with integration might be to pay more respect to patients' values and requests, and by doing so, increase participation in choices of health care and treatments' (MOT 2009/10: So228).

Suggested integration takes different forms, from inclusion of CAM treatments in public care and the public health insurance to collaboration between specific groups of professionals (such as doctors and CAM practitioners) and integration of CAM knowledge within the general 'research community'. These goals are also closely linked to public health issues and to how users, patients, and the general population might benefit from the inclusion of CAM in public and/or conventional healthcare, for example, by collaboration between professionals:

> Because citizens have great trust in complementary treatments, we find it to be an eligible and important development to establish conditions for integration and increased collaboration between school medicine and alternative treatments. (MOT 2001/02: So605)

Other recurrent goals, which are linked to political problems on lack of knowledge and research, focus on more CAM research, increased funding of research, and establishment of a research (or knowledge) centre. The last goal was high on the agenda for two decades, from the early 1990s to 2009. In many of the motions, the politicians discussed such a centre in terms of integrative medicine and that it should have the capacity to combine competences from conventional medicine and CAM practitioners. For example: 'Here research is going to take place, in school medicine but also in collaboration with CAM-practitioners. The goal is to take advantage of the competence in the CAM area, which cannot be systematised today because it does not have access to the research field' (MOT 2002/03: So365). Other expectations on such a centre were that it should serve the role for coordinating higher education in CAM, inform patients and healthcare professionals as well as official agencies about treatments and research, and facilitate clinical CAM research. In several of the proposals these goals are connected to problems for individuals to access relevant information. For example, representatives of *Socialdemokraterna* focused on the limited resources of voluntary initiatives and argued for a publicly funded centre:

> Today, Sweden has no centre for knowledge and education on alternative treatments. Citizens try to find information in other ways, e.g. by KAM, The Committee for Alternative Medicine. KAM, as a voluntary association with no public support, has, however, limited resources to support information for citizens. (MOT 2006/07: So413)

In 2006 the Osher Center for Integrative Medicine was established at the Karolinska Institute, the top-ranked medical university in Sweden. The main funding was from the private Osher Foundation, although the university co-funded it (which, indirectly, was done with public means). Since this establishment, the goal of a national CAM research centre has faded away from the political debate.

Closely linked to the goal of a research centre is a suggested register of CAM practitioners. This is, by far, the most frequent political goal from the mid-1990s to 2013. This is also one of the most complex political issues in the debate in terms of how it has been dealt with in a large number motions, reports from the Committee of Social Affairs, and in several public investigations (the main report from the Committee on Alternative Medicine, SOU 1989:60, the so-called *AKM-Inquiry*, SOU 2004: 123, and the so-called *Eligibility Inquiry*, SOU 2010:6). In general, the goal of a register has been promoted by representatives of *Miljöpartiet* and *Socialdemokraterna* and in some cases by *Kristdemokraterna*. In several of the motions the idea is that a register that is chronologically linked to the establishment of a research or knowledge centre. For example, representatives of *Socialdemokraterna* wrote: 'It is urgent that such a register be established. A national register should be a first step towards a national information and knowledge centre, where competence in complementary and alternative medicine can be gathered as well as research data' (MOT 2007/08: So416). In other cases, the register is presented as an independent goal motivated by concerns about patient security and difficulties for patients and users to access relevant information. In some of the motions the idea of a register is also connected to ideas on standardised requirements of education and coordination of titles. Two of the most active representatives of *Socialdemokraterna* argued as follows in one of several motions on the topic:

> By a national register for complementary and alternative practitioners will the same treatment/therapy have the same requirements concerning education, which is not the case today. Thus, patients' choices will be easier because the same concepts will be used for the same treatments. (MOT 2006/07: So413)

Because of the empirical material—motions written by one type of actor—interessement or interposition of CAM might seem a bit implicit. What we can see in these documents is what is prioritised as goals, and how they are motivated, but not any counter arguments.

Enrolment of Credible Actors and Mobilisation of Research and Ideals on Freedom of Choice

In the process of defining political problems and proposing various goals and solutions, the political representatives have enrolled a number of credible actors, such as governmental agencies, professional associations, universities, hospitals, well-known individuals, law texts, and reports. These actors, in turn, have been mobilised to support different kind of values, ideas, and claims. From the material, it is clear that these actors are not restricted to traditional actors, in terms of individuals or associations, but that they take many symbolic and de-personalised forms (cf Law 1992).

By far the most commonly mobilised claim is the popularity and extensive, or increasing, use of CAM. This claim is used through the whole time period by representatives of all political parties and is often formulated in very general terms:

A large share of the population uses complementary or alternative medical treatments along with [conventional] health care. This may include visiting chiropractors, osteopaths and acupuncturists. (MOT 2010/11: So573)

Many of the main actors support this type of claim with findings from reports from county councils and/or researchers and universities:

More and more people are interested in complementary treatments. An investigation by Linköping University in 2001 showed, among other things, that people have great faith and confidence in complementary efforts... (MOT 20013/14: So625)

This way of drawing links to investigations and reports, and to authorities such as universities, is not delimited to this issue but is found in many arguments about the efficacy and safety of CAM treatments. Again, this is often formulated in general terms to indicate the existence of scientific studies and/or positive results, including 'Well documented studies' (MOT 1992/93: 190), 'A recurrent factor that is highlighted in studies of complementary medicine is...' (MOT 2007/08: So244), and 'There is rich documentation of scientific studies, which show positive effects of integrative, complementary treatments to school medicine' (MOT 2007/08: Sk382). There are examples in which specific studies, results, and researchers and institutes are enrolled in the debate but compared to the general pattern these are notable exceptions. In a few motions there are links to international research, named researchers, and universities like the University of Florida and Harvard School of Medicine. In others, the politicians draw links to Swedish research and enrol actors such as the Osher Center for Integrative Medicine at the Karolinska Institute, Linköping University, KTH Royal Institute of Technology, and *Vidarkliniken* (a private but publicly supported anthroposophic hospital south of Stockholm). Some of these actors, such as the national and international universities, signify relatively general and conventional scientific legitimacy in being well known to wide audiences as trusted and well-reputed scientific institutions. Other actors, such as the Osher Center, *Vidarkliniken*, and named Swedish researchers, probably signify a slightly different legitimacy by indicating the existence and establishment of CAM in scientific and medical contexts.

In the debate, there are also other kinds of actors enrolled. During the years from 2002 to 2008, some of the most recurrent actors were the WHO, the WHO document *Traditional Medicine Strategy 2002–2005*, and the WHO resolution *EB:111.R12 on Traditional Medicine*.

These actors were enrolled both to back up arguments on the extensive use of CAM and to support integration and patient security (e.g., by establishing a research centre, a register of practitioners, or more general quality assurance). For example, some of the most active representatives of *Socialdemokraterna* enrolled the WHO and its specific strategy:

> In its strategy for 2002–2005, the WHO describes how every member state should strive for increased integration between school medicine and complementary and alternative medicine. To deepen co-operation, in accordance with the global plan of the WHO, it is important that HSL [the general health care act] and Lysen [the law on professional practice in the health care sector] be adjusted to the new conditions. (MOT 2005/06: So590)

In a similar manner, several other official agencies (such as the Swedish Agency for Health Technology Assessment and Assessment of Social Services, the National Board of Health and Welfare, and the Medical Product Agency), associations (such as KAM, the voluntary committee on CAM in Sweden, and NSK, its Nordic counterpart), laws (especially the general healthcare act), and public inquiries (such as the so-called AKM-Inquiry) are enrolled in the debate. A striking aspect is that enrolled actors, such as named researchers, universities, and official agencies, are expected to speak for themselves in the motions. They are seldom introduced or described. To some extent this is expected because of the context of the motions. One could expect the main audience of the documents (members of the parliament and members of the political committees in the parliament) to be familiar with Swedish universities, official agencies, and general regulations. But in other cases, it is less self-evident. For example, when introducing named researchers, this is usually supported by basic information on affiliation but with very limited information on the researcher's specific competence or research area.

Another striking pattern is the mobilisation of ideals on freedom of choice. Especially in the motions by liberal and conservative representatives, there are recurrent links between specific political problems (e.g., on costs, taxes, general availability of treatments, and lack of holistic perspectives) and notions of freedom of choice and active patients or consumers. As indicated earlier, many of the motions highlight that patients and users have the right, and in some cases the preference to choose their treatments. This is often supported by enrolment of the general health-care act but also by scientific reports and public inquiries on the extensive use of CAM. For example, a representative of *Centerpartiet* stated: 'The right of the patient to choose therapy is also established in the Swedish health care act' (MOT 1991/92: So107). Closely connected to these arguments is the idea that patients or consumers have the capacity, but also the responsibility, to decide on their own healthcare. In some motions these ideas are formulated in relatively soft terms, that many people in contemporary society have an interest in promoting their health and searching for alternatives to conventional medicine. In others, they are formulated in explicit ideological terms, that people need to take more responsibility for their health and healthcare choices.

Discussion

In this chapter, I have analysed the political debate on CAM in the Swedish parliament with help from an actor network approach. In general, the political translation of CAM, in terms of what kinds of networks have been stabilised, has been in favour of the phenomenon. The main actors, in this case the parliamentary politicians, have argued for interventions to facilitate CAM use or CAM practice. Only a few motions include proposals intended to limit or restrict CAM, although risks, especially for users and patients, have been highlighted in many more.

To summarise some of the main findings, the translations consist of two main types of problematisations. In the first, the political problems are related to public health issues such as long-term sick leaves, increasing societal costs, and lack of preventive healthcare. Here, CAM is presented as a contribution to general healthcare and might support individuals and society, often along with other types of treatments. This type of problematisation is also almost exclusively linked to liberal and conservative parties, such as *Centerpartiet* and *Moderaterna*. It is also quite obvious that CAM is not the main focus here but more of a bonus or a side track that will contribute to resolving the larger issues. In the second, the problems are focused on CAM itself and on more specific circumstances affecting CAM use or practice. This type of problematisation is the most common in the material and also the most diverse. Here we find a number of broad themes, such as unequal conditions, professional practice, legal constraints, lack of knowledge and research, and various forms of risk. This type of problematisation is expressed by representatives of all political parties in the debate, no matter their ideological orientation.

When following the links from the political problems, we also find a number of goals and suggested solutions. To some extent, these can be defined in the same way as the political problems, either focusing on public health or on CAM itself, but they also overlap. The goals connected to public health are in most cases very general, either focusing on better health or decreased costs at a societal level or on more freedom and/or more individual responsibility in healthcare choices. In contrast, most CAM goals are much more specific. Here we find proposals on increased integration of CAM and conventional medicine, for example, concerning professional practice, establishment of a research or knowledge centre, and a register of CAM practitioners. Several of these goals have also been on the agenda for many years by different political parties representing different ideological standpoints.

When analysing the material in more detail, and also considering what is mobilised and enrolled by the politicians, several interesting aspects appear. First of all, it is clear that this is a relatively liberal, and to some extent neoliberal, debate. Although neoliberalism is a tricky, and often poorly defined, concept (Boas and Gans-Morse 2009; Thorsen 2011), it is often associated with ideals on free markets, to organise exchanges of services and goods. As a consequence, it is also associated with reforms on privatisation, deregulation, decentralisation, and tax reductions, which are assumed to have positive effects on the economy by not restricting market mechanisms. It is also an ideology giving priority to individual freedom, active choices, and personal responsibility (e.g., Friedman 2009;

Friedman and Friedman 1990). This particular debate is not only dominated by representatives of liberal and conservative parties, who have written about 60 per cent of the motions, but it is also characterised by typical neoliberal ideas. These ideas are connected to a number of political problems and goals, both concerning general public health and more specific CAM issues (e.g., on the right to choose healthcare and/or CAM and fair competition for CAM practitioners). Although the neoliberal ideas are most frequent and elaborated in the motions by *Centerpartiet* and *Moderaterna*, they are found in motions from almost all political parties in the debate. This could be related to general arguments about the neoliberalisation of society or to more specific ones about neoliberalisation of health and healthcare systems (e.g., McGregor 2001). Several scholars have also discussed neoliberalism in relation to CAM and how neoliberal discourses on consumerism are congruent with common CAM ideals on self-management, active choices, and personal responsibility (e.g., Brenton and Elliott 2014; Broom et al. 2014; Fries 2008). But this is only one side of the debate. In parallel, we can detect general ideals on social equality and fairness in motions from representatives of almost all political parties. For example, several of the liberal and conservative representatives problematise access to CAM in terms of inequality and social class, which could be surprising. But, as indicated earlier in the chapter, this probably needs to be understood in relation to long traditions of universalistic and egalitarian healthcare policies in Sweden.

Another important finding is how the debate follows scientific and biomedical norms. Although there are some striking counter examples, such as when the politicians destabilise this norm (e.g., by suggesting black-box approaches and the expansion of the view on what is considered as evidence), the general pattern is that science and conventional medicine are more or less taken for granted. The politicians recurrently mobilise reports and scientific studies, although in very general terms, to show the popularity, extensive use, and positive results of CAM. They also enrol a number of actors, such as universities, hospitals, and researchers, which are associated with the scientific and medical establishment, to support their arguments. Several of the goals, such as the establishment of a research or knowledge centre and a register of practitioners, also indicate a strong biomedical norm and that the general goal is to get

CAM accepted by various establishments, not necessarily on its own terms. In the motions there are also many distinctions expressed by the politicians, indicating the ambiguous position of CAM, for example, by using formulations like 'so-called alternative medicine' and by highlighting the fine line between CAM and quackery.

There are certainly more aspects to explore in this political debate, both concerning the reception of the motions (especially in the parliamentary committees) and follow-up on which motions have resulted in political interventions (e.g., changes in regulations or increased funding), and more focus should be put on quantitative aspects of the patterns indicated in the analysis earlier. It would also be very interesting to explore other national debates on CAM, or the debate in the EU or in the WHO, to see whether or not these political translations of CAM are general or are tied to specific national characteristics (such as the general outline of the healthcare system or the status of CAM).

Note

1. Several of these parties have changed their names during the debate or have longer full names. In the chapter, I have chosen the name used in everyday language and/or dominating during the time period in focus.

References

Angell, M., & Kassirer, J. P. (1998). Alternative medicine – The risks of untested and unregulated remedies. *New England Journal of Medicine, 339*(12), 839–841.

Bergqvist, K., Yngwe, M. A., & Lundberg, O. (2013). Understanding the role of welfare state characteristics for health and inequalities – An analytical review. *BMC Public Health, 13*(1), 1234.

Boas, T. C., & Gans-Morse, J. (2009). Neoliberalism: From new liberal philosophy to anti-liberal slogan. *Studies in Comparative International Development, 44*(2), 137–161.

Brenton, J., & Elliott, S. (2014). Undoing gender? The case of complementary and alternative medicine. *Sociology of Health & Illness, 36*(1), 91–107.

Broom, A., Meurk, C., Adams, J., & Sibbritt, D. (2014). My health, my responsibility? Complementary medicine and self (health) care. *Journal of Sociology, 50*(4), 515–530.

Callon, M. (1986). Some elements of a sociology of translation – Domestication of the scallops and the fishermen of St-Brieuc Bay. *The Sociological Review, 32*(1_suppl), 196–233.

CAMDOC Alliance. (2010). *The regulatory status of complementary and alternative medicine for medical doctors in Europe*. Retrieved November 13, 2017, from http://www.camdoc.eu/Pdf/CAMDOCRegulatoryStatus8_10.pdf.

Clarke, D. B., Doel, M. A., & Segrott, J. (2004). No alternative? The regulation and professionalization of complementary and alternative medicine in the United Kingdom. *Health & Place, 10*(4), 329–338.

Esping-Andersen, G. (1990). *The three worlds of welfare capitalism*. Princeton, NJ: Princeton University Press.

Ferrera, M. (1996). The 'southern model' of welfare in social Europe. *Journal of European Social Policy, 6*(1), 107–111.

Fisher, P., & Ward, A. (1994). Complementary medicine in Europe. *British Medical Journal, 309*(6947), 107–111.

Friedman, M. (2009). *Capitalism and freedom: Fortieth anniversary edition*. Chicago: University of Chicago Press.

Friedman, M., & Friedman, R. D. (1990). *Free to choose: A personal statement*. Boston: Houghton Mifflin Harcourt.

Fries, C. J. (2008). Governing the health of the hybrid self: Integrative medicine, neoliberalism, and the shifting politics of subjectivity. *Health Sociology Review, 17*(4), 353–367.

Graneheim, U. H., & Lundman, B. (2004). Qualitative content analysis in nursing research: Concepts, procedures and measures to achieve trustworthiness. *Nurse Education Today, 24*(2), 105–112.

Latour, B. (1996). *Aramis, or, the love of technology*. Cambridge, MA: Harvard University Press.

Latour, B. (2005). *Reassembling the social: An introduction to actor-network-theory*. Oxford: Oxford University Press.

Law, J. (1992). Notes on the theory of the actor network – Ordering, strategy, and heterogeneity. *Systems Practice, 5*(4), 379–393.

Magnussen, J., Vrangbaeck, K., Saltman, R. B., & Martinussen, P. E. (2009). Introduction: The Nordic model of health care. In J. Magnussen, K. Vrangbaeck, & R. B. Saltman (Eds.), *Nordic health care systems – Recent reforms and current policy challenges* (pp. 3–20). Maidenhead: Open University Press.

McGregor, S. (2001). Neoliberalism and health care. *International Journal of Consumer Studies, 25*(2), 82–89.

Palier, B. (2006). *Hälso- och sjukvårdens reformer – En internationell jämförelse.* Stockholm: Sveriges Kommuner och Landsting.

Saks, M. (1999). The wheel turns? Professionalisation and alternative medicine in Britain. *Journal of Interprofessional Care, 13*(2), 129–138.

Singh, S., & Ernst, E. (2008). *Trick or treatment? Alternative medicine on trial.* London: Bantam.

Thorsen, D. E. (2011). The neoliberal challenge – What is neoliberalism. *Contemporary Readings in Law and Social Justice, 2*(2), 188–214.

Welsh, S., Kelner, M., Wellman, B., & Boon, H. (2004). Moving forward? Complementary and alternative practitioners seeking self-regulation. *Sociology of Health & Illness, 26*(2), 216–241.

Werneke, U., Earl, J., Seydel, C., Horn, O., Crichton, P., & Fannon, D. (2004). Potential health risks of complementary alternative medicines in cancer patients. *British Journal of Cancer, 90*(2), 408–413.

Wiesener, S., Falkenberg, T., Hegyi, G., Hök, J., di Sarsina, P. R., & Fønnebø, V. (2012). Legal status and regulation of complementary and alternative medicine in Europe. *Forschende Komplementärmedizin, 19*(2), 29–36.

8

Safety as 'Boundary Object': The Case of Acupuncture and Chinese Medicine Regulation in Ontario, Canada

Nadine Ijaz and Heather Boon

In this chapter, we apply a theoretical concept from science and technology studies, that of the *boundary object*, to the field of professional regulation as it pertains to traditional, complementary and alternative medicine (TCAM). With reference to our recent case study of acupuncture and Chinese medicine regulation in the province of Ontario, Canada, we use the 'boundary object' concept as a mechanism to highlight the disproportionate role that safety-related discourse may play in TCAM professional regulatory projects. We then discuss possible implications of our observations with respect to TCAM professionalisation studies more broadly.

Boundary Objects and TCAM Research

The *boundary object* concept was first theorised by Star and Griesemer (1989) and relies on the *social worlds framework*, elaborated over multiple decades within the symbolic interactionist tradition of sociology and

N. Ijaz (✉) • H. Boon
Leslie Dan Faculty of Pharmacy, University of Toronto,
Toronto, ON, Canada

widely used in studies of science and technology (Clarke and Star 2008). Social worlds are conceptualised as 'shared discursive spaces' in which 'multiple collective actors' engage in particular primary activities, at specific locations or sites, in particular ways and ultimately aim to promote or propagate some aspects of these activities (p. 114). 'Over time,' note Clarke and Star (p. 113), 'social worlds typically segment into multiple worlds, intersect with other worlds ... and merge.' They use the term 'arena' to describe an ecology in which multiple social worlds organise 'around issues of mutual concern and commitment to action' (p. 113). The social worlds framework has been extensively used to study occupations and professions, as well as a wide range of other groups and settings.

In their 1989 case study of the Berkeley Museum of Vertebrate Zoology, Star and Griesemer advanced social worlds theory by introducing to it the boundary object concept. They characterised boundary objects, which may be 'abstract or concrete,' as having 'different meanings in different social worlds,' while preserving a structure 'common enough to more than one world to make them recognisable, a means of translation ... [for] developing and maintaining coherence across intersecting social worlds' (Star and Griesemer 1989: 393). Examples of boundary objects in Star and Griesemer's original study included 'species and subspecies of mammals and birds,' as well as 'the habitats of collected animal species,' which carried distinct meanings across the social worlds of (among others) the museum's 'research scientists, curators, amateur collectors, private sponsors and patrons' (p. 392). Although members of the aforementioned social worlds shared a common goal of 'preserving California's nature' in Star and Griesemer's study (p. 408), they brought to this endeavour a range of different perspectives and approaches, made evident in their distinct conceptualisations of, and engagement with, the identified boundary objects.

Star and Griesemer's original boundary object concept has been applied and theoretically nuanced across a range of scholarly fields, including in TCAM-related research (Derkatch 2008; Keshet et al. 2013; Owens 2015). In contrast to Star and Griesemer's early characterisation of boundary objects as operating within mutually advantageous collaborative settings, TCAM scholars' application of the boundary object concept has specifically addressed the differential power dynamics typically at play in TCAM-biomedical encounters. Owens, for example, points to the effective deployment of the *sterile needle* as a boundary object from within the social world of American acupuncturists, who sought to facilitate traditional acupuncture's increased entry into the politically dominant social world of mainstream US healthcare. She notes (2015: 21):

> The sterile needle 'worked' as a boundary object during this period due to its cohesion with two major trends in the early 1990s: the concern over infectious disease transmission through needles and the increased call for evidence-based medicine.

In this chapter, we similarly use the boundary object concept to explore acupuncture's increased integration into mainstream healthcare, but, in this case, with reference to professional regulation. In our analysis, we shift focus from the needle itself to the concept of *safety* as a *rhetorical* boundary object, echoing Derkatch's work (2008) about evidentiary debates around TCAM. There, Derkatch theoretically extends the boundary object concept to include *rhetorical strategy*, referring to the concept of *efficacy*, one of evidence-based medicine's core principles. With reference to the reification of randomised control trials in biomedicine, Derkatch (2008: 379) analyses *efficacy* as a shape-shifting, rhetorical boundary object through which 'a given health practice or study' may be positioned 'within or beyond the borders of science.' As Derkatch notes within the context of research:

> *Efficacy*, and its sister term, *safety*, are cited, mantra-like, throughout the medical literature as the chief motivations behind research ... [A]s keywords, safety and efficacy are so flexible that they can function as gatekeepers. (381)

In this work, we use a similar theoretical approach as Derkatch, this time to demonstrate how evidence-based medicine's cardinal virtue of *safety* may act, somewhat problematically, as a central discursive boundary object in defining regulatory parameters for TCAM practices and practitioners. With reference to the case of acupuncture and Chinese medicine regulation in Ontario, Canada, and to the arena of intersecting social worlds at play in that process, we point to three areas in which *safety* has played a key discursive role as a regulatory boundary object: (a) in establishing the need for acupuncture's regulation, (b) in formulating training standards across the professions and (c) in defining policy to address the distinct ethnolinguistic features of the Chinese medicine profession.

The data we interpret in this study were collected as part of a qualitative case study we conducted on the statutory regulation of acupuncture and traditional Chinese medicine in Ontario, Canada. Case study data included an extensive body of public documents from the period 1984 through 2017, including consultative documents from regulators, transcripts of court proceedings and government hearings, minutes of public meetings, regulations, public petitions, statements by public officials, websites of professional organisations and media reports. We also conducted 32 qualitative interviews with key informants including Chinese medicine and acupuncture community leaders and practitioners, and state officials, who had been involved in the Chinese medicine/acupuncture regulatory process.

In this chapter, we engage with boundary object theory to reinterpret previously reported findings from this case study (Ijaz et al. 2015, 2016; Ijaz 2017). More specifically, we apply the boundary object lens to discuss the prominence of safety discourse in the case under study, permitting a metalevel interpretation of our previously-reported study findings. This chapter references previous study findings as well as primary documents in some cases but does not cite any interview-based findings directly as they have been reported elsewhere. We now turn to our analysis.

Shifting Safety Discourse Across Social Worlds: Establishing the Need for Acupuncture's Regulation

Ontario's Chinese medicine practitioners had lobbied for statutory self-regulatory status over three decades before the profession—and with it, the practice of acupuncture—were regulated in 2013. Until that time, the insertion of acupuncture needles for therapeutic purposes was not subject to any statutory limitations. In 1984, the Ontario government—one key social world in our study—undertook to redesign its health professional regulatory framework in an effort to 'level the playing field' across a range of healthcare occupations, by governing all regulated groups under a single piece of umbrella legislation. Primary among the province's nine identified criteria for self-regulation in 1984 was demonstration of a substantial potential 'risk of harm … to individual patients' (O'Reilly 1999). In other words, the Ontario government constituted *safety* as a key gatekeeping factor in determining which healthcare practices or occupations required regulatory boundaries around them.

At the time, Chinese medicine practitioners—another social world at play in our analysis—were among over 100 healthcare occupational groups requesting to be newly regulated. However, the provincial government determined that acupuncture—one of Chinese medicine's central practices—was 'not inherently hazardous' (HPRAC 1996: 1), that is, not sufficiently risky to warrant regulatory controls. The practice of acupuncture thus remained in the public domain, and Ontario's Chinese medicine practitioners remained unregulated. However, the Ontario government's stance as to acupuncture's associated risk profile would change twice more over the decades leading up to the province's 2013 acupuncture and Chinese medicine regulations. During this period, the arena of intersecting social worlds engaged with the issue of acupuncture's statutory regulation would become progressively larger and more differentiated into complex and intersecting sub-groupings.

In 1995, the Ontario government received three formal requests for new regulations involving the practice of acupuncture from three separate groups (each of which we characterise as a distinct social world): one from a Chinese medicine practitioner association, another from the province's naturopathic profession, and the third from a provincial coalition of acupuncture-practising biomedical health professionals. Whereas the Chinese medicine group requested that a *profession of Chinese medicine* be regulated (with acupuncture as a central therapeutic intervention), the other two groups were exclusively concerned with seeing the *practice of acupuncture* regulated as a practice within their own professions' broader scopes.

Ontario's health minister tasked an arm's-length provincial body, the Health Professions Advisory Council, with studying these three requests. The Council decided to focus a single study on what was shared across these requests: the question of acupuncture regulation (HPRAC 1996).

Noting that 'risk of harm' constituted 'the threshold for regulating a new activity' under Ontario's health professional regulatory structure (HPRAC 1996: 4), the Council undertook a 'public review … to generate a fuller understanding of acupuncture including its risk of harm' (p. 8). Among the stakeholders who contributed written documents and oral presentations during this review were representatives of the social worlds identified earlier. How to characterise acupuncture's safety profile was central among the core questions the Council posed of stakeholders. Stakeholders represented a range of individuals, as well as representatives of multiple social worlds including medical doctors, Chinese medicine practitioners and naturopaths, as well as chiropractors, nurses and physiotherapists. What was shared across these worlds was a common interest in seeing acupuncture regulated in the province, discursively expressed as a characterisation of acupuncture as sufficiently unsafe to warrant statutory controls.

In this light, the Council determined that acupuncture did indeed carry inherent risks when performed by 'untrained or incompetent practitioners' (HPRAC 1996) and recommended that acupuncture be regulated in the province. The Council's 1996 report emphasised that there had been 'considerable agreement among respondents that acupuncture is philosophically rooted in [traditional Chinese medicine]' (p. 10). This was, ultimately, a position the Council also took, advising that some degree of Chinese-medicine-based training should be a regulatory requirement for its *safe* practice. The 'needling practices' of health professionals seeking to use acupuncture needles from an exclusively biomedical perspective, the report concluded, should be separately evaluated and governed. These recommendations, which set out—using safety as a central discursive object—to construct regulatory boundaries around acupuncture that validated indigenous Chinese medical knowledge as legitimate science (see Ijaz et al. 2016), were, however, shelved rather than implemented.

In 2001, a renewed political will to regulate acupuncture and Chinese medicine emerged in the province; the same provincial Council (which had undergone a significant turnover of members) undertook a second study of the issue. As in 1996, the Council concluded that acupuncture and Chinese medicine should be regulated in order to protect the public from potential harms. Similar stakeholders were involved in this second investigation and again used safety-based discourse to substantiate a commonly held view among the occupational groups involved that acupuncture should be regulated in the province. The specifics of the risk discourses deployed differed, however, across occupational groups, reflecting the ways in which safety as boundary object carried contrasting discursive subtexts across social worlds.

Some, such as Ontario's physiotherapists and podiatrists, bolstered their safety-based argumentation in support of acupuncture's regulation by turf-related claims over the practice, as well as efficacy-based discourse geared to invalidating the epistemic claims of Chinese-medicine-based practitioners. For example:

Acupuncture [should be] a controlled act because there is a risk of harm. Acupuncture is within the scope of practice of physiotherapy to treat pain and neuromuscular disorders. The [Ontario Physiotherapy Association] questions whether the regulation of [traditional Chinese medicine] and acupuncture under the [Regulated Health Professions Act] would amount to endorsement of its efficacy. (HPRAC 2001 Appendix H: 7)

Chinese medicine practitioners, by contrast, used safety discourse to argue that their government should limit the practice of acupuncture to those with some Chinese-medicine-based training. 'The improper practice of acupuncture may cause side effects,' they argued, alluding to argumentation that had been foregrounded in the Council's 1996 report, which strongly distinguished the practice of biomedical needling from traditional acupuncture:

Ultimately, the Council sided with biomedical stakeholders, noting that it ... did not receive convincing evidence that adhering to any philosophical or theoretical basis for the procedure affected the risk of harm (and hence the need for regulation) for acupuncture. (HPRAC 2001: 20)

Chinese medicine knowledge, the Council's 2001 report discursively concluded (in contrast to its 1996 recommendations), was irrelevant to the *safe* performance of acupuncture, a practice the Council now redefined in biomedical terms as strictly involving the physical insertion of needles 'below the dermis' (HPRAC 2001).

As we have elsewhere discussed at length (see Ijaz et al. 2016), these later recommendations were conceptually predicated on a discourse of safety that privileged biomedical science in policy, implicitly excluding Chinese medicine's indigenous knowledge perspectives from within the boundaries of state-recognised knowledge. Notably, Ontario's eventual acupuncture regulations would closely reflect the exclusively biomedical epistemic position underpinning the 2001 report's recommendations. In separating acupuncture from its traditional Chinese roots, these regulations' conceptual underpinnings exemplify the cultural misappropriation of traditional knowledge. Such misappropriation, we find, was made possible through the state's adoption of risk-based discourses by stakeholders from biomedically trained occupational social worlds.

That said, the province's concurrent regulation of Chinese medicine practitioners as one acupuncture-practising group could also be argued to raise this group of traditional medicine practitioners' sociocultural status, somewhat complicating biomedicine's hegemonic position within the broader healthcare system. Regardless of such multidimensional power dynamics, our analysis of safety as a discursive boundary object in the state's establishment of whether, and how, to regulate acupuncture makes three points clear. First, safety is not a neutral concept but rather a principle upon which a range of epistemic perspectives and political motives may be superimposed from across diverse social worlds. Second, and related, the safety principle may be deployed as state discourse to give greater or lesser weight to particular epistemic or political stances. Finally (see Ijaz et al. 2016), the subjugation of traditional/indigenous knowledges to biomedical evidentiary perspectives is a historically situated phenomenon, rooted in European colonisation (Harding 1998; Shiva 1997; Ijaz et al. 2016). As such, state risk discourses around TCAM professional regulation may serve—as seen in Ontario's case—to contest and/or advance traditional medicine's neocolonial misappropriation, whether intentionally or not.

However, as we now discuss, it is not only in establishing TCAM practices' eligibility for inclusion within professional regulatory structures that the safety principle may play the role of boundary object but also with respect to practice standards and professional entry requirements implemented.

Differential Application of the Safety Principle: Acupuncture Training Standards Across the Professions

In its 2001 study report recommending the future regulation of acupuncture, Ontario's Health Professions Advisory Council had proposed that five professions—a new Chinese medicine profession, as well as dentistry, medicine, naturopathy and nursing—be authorised to perform the practice within their scope moving forward. It furthermore recommended that these professions 'be required … to establish through regulation the appropriate educational standard needed to provide *safe and effective* [our emphasis] acupuncture treatment' (HPRAC 2001). Any other professions seeking similar 'authority to perform acupuncture,' the report advised (p. 23), should be required to formally apply for 'an expansion of scope of practice,' and similarly produce appropriate training standards.

It would initially appear that the Council constructed safety *and* efficacy as core boundary objects around which individual professions might develop standards for acupuncture. However, given the evidentiary conditions of the time period, the Council also noted that 'the strongest evidence available to show that acupuncture is efficacious for the treatment of certain conditions is empirical evidence' (HPRAC 2001: 20). As such, the Council implied that safety would be the primary locus around which a limited number of Ontario professions might craft future acupuncture training standards. However, as we now discuss, when the province's acupuncture regulations eventually came into effect, the concept of safety would serve less as a tangible guide to standards production and more as a discursive principle differentially applied across the province's acupuncture-practising occupational social worlds.

In 2006, the Ontario government announced that it would (a) add acupuncture to its list of healthcare activities restricted to regulated professionals and (b) regulate a new Chinese medicine profession, under whose scope acupuncture would specifically fall. As recommended in the 2001 report, the province's dentists, medical doctors, naturopaths and nurses would also be permitted to perform the practice. Diverging from its 2001 recommendations, the province also created a regulatory exemption through which the province's chiropractors, physiotherapists, occupational therapists, massage therapists and chiropodists would be automatically authorised to include acupuncture within their existing scope. Within Ontario's system of self-regulation for health professionals, individual professions are tasked with developing their own practice standards within their statutory scopes. Across the ten professions authorised to perform acupuncture, four disparate types of acupuncture training standards were ultimately implemented. Viewed as a whole, these standards tell a story about risk, professional regulation and inter-occupational stratification across social worlds. This story echoes in regulatory context Derkatch's observation (which we discuss further on), made in the context of research, that 'biomedical studies so routinely fail to meet the same standards to which CAM studies are held' (2008: 379). More specifically, we draw attention to these standards' relationship with (a) their associated professions' respective positioning within the broader arena or health systems ecology (see Abbott 2005), (b) the safety principle, previously construed by the Ontario government as a key regulatory boundary object aimed at governing professional authority over acupuncture and (c) the question of medical epistemology.

As the only profession within whose scope acupuncture constitutes a primary component, the competency-based standards for acupuncture implemented by Ontario's Chinese medicine profession would be the most rigorous in the province, equivalent to approximately 2000 hours of training. These standards—which emphasise traditional Chinese medical theory and practice but include training in the biomedical sciences—align substantially with the World Health Organization's training guidelines for traditional acupuncture practitioners (WHO 1999) and with parallel standards governing traditional acupuncture practitioners across other jurisdictions (see Birch 2007).

The acupuncture training requirements implemented across three other Ontario complementary medicine professions (naturopathy, massage therapy and chiropractic) mandate that practitioners wishing to perform acupuncture document, at a minimum, a training standard that adheres roughly to the 200-hour World Health Organization guidelines for health professionals using acupuncture as an adjunct modality within their broader scope (WHO 1999). Echoing the recommendations of the Ontario government's 1996 report on acupuncture, two of these three professions—chiropractic and naturopathy—furthermore require that their members' acupuncture training includes Chinese medicine theoretical approaches.

Like the aforementioned complementary medicine professions, two of the province's three allied (biomedical) health professions, physiotherapy and occupational therapy, keep a register of their acupuncture-practising members.[1] However, while being listed on such a roster requires that these allied health professionals document 'some' theoretical and practical learning in the field of acupuncture, the specifics of such training (i.e., the number of hours, competencies, epistemic basis of training, skill of instructor) are left entirely at the individual practitioner's discretion. Further in this vein, the province's three longest-standing biomedical health professions (medicine, nursing and dentistry) have articulated no acupuncture standards whatsoever for their members and do not keep a roster of practitioners who elect to use acupuncture with patients. It is clear that the approach taken by both allied and biomedical health professionals diverges considerably from the province's safety-related recommendations in both 1996 and 2001.

As self-regulating entities, none of the province's acupuncture-authorised professions would have been externally mandated to enforce particular acupuncture standards for its members. That said, the way each of these professions *responded* to being authorised to include acupuncture within its scope is suggestive of a self-imposed disparity in standard-setting practice that reflects each profession's position in an inter-professional hierarchy. It is difficult to rationally justify why those practitioners registered as members of an allied health profession (e.g., physiotherapists) would require less documented training in order to *safely* perform acupuncture than regulated complementary medicine practitioners (e.g., chiropractors). Nor is it reasonable to suppose that nurses or medical doctors might be more adept at self-assessing their own competency in the field of acupuncture than, for example, occupational therapists or naturopathic physicians.

Chinese medicine practitioners' significantly higher acupuncture training standards may be understood as central to their claim as specialists in the field, defining them as a new profession in the province. However, the inter-professional stratification in acupuncture training standards evident across the other nine professions authorised to perform the practice may represent a kind of differential posturing through which more marginal groups seek to demonstrate their professional rigour (and their explicit adherence to the safety-based standards that are hallmarks of today's dominant 'evidence-based medicine' approach) more proactively than do more dominant groups.

Such an observation in a regulatory context echoes the known boundary-crossing strategies of CAM research scientists, who 'exhibit a kind of hyper-performance' (Derkatch 2008) of established biomedical research methods to establish their credibility. As Polich et al. (2010) similarly note in their empirical study of CAM research (pp. 114–115):

> Methodological rigour carried a special potency for [TCAM researchers], one extending beyond what is typical for more conventional scientific research … [They] strategically employed a scientific vocabulary in an effort to give unconventional research a more conventional guise … [T] CAM researchers also responded to professional scepticism by definitively asserting their scientific credentials.

Recalling the discursive link between safety and epistemology addressed earlier on, we furthermore note that among those relatively marginal TCAM professions that elected to implement clear acupuncture training standards, the majority included at least some Chinese medicine theory among their required competencies. By not implementing clear acupuncture standards for their members, by contrast, the province's more established allied and biomedical health professions conveyed an implicit message that their existing (biomedical) knowledge base represented a sufficient epistemic and practical basis for the safe performance of acupuncture. This act of omission, we suggest, echoing our earlier findings about the province's policy recommendations for acupuncture prior to its regulation, represents another form of traditional knowledge misappropriation that may again be situated within the historical context of European colonial dominance. Regardless, as a regulatory boundary object, it is clear that the safety concept has been differentially interpreted and applied across the social worlds of Ontario's acupuncture-practising professions, as expressed in their associated training and practice standards. It is noteworthy that those professions for which evidence-based medicine is widely characterised as axiomatic are those that would, in their response to being authorised to include acupuncture within their scope, be least likely to exemplify evidence-based medicine's cardinal safety principle in their acupuncture training standards. As noted earlier, Ontario's professional self-regulatory model was redesigned in 1984 in an attempt to level the playing field across regulated occupational groups by granting them each equal access to professional status under the same piece of legislation. However, our findings suggest that these groups continue to *self-govern* both in response to, and in preservation of, long-standing (historical and neocolonial) power dynamics between them. The malleable safety principle, as manifest in training standards—and other professional entry requirements, as we now discuss—clearly represents a boundary object that helps to illuminate these power relationships.

Safety, Language and Chinese Medicine Professional Entry: Regulatory Mimicry

Derkatch (2008) and Polich et al. (2010) have observed that TCAM researchers' vigilant application of biomedical research methods, in pursuit of greater credibility, commonly extends to situations where such methods (as the randomised control trial) are known to poorly accommodate the therapies being studied. A similar pattern seems apparent within the context of professionalising TCAM occupations worldwide, wherein these groups increasingly reshape themselves to include more biomedical subjects in their educational curricula (e.g., Flesh 2013), despite—in many cases—being at odds with the occupations' own epistemic foundations. We have also found such a phenomenon to be evident—if not exemplified—in our previous study of English-language proficiency requirements implemented by traditional acupuncture and Chinese medicine regulators and certification bodies in two Canadian provinces (Ontario and British Columbia), two-thirds of American states and across Australia (Ijaz 2017). In these jurisdictions, we observe a tendency from within the occupational leadership to institute professional entry requirements that echo those implemented in biomedical professions, despite contextual factors that render such requirements very difficult to meet for some of the occupation's most experienced members. Notably, safety-related discourse again appears as a key boundary object invoked by a range of actors to justify these requirements.

Across the aforementioned jurisdictions, a significant proportion of traditional acupuncture and Chinese medicine practitioners are immigrants from East Asian countries, some of who conduct their clinical practices primarily in an East Asian language. A small percentage of such practitioners—who are typically over the age of 50—are also known to have low English-language proficiency. As part of our study (Ijaz 2017), we interviewed 28 key informants involved in, or affected by, the various linguistic policy approaches discussed. Informants included regulators and other state actors, as well as traditional acupuncture practitioners (about half of whom were East Asian immigrants). In analysing the range of stakeholder views relating to these policies, we found safety-related discourses to have played a prominent role on both sides of a significantly polarised debate.

Attesting to the segmentation that may occur within particular social worlds, there were both 'state actors and practitioners of diverse demographic [ethnic] makeup on either side' of the debate over regulatory English-language proficiency requirements (Ijaz 2017: 114). Those who supported English-only policies emphasised safety as their primary concern, arguing that 'non-English proficient practitioners create unnecessary patient risks … particularly in emergency situations' and in the 'context of interprofessional communication' (p. 114). Those opposing such policies, by contrast, argued that 'English-only policies create more significant risks' by driving underground 'some of the most experienced' immigrant practitioners, thus

> removing statutory accountability and recourse mechanisms for patients who might otherwise be harmed ... and compromis[ing] delivery of safe [legal] care for East Asian immigrant patients lacking English fluency. (Ijaz 2017: 114)

In Ontario's context in particular, we demonstrated that language proficiency requirements for traditional acupuncture practitioners that construct low English proficiency as a deviant trait in need of remediation may lead to the premature retirement and/or underground practice of significant numbers of senior immigrant practitioners with decades of clinical experience (Ijaz 2017). Such outcomes are not only of concern in terms of their impacts on these individual practitioners but threaten the integrity of the profession as a whole. Indeed, as has been widely recognised, the oral transmission of traditional medical knowledge from senior to junior practitioners through a mentorship relationship is an important historical, and ongoing, form of indigenous knowledge preservation (WHO, WIPO and WTO 2013) including in East Asian medicine (Hsu 1999). When patient safety is constructed by policymakers as the primary boundary object surrounding linguistic regulatory entry requirements for traditional East Asian medicine practitioners in English-dominant jurisdictions—as was evident in our study of the Ontario case—core historical and contextual features of the occupational groups being regulated are perilously overlooked.

What is notable in several North American jurisdictions is that English-proficiency requirements have been implemented *from within* Chinese medicine and traditional acupuncture regulatory or certification bodies. In Ontario as in the United States, many of the decision-makers involved in these policy projects have been practitioners from within the Chinese medicine social world who seemed aware that (a) the occupational group had distinct demographic features that might render English proficiency a challenging professional registration requirement to meet and (b) there was widespread opposition to language proficiency requirements from within the practitioner community itself.

In the same way as TCAM researchers commonly mimic or adopt poorly fitting biomedical methods to fortify their studies' mainstream credibility, our findings suggest that regulators and certification bodies governing marginal health occupations—including those comprised of cultural insiders—may be strategically using safety-based discourse as a mechanism through which to justify a mimicry of biomedical professions' registration requirements, in order to secure their own groups' tenuous regulatory status. Although safety is certainly not an irrelevant regulatory consideration with respect to linguistic entry requirements for traditional East Asian medicine practitioners, there are other important issues that appear to receive insufficient attention when safety-as-boundary-object dominates the regulatory debate.

Beyond a Discourse of Safety: Regulating TCAM Professionals in the Public Interest

Our discussion to this point shows the concept of patient safety to be a central discursive boundary object in the regulation of acupuncture and Chinese medicine in Ontario. We have pointed to three distinct regulatory issues in which actors from across a range of social worlds variously invoked the safety concept to either preface or substantiate a particular policy position. As discussed, safety was the primary discursive consideration at play in the province's initial decision to leave acupuncture and the profession of Chinese medicine unregulated and subsequently to regulate both practice and profession. The rationale offered for the specific regulatory model to be applied was also framed in safety-related terms. Similarly, the Ontario government pointed to safety as a measure of primary importance in creating future acupuncture-related standards across the Ontario professions performing the practice. Finally, Ontario's new Chinese medicine regulator positioned safety among the primary rationales behind the linguistic professional entry requirements it implemented as the new regulations came into effect.

As a regulatory boundary object, the concept of safety took several guises across distinct social worlds, playing multiple roles in the drama surrounding the regulation of acupuncture and Chinese medicine in the province. For instance, state actors' discursive emphasis on patient safety masked issues not directly safety-related. This was evident between 1984 and 1996, when the Ontario government changed its official stance as to whether acupuncture was sufficiently risky to regulate, although it is clear that the practice itself (and its associated risks) would not have substantively changed over this period. The notion of safety was also deployed to construct regulatory boundaries surrounding acupuncture that would ultimately preserve biomedicine's epistemic and positional authority in the province's regulatory structures. In 2001, for example, the province would use the notion of safety to justify acupuncture's regulatory separation from its Chinese medical and cultural roots, re-conceptualising the practice in exclusively biomedical terms.

The Ontario government would, that same year, use safety-based grounds to call for stringent future training requirements across the province's acupuncture-practising professions. However, it would become clear as the regulations came into effect in 2013 that those professions occupying more marginal positions within the province's overall interoccupational hierarchy would be more likely to implement training standards for their members that directly addressed the principle of patient safety in practice. The propensity of marginal occupational groups to adopt professional entry standards typical across biomedical professions—regardless of whether such requirements in fact met the specific needs of their members—was furthermore evident in the case of Ontario's Chinese medicine professional linguistic entry requirements.

Scholars of the professions have long analysed the jurisdictional 'turf' struggles over scope and standards that typify the transition from occupation to profession, frequently via statutory regulation (Parkin 1974, 1979; Murphy 1988; Collins 1979, 1990; Abbott 1988). There is, similarly, a body of sociological literature that addresses risk as a central thematic and discursive focus in policymaking across industrialised countries, including in the context of healthcare (Allen et al. 2016) and health professional regulation (Phipps et al. 2011). What our work here highlights are some of the specific ways in which safety discourse may be deployed within a policy context characterised by differential power relations. In particular, in relation to TCAM professional regulation, we have drawn attention to some ways in which historical colonial power relations may be reproduced through the mechanism of safety as discourse.

In the same way that Derkatch has characterised 'efficacy' as a rhetorical boundary object surrounding complementary and alternative medicine research, we argue that 'safety'-related discourse may be playing a gatekeeping role in the statutory regulation (and ongoing sociopolitical subjugation) of TCAM practitioners and practices. In the context of research, Derkatch (2008: 382) has argued that the efficacy concept can be poorly suited to researching complementary and alternative medicine interventions:

> CAM practices do not fit well within an efficacy model; they are much more amenable to effectiveness studies because such studies can better accommodate the sorts of patients, symptoms, treatments, and outcomes typical of CAM … But many critics of CAM hold efficacy, not effectiveness, up as the criterion for evaluating CAM, even though much significant biomedical research is effectiveness-based.

We do not contest that safety should be given careful consideration in the professional regulation of TCAM practitioners or practices. However, the safety concept is malleable, capable of supporting a range of epistemic stances and, in our study, shown to be unevenly applied in ways that mask a range of regulatory issues and power dynamics across the range of health professions. As such, we propose that those involved in crafting professional regulations for TCAM practitioners and practices make efforts to identify and directly address these other issues and dynamics, so that a slippery rhetoric of safety does not inappropriately dominate the policy process.

We have elsewhere proposed a principle-based public interest framework intended to inform TCAM professional regulations, which may assist those undertaking such a pursuit (Ijaz 2017). Situated within post-colonial theoretical parameters, our framework addresses the set of distinct regulatory challenges that accompany TCAM professional regulation, warranting an *equity*-driven policy approach: one that attends fairly to contextual factors surrounding TCAM professional regulation, rather than simply reproducing regulatory models implemented for biomedical professions. *Traditional knowledge protection* is one such key factor of unique importance within a TCAM professional regulatory context. Healthcare *quality* and *accessibility* are other core principles, positioned on equal footing with *safety* as essential public interest parameters. Regulators' application of our framework, we hope, may be one mechanism by which the disproportionate *discursive* emphasis on safety seen in our Ontario study may be prevented in other TCAM professional regulatory contexts.

That said, this chapter's distinct contribution lies in its demonstration of multiple means by which a discourse of safety may dominate a TCAM professional regulatory project in ways that ultimately reinforce biomedicine's epistemic and institutional authority. As our analysis demonstrates, this type of reinforcement of dominant power dynamics may occur even as these same power relations are contested by the inclusion or entry of traditional medicine practices and professions into healthcare systems from which they would have previously been excluded. This type of hybrid phenomenon, characterised by multidirectional power relations amidst the blending of healthcare systems and approaches that were once considered distinct, is an area ripe for additional research.

Note

1. The province's third acupuncture-authorised 'allied health profession,' chiropody, has advised our research team that it continues to work on establishing an approach to acupuncture training standards for its members. No standards, or rostering requirement, are currently in place.

References

Abbott, A. (1988). *The system of professions: An essay on the division of labor.* Chicago: University of Chicago Press.
Abbott, A. (2005). Linked ecologies: States and universities as environments for professions. *Sociological Theory, 23*(3), 245–274.

Allen, D., Braithwaite, J., Sandall, J., & Waring, J. (Eds.). (2016). *The sociology of healthcare safety and quality*. London: Wiley Blackwell.

Birch, S. (2007). Reflections on the German acupuncture studies. *Journal of Chinese Medicine, 83*, 12–17.

Clarke, A., & Star, S. (2008). The social worlds framework: A theory/methods package. In E. J. Hackett, O. Amsterdamska, M. Lynch, & J. Wajcman (Eds.), *The handbook of science and technology studies* (3rd ed., pp. 113–137). Cambridge, MA: MIT Press.

Collins, R. (1979). *The credential society*. New York: Academic Press.

Collins, R. (1990). Changing conceptions in the sociology of the professions. In M. Burrage & R. Torstendahl (Eds.), *The formation of professions: Knowledge, state and strategy* (pp. 11–23). London: Sage Publications.

Derkatch, C. (2008). Method as argument: Boundary work in evidence-based medicine. *Social Epistemology, 22*(4), 371–388.

Flesh, H. (2013). A foot in both worlds: Education and transformation of Chinese medicine in the United states. *Medical Anthropology, 32*(1), 8–24.

Harding, S. (1998). *Is science multicultural? Postcolonialisms, feminisms and epistemologies*. Bloomington, IN: Indiana University Press.

HPRAC. (1996). *Advice to the minister of health: Acupuncture referral*. Ontario: Government of Ontario.

HPRAC. (2001). *Traditional Chinese medicine and acupuncture: Advice to the minister of health and long-term care*. Ontario: Government of Ontario.

Hsu, E. (1999). *The transmission of Chinese medicine*. Cambridge: Cambridge University Press.

Ijaz, N. (2017). *Regulating traditional medicine professionals in the public interest: A case study of Chinese medicine and acupuncture regulation in Ontario, Canada*. PhD Thesis, University of Toronto, TSpace, 2017.

Ijaz, N., Boon, H., Muzzin, L., & Welsh, S. (2016). State risk discourse and the regulatory preservation of traditional medicine knowledge: The case of acupuncture in Ontario, Canada. *Social Science and Medicine, 170*, 97–105.

Ijaz, N., Boon, H., Welsh, S., & Meads, A. (2015). Supportive but 'worried': Perceptions of naturopaths, homeopaths and Chinese medicine practitioners through a regulatory transition in Ontario, Canada. *BMC Complementary and Alternative Medicine, 15*, 312–325.

Keshet, Y., Ben-Arye, E., & Schiff, E. (2013). The use of boundary objects to enhance interprofessional collaboration: Integrating complementary medicine in a hospital setting. *Sociology of Health and Illness, 35*(5), 666–681.

Murphy, R. (1988). *Social closure: The theory of monopolization and exclusion.* Oxford: Clarendon Press.

O'Reilly, P. (1999). *Health care practitioners: An Ontario case study in policy making.* Toronto: University of Toronto Press.

Owens, K. (2015). Boundary objects in complementary and alternative medicine: Acupuncture vs. Christian science. *Social Science and Medicine, 128,* 18–24.

Parkin, F. (1974). Strategies of social closure in class formation. In F. Parkin (Ed.), *The social analysis of class structure* (pp. 1–18). London: Tavistock.

Parkin, F. (1979). *Marxism and class theory: A bourgeois critique.* New York: Columbia University Press.

Phipps, D. L., Noyce, P. R., Walshe, K., Parker, D., & Ashcroft, D. M. (2011). Risk-based regulation of healthcare professionals: What are the implications for pharmacists? *Health, Risk and Society, 13*(3), 277–292.

Polich, G., Dole, C., & Kaptchuk, T. (2010). The need to act a little more 'scientific': Biomedical researchers investigating complementary and alternative medicine. *Sociology of Health and Illness, 32*(1), 106–122.

Shiva, V. (1997). *Biopiracy: The plunder of nature and knowledge.* Toronto: Between the lines.

Star, S., & Griesemer, J. (1989). Institutional ecology, 'translations' and boundary objects: Amateurs and professionals in Berkeley's museum of vertebrate zoology, 1907–1939. *Social Studies of Science, 19*(3), 387–420.

World Health Organization. (1999). *Guidelines on basic training and safety in acupuncture.* Geneva: World Health Organization.

World Health Organization, World Intellectual Property Organization and World Trade Organization. (2013). *Promoting access to medical technologies and innovation: Intersections between public health, intellectual property and trade.* Geneva: World Health Organization.

Part III

Making CAM Knowledge: Evidence and Expertise

9

Conversions and Erasures: Colonial Ontologies in Canadian and International Traditional, Complementary, and Alternative Medicine Integration Policies

Cathy Fournier and Robin Oakley

Introduction

Canada and other high-income countries are increasingly integrating traditional, complementary, and alternative medicine (TCAM)[1] into their public healthcare structures in response to increased public use. We conducted a qualitative document analysis exploring the nature of TCAM's integration into public healthcare in Canada and globally by analysing TCAM-related documents from the World Bank, the World Health Organization (WHO), and Health Canada (Canada's national health department), the latter of which cannot properly be understood without also exploring the handling of TCAM by the first two global institutions.

C. Fournier (✉)
Wilson Centre, University of Toronto, Toronto, ON, Canada

R. Oakley
Dalhousie University, Halifax, NS, Canada

© The Author(s) 2018
C. Brosnan et al. (eds.), *Complementary and Alternative Medicine*, Health, Technology and Society, https://doi.org/10.1007/978-3-319-73939-7_9

Canada, a former British colony, provides a rich context to explore the integration of TCAM with biomedicine because of the expanded incorporation of TCAM into public healthcare, increasing privatisation of healthcare, and a growing interest and use of TCAM by the public as out-of-pocket expenditures (Silnicki 2013; Armstrong and Armstrong 2009; Bodecker and Kronenberg 2002). Public healthcare in Canada is predominantly biomedical in nature, has a dominant curative healthcare sector influenced by large private biomedical monopolies that are paid with public funds (Leys 2009), and is also embedded in a liberal state apparatus that is friendly to monopoly capital (Navarro and Shi 2001; Oakley and Grøsneth 2007; Oakley et al. 2013). Consequently, healthcare in Canada has a poorly developed preventative sector, and chronic disease after the age of 40 is the norm (Betancourt et al. 2014; Morgan et al. 2007). Combined with this are the assimilationist principles of the Indian Act in Canada (1976), which rendered it illegal for Indigenous Peoples[2] to use their traditional approaches to medicine and healing at various points in the nation's history (Robbins and Dewar 2011). As a result, many indigenous healing practices were driven underground (Oakley forthcoming; Manitowabe and Shawande 2013; Robbins and Dewar 2011) or were simply too time-consuming or difficult to engage in due to lack of time or non-availability of ingredients, such as plant-based medicines (Kelton 2007; Manitowabe and Shawande 2013). Add to this a large immigrant population that regularly use TCAM in their homes (Barimah and van Teijlingen 2008; Quan et al. 2008), and Canada proves a potboiler of medical pluralism and a rich context to explore TCAM.

TCAM in Canada

The integration of TCAM in biomedical healthcare settings, sometimes referred to as integrative medicine, is increasingly part of the healthcare landscape in Canada and other high-income countries (Adler 2008; Gale 2014; Hollenberg and Muzzin 2010). TCAM is typically defined as a heterogeneous group of healthcare practices that fall outside the rubric of biomedicine (Tovey et al. 2004). Examples of TCAM practices in Canada include massage, indigenous healing practices/medicines, Yoga, Ayurveda, traditional Chinese medicine, and herbal medicine (WHO 2013a; Statistics Canada 2017).

In Canada, approximately 70 per cent of the population use some form of TCAM, and Canadians spent an estimated 8.8 billion CAD in 2015–2016 on TCAM therapies (Esmail 2017; Statistics Canada 2017). As TCAM is not currently covered under public healthcare in Canada, these costs were paid for out of pocket (Esmail 2017).

In 2002, Health Canada funded a steering committee to facilitate a workshop on the integration of TCAM in undergraduate medical education. This workshop was initiated to help to develop a 'national vision' for TCAM in undergraduate medical education, emphasising the 'need' to include it for two main reasons (Health Canada 2003c). Firstly, their report stated that patient safety is threatened because of increased concurrent use of TCAM and biomedicine, and with it the increased potential for adverse reactions between pharmaceuticals and herbal medicines, particularly as many patients do not disclose concurrent TCAM use to their physicians for fear of disapproval (Ventola 2010). The response to this has been a push towards developing physicians' understanding of TCAM therapies in order to oversee patient TCAM use, to ensure public safety (Health Canada 2003c). The second reason Health Canada promoted the integration of TCAM into undergraduate medical education was so physicians could become a reliable source of information about TCAM for their patients (Health Canada 2003c), thus potentially expanding their role as 'overseers' and gatekeepers of patients' TCAM use.

The 'integration' of TCAM practices into biomedical settings has been articulated as part of an ingrained pattern of indigenous knowledge expropriation, assimilation, and in some cases, even conversion or erasure (see Barry 2006; Baer and Coulter 2008; Hollenberg and Muzzin 2010; Kincheloe 2006; Sefa-Dei et al. 2000; Shiva 2000; Smith 1999; Semali and Kincheloe 1999; Harding 1998; Yalamala 2013). In their exploration of epistemological challenges related to the integration of TCAM in four major urban hospitals in Canada, Hollenberg and Muzzin (2010) argue, for example, that there are underlying problems with integrating biomedicine and TCAM that have been ignored and undertheorised. Using an anti-colonial framework, their findings suggest that integrative medicine contributes to a 'monolithic worldview', resulting from paradigm 'appropriation and assimilation' (2010: 34), which can be traced back to the devaluation of indigenous knowledges that occurred during the colonial period in Canada. They contend that in the Western, biomedical context, TCAM's indigenous epistemologies as they relate to various forms of bodywork, indigenous healing, and plant-based medicine, for example, are being reinterpreted to fit into a Eurocentric biomedical paradigm of health and illness or, as McKenna theorises, moulded to fit into a neoliberal and biomedical homogeneity (2012), a sentiment referred to by Navarro and Shi as the logic of capital/market (2001). Likewise, King (2002) suggests that the 'language of integration' contributes to rhetoric of inclusivity and medical pluralism that is largely unrealised, making the incorporation of TCAM into biomedical settings seem more egalitarian than it actually is (see also Baer 2004).

Integration is taking place within the context of an emerging disease paradigm. The emerging disease worldview is a perspective on international health that is concerned with the development of the global medical-industrial technological complex (e.g., increasing the global capitalist market by increasing the market for pharmaceuticals) (King 2002). It is a form of selective healthcare (Yalamala 2013) preoccupied with market interests and the commodification and standardisation of traditional health systems (Leys 2009; Towghi 2004; King 2002; Navarro 1976, 2007). Although King and colleagues are writing about the US, the parallels to Canada, with the increasing focus on market interests, and the commodification of healthcare, are striking (e.g., Armstrong and Armstrong 2009; Jacklin and Warry 2004).

Biomedicine and Capitalism

The integration of TCAM in Canada cannot be understood without exploring the dominant paradigm in public health in Canada today: biomedicine. By the twentieth century, biomedicine surfaced as a 'profit-making venture' in the West, and 'its self-confident worldview [was] firmly established…' (Baronov 2008: 236). During this time, biomedicine was considered the dominant form of medicine (Moore and McLean 2010; Baronov 2008) and the benchmark by which all other forms of medicine were to be evaluated (see Khan 2006; Baer 2004).

Biomedicine, with its profit-making potential, and focus on microscopic pathogens as the cause of disease, aligned well with capitalism, as it exonerated socio-economic disparities as a health determinant (Baer 2004; Gordon 1988; Martin 2001). Brian McKenna even suggests 'that in the drama of [bio]medicine, the doctor helps perform the hard work of a neoliberal culture by reproducing the conditions for "wage slavery" of the worker/citizen...' (2012: 98). Health itself tends to be measured in terms of productivity; symptoms of poverty and hunger may be reconceptualised as medical conditions and treated with biomedicine, rather than shifting the distribution of wealth and access to resources (Scheper-Hughes 1992).

Biomedicine's association with science, or what is referred to by some scholars as science under capitalism, or even pseudoscience (McKenna 2010; Leys 2009; Nanda 2001; Navarro 1976, 2007), limits 'the ontological world of health and healing to observable and measurable physical phenomena' (Baronov 2008: 241). Highlighting this aspect of biomedicine holds important implications for the content of TCAM as it is integrated into health systems and biomedical education. For example, how might humoral systems of medicine, with their focus on human balance with nature, food intake, and social relations having primary impact on health (Horden and Hsu 2013; Nayak 2012), retain their holistic focus within biomedicine's reductionist framework for understanding dysfunction and disease, without being profoundly reinterpreted?

Sax and Nair (2014) call biomedicine the most successful Western export in the world, even more successful than capitalism. Yet often missing from these types of discussions is that biomedicine itself is a form of 'traditional' medicine in the modern Western context (see Leslie and Young 1992). Further, these discussions obscure the various forms of other 'traditional' medicines that have been incorporated into biomedicine over time (Boomgaard 2003; Adams et al. 2013; Harris 2010; Horden and Hsu 2013; Nabipour et al. 2009; Siraisi 1987; Zargaran et al. 2013) and how they have influenced biomedicine (Fournier 2016). As such, perhaps 'traditional' forms of medicine could be considered biomedicine's most successful import. Currently, TCAM tends to be presumed irrational and superstitious in relation to biomedicine (Adams 2002; Arnold 1988; Moore and McLean 2010; Zhang 2007; Zhan 2001), while biomedicine is often essentialised as purely Western, rational, scientific, and universalistic. Biomedicine is viewed as entrenched within a Eurocentric science that is valued as the ultimate and only science (Harding 1998, 2011; Hollenberg and Muzzin 2010). Vincanne Adams (2002), in her study examining the nature of postcolonial science, argues that scientific knowledge, including medical knowledge, is embedded in market capitalism and serves to produce a globalised 'medical truth'. Biomedicine and TCAM share many qualities that are often overlooked, such as empiricism, and dynamic evolution (Aikenhead and Ogawa 2007), yet tend to be characterised as radically different.

Methodology

This study engaged with the ontological content of the integration of TCAM into public health systems by contextualising and 'studying through' (Wedel et al. 2005) TCAM policy-related documents, memos, and reports from the World Bank, the WHO, and Health Canada. 'Studying through' can bring into focus how overarching, dominant global institutions, such as the WHO and World Bank, and national governing institutions, such as Health Canada, influence the everyday world (Wedel et al. 2005), in this case, the nature of TCAM's integration into biomedical education. As Wedel et al. (2005) note:

> [a]nthropology offers a social organizational approach that illuminates the structures and processes that ground, order, and give direction to policies. An ethnographer explores how individuals, organizations, and institutions are interconnected and asks how policy discourses help to sustain those connections even if the actors involved are never in face-to-face (or even direct) contact. 'Studying through'—the process of following the source of a policy—its discourses, prescriptions, and programs—through to those affected by the policies does just that. (p. 39)

Policies have the capability to impose conditions on micro and macro-processes, and can thus be understood as a form of governance—a form of power that 'acts on and through the agency and subjectivity of individuals as ethically free and rational subjects' (Shore and Wright 2003: 6).

As such, investigating the language employed by the World Bank, the WHO, and Health Canada allowed us to suggest their hegemonic role in influencing health policy and initiatives related to TCAM, and biomedical education (Khan 2006; Nichter and Lock 2002), while exploring the *why* and *how* questions. The WHO, World Bank, and Health Canada sites were chosen because these are all governing institutions that exert tremendous influence on health policy, and how health and healthcare systems are run both covertly and overtly (Attaran et al. 2006; Brown and Bell 2008; Ruger 2005, 2007; Bodecker and Kronenberg 2002).

Following Krippendorff (2013), a qualitative, text-based content analysis was employed to analyse sample documents selected from the WHO, World Bank, and Health Canada websites. We relied on a deductive approach to coding (Krippendorff 2013; Berg 2009; Bernard 2006), and used a thematic scheme informed by our theoretical perspective to explore our research questions, and we developed analytical/theoretical codes based on preliminary readings of these web-based documents (Krippendorff 2013; Berg 2009; Bernard 2006). We ensured that the research design remained flexible enough for new ideas and themes to emerge on their own as we analysed the materials (Krippendorff 2013). To ensure rigour, we did an initial count of key words and phrases of the sample documents to help ground our readings and thematic codes (Krippendorff 2013).

We examined 120 web-based documents in total. The criteria for inclusion were documents such as memos, reports, and policy-related documents found on the organisation's website that included the terms 'complementary and alternative medicine', 'complementary and alternative healthcare', 'traditional medicine', 'indigenous medicine', 'traditional and complementary and alternative medicine', and 'integrative medicine'. Our inquiries focused on thematic continuities and differences between the powerful governing institutions of the World Bank, WHO, and Health Canada in terms of their constructions of how TCAM and biomedicine should be integrated. This chapter addresses the question of what is stripped away in the framing or conceptualisation of TCAM in these policy documents, what vocabulary and terms are used, and what worldview is represented.

Thematic codes were created deductively after numerous readings of each document, using manual coding and Excel charts of terms that were repeated multiple times. Some of the codes included regulation, categorisation, surveillance, science/scientific proof, evidence-based medicine, standardisation, surveillance and public safety, gatekeeping, and science versus charlatanism. An overarching theme that emerged from the data (see Berg 2009) was the naturalisation of biomedicine as the valid benchmark to assess all other forms of medicine and a prevalent devaluation of all forms of TCAM. Another set of themes involved a preoccupation with standardisation to exert control over the forms of TCAM that would become part of the public healthcare system and also to control or contort them in ways that corresponded with biomedicine.

Limitations

There are limitations to this study. We explored an evolving phenomenon through an analysis of web-based policy-related documents, memos, and reports. As such, the materials we examined were limited to those publicly accessible on websites. These documents are not static. New documents may be added, and links became inactive or archived during the course of the study. For example, during the course of this study, 2013–2016, TCAM-related documents from both the WHO and Health Canada were archived and are no longer available without special request.

Analysis of the Documents

TCAM and the World Bank: Surveillance, Standardisation, Commodification, and Scientific Proof

The World Bank supports a global institutionalisation of TCAM, and in 1996, it created a 'knowledge bank' and branded itself as the protector cum mediator between ideas and financial resources in relation to an array of traditional/indigenous knowledges on a global level.

The World Bank, as well as the WHO, groups TCAM as indigenous forms of medicine, many of which derive from local, traditional, or indigenous knowledges (Massey and Kirk 2015), particularly in reference to low-income countries.

The World Bank has consequently undertaken the 'challenge to learn from the practices of communities so as to leverage the best in global and local knowledge systems' to improve global health (World Bank 2004c), and in response initiated the Indigenous Knowledge for Development Program (IKDP), a series of papers related to managing and, we argue, potentially exploiting indigenous knowledge for profit by industries such as Big Pharma (see Adams 2002). While challenging Eurocentrism and neocolonial ontologies, Linda Tuhiwai Smith (1999) and others (see Robbins and Dewar 2011; Kincheloe 2006; Shiva 2000) argue that initiatives such as these are a form of neocolonialism and knowledge appropriation disguised as acts of humanitarianism (also see Ruger 2005; King 2002). The World Bank IKDP claims to empower 'poor people', by helping them 'capitalise' on the profit-making potential of indigenous knowledge(s), and traditional medicine (World Bank 2004c). The documents reviewed deploy moralised phrases such as 'empowering' indigenous communities towards their own 'development' in the context of globalisation and 'helping countries capitalise' on indigenous knowledge. The reference to the term 'capitalise' suggests a push to commodify indigenous knowledge (King 2002; Baer et al. 2003). Further, Mehta (2001) calls the World Bank and its IKDP an 'emerging knowledge empire', implying that instead of knowledge circulation flowing equally in both directions, more 'legitimate' Eurocentric forms of knowledge are transferred from those who 'know' to those that 'don't know' (Mehta 2001: 190).

The sample documents from the World Bank, which included policy documents, memos, and reports, thematically construct TCAM practitioners as having poor or untrustworthy biomedical knowledge, leading to dangerous practices (World Bank 2004a, 2013b). They claim that the main reason TCAM is excluded from 'modern' national health systems is the lack of documentation of 'scientific' proof of safety, a claim which denies any political or economic motivation for its marginalisation and exclusion (Adams 2002). It also erases the textual record of medical manuscripts by well-known practitioners in China, India, and the Middle

East, such as the well-known *Yellow Emperors Classic of Internal Medicine*, one of the most important ancient Chinese medicine texts written between 475 BC and 221 BC and during the Han dynasty period, 206 BCE–220 CE (see also Horden and Hsu 2013; Adams et al. 2013; Hsu and Harris 2010; Quah 2003).

Within the World Bank materials we examined, there was a focus on the profit-making potential of indigenous knowledge through the 'discovery' of active ingredients in medicinal plants that have been around and used for thousands of years. Some scholars have argued that integrating traditional medicine into biomedicine can facilitate this profit motive, thus increasing concerns over knowledge appropriation (Martin-Hill 2003; Timmerman 2003). These so-called discoveries are then being used for new pharmaceuticals (World Bank 2004b). As such, these 'discoveries' become the property of the major industries involved, mainly pharmaceutical companies framed as a humanitarian push to find new drugs (Sundar Rajan 2007; Gautam et al. 2003: King 2002).

Although the World Bank has declared that TCAM knowledge is a viable and valuable avenue for 'development', and there are World Bank–supported efforts for the adoption of policies for the protection of indigenous knowledges, the policy related to public health and the 'health for all' campaigns enables the appropriation of indigenous knowledges for the benefit of any member states of the World Trade Organization (World Bank 2004c). To illustrate:

> …to encourage the discovery of new drugs derived from Indigenous Knowledge and to reward its custodians, the [Alma Ata] Declaration pledged a commitment from industrial countries to provide incentives to their enterprises and institutions to promote and encourage technology transfer to least developed countries. This could help build up the research and development (R&D) capacity of national drug laboratories to undertake clinical trials on herbal treatments derived from Indigenous Knowledge. A partnership could develop between the local healers and scientists to share their knowledge of medicinal plants and the subsequent economic gains derived from the end-products. (World Bank 2004a: 3)

The World Bank claims to be promoting the development of partnerships between powerful industry, scientists, and local healers, promising that it would benefit everyone involved but because of the unequal relationship between lower- and higher-income countries, largely due to colonisation, there are concerns that these partnerships may not benefit poorer countries (Adams 2002; Biehl and Petryna 2013; Mgbeoji 2006).

The discourses in the World Bank sample documents employ a language of inclusion and regard for TCAM in some places but then contradict this position in others. For example, they state that TCAM is a valuable resource, yet then say that it must use modern Western medicine's means of diagnosis, such as laboratory testing and MRIs in order to improve safety and efficacy (World Bank 2004b). Yet an MRI or other modern laboratory tests do not diagnose social factors, such as poverty or oppression, as the cause of illness, nor are they equipped to show a blockage of qi, supernatural powers, or the disharmony between humans and nature as a diagnosis or having impact on health. These are fundamental ways of understanding disease in many TCAM practices, such as traditional Chinese medicine, Ayurveda (Patwardhan et al. 2005), and indigenous healing practices in Canada (Maar and Shawande 2010; Manitowabe and Shawande 2013).

The terms 'consumer', 'regulation', and 'standardisation' are also frequently used to discuss how the World Bank is endeavouring to teach TCAM practitioners what to do as per the privatisation processes ongoing in Canada, and North America as a whole, with a preoccupation on profits and markets (see King 2002; Navarro and Shi 2001). On close examination, the language used in many of the discussions illuminates how biomedicine is naturalised as the most advanced form of medicine from which TCAM should be measured. To illustrate:

At all levels, modern medicine is an evolving medicine that is open to knowledge and progress through continuous research.... In contrast to this dynamic Cartesian medicine [biomedicine], one must admit that from its nature, traditional medicine does not aim at progress. It is not open to innovation, renewal and the progressive modifications of its principles, means, and methods. Tradition keeps it static and inward looking, subjected

to the passivity of empiricism set rigidly by the elders and followed faith-
fully by apprentices. (World Bank 2004a: 3)

It has also been suggested that:

In order for traditional medicine to integrate and work with globalisation,
traditional medicine must reassess and open itself to the requirements of
scientific rationality, convert itself in its diagnostic and therapeutic
approach methods as well as in its deontology. It will thus ensure its influence, productivity, and progress as well as enhance its therapeutic efficiency
and competitiveness. (World Bank 2004a: 4)

These statements highlight presumptions made about TCAM on a
fundamental level, that they are stuck in the past, never changing, and
about the naturalisation of biomedicine as the only 'real scientific medicine'. Furthermore, the statements illustrate how regulation and standardisation of TCAM will require a form of biomedicalisation of TCAM
practices.

The WHO and TCAM: Surveillance, Standardisation, and Scientific Proof

The WHO has declared the need to establish its role in a global TCAM
strategy to address the increased use of TCAM. Identifying 'an urgent
need' for national and international policies for the regulation and standardisation of TCAM, as well as the establishment of surveillance systems
to help control adverse events related to TCAM use, the WHO states that
developing national and international policy is a 'sound basis for defining
the role of TCAM' (WHO 2004, 2013a).

The WHO plays a key role in establishing these national and international standards (Prah and Yach 2009). The WHO is also a key player in
managing TCAM-related information and promoting evidence-based
TCAM use (Xue 2008). It has also identified what it sees as a lack of
training for TCAM providers, as well as a lack of training about TCAM
for biomedical healthcare providers (WHO 2002, 2013b). WHO

documents also discuss what they call a lack of communication and collaboration between TCAM and biomedical healthcare practitioners (WHO 2002, 2013b). As such, one of the WHO's goals for 2002–2005, and again for 2014–2025, is for biomedical practitioners to have basic training in TCAM. While the WHO publicly acknowledges the potential value of TCAM in addressing health issues, especially chronic disease, locally and around the globe, the underlying theme of control, standardisation, and categorisation, informed by the biomedical paradigm, and market interests, surfaces in their TCAM policy documents. This is consistent with themes that emerged in the World Bank sample documents. Further, although both the World Bank and the WHO admit to the tension between finding 'scientific' proof of efficacy in TCAM, and the hundreds of years (actually thousands of years in some cases) of so-called mere 'anecdotal evidence', these discussions, while promising, are fleeting. Additionally, the fact that indigenous knowledges have contributed or been the basis of many modern scientific discoveries (Patwardhan et al. 2004) is largely neglected.

Another WHO-purported goal is to get member states to cooperate in the promotion of traditional medicine for healthcare (WHO 2013a, b). The collaboration aims to:

> support and integrate traditional medicine into national health systems in combination with national policy and regulation for products, practices and providers to ensure safety and quality; ensure the use of safe, effective and quality products and practices, based on available evidence; acknowledge traditional medicine as part of primary health care, to increase access to care and preserve knowledge and resources; and ensure patient safety by upgrading the skills and knowledge of traditional medicine providers. (WHO 2013a: 2)

While efforts to upgrade and standardise TCAM education to foster increased collaboration between TCAM practitioners and biomedical practitioners may be beneficial, it alludes to health systems based on equality, and underlying power relations remain unacknowledged, which may impact the very integrity of TCAM practices as they are 'integrated' into national health systems (Tsing 2000).

The WHO also endorses a 'policy and action checklist' approach to follow in order to foster informed and 'proper' use of TCAM, to make sure that TCAM practitioners are following a set of guidelines underpinned by the biomedical paradigm. This checklist approach follows regulatory frameworks for biomedical practitioners. For example, the WHO endorses a checklist which includes establishing registration and licensing of providers; identifying safe and effective therapies and products; developing training guidelines for the most commonly used therapies; strengthening and increasing organisation of TCAM providers; and strengthening cooperation between TCAM providers and other healthcare providers (WHO 2004).

Both the World Bank and the WHO are also interested in developing TCAM typologies, classifying TCAM into subdivisions used in biomedicine, such as 'generalists' and 'specialists' (WHO 2010). They propose 'benchmarks' for training such as a hierarchical categorisation of training into Type I, II, and III depending on where the practitioners have been trained (WHO 2010). While preventing misuse and misrepresentation by TCAM practitioners as to potentially unfounded claims for curing illnesses is important, the concern is that these benchmarks put in place to safeguard against improper practicing and use of TCAM will be problematic if their main impact is simply to legitimise a Eurocentric biomedical model of knowledge and practice (Barry 2006; Evans 2008; Martin-Hill 2003; Smith 1999).

Health Canada and TCAM: Public Safety and Surveillance

Health Canada has also turned its attention towards developing policies that will ensure the 'safe and effective use of [T]CAM therapies' and is concerned with defining an 'acceptable level of evidence' to ensure this (Health Canada 2003a). Similar to the World Bank and the WHO, it is focused on defining, standardising, and categorising TCAM therapies in order to facilitate this process. It is pushing to establish and enforce a uniform terminology within TCAM practices, a terminology derived from biomedically informed categories. For example, it has come up with nine categories of TCAM products and practices: (1) Natural Health Products, (2) Traditional Chinese Medicine, (3) Naturopathic Medicine, (4) Chiropractic, (5) Homeopathy, (6) Therapeutic Bodywork, (7) Mind-Body Practices, (8) Expressive Therapies, and (9) Energy Therapies. These nine categories reduce and reinterpret or contort TCAM therapies into tidy compartments dividing mind/body and energy and also exclude a whole range of other non-biomedical practices (e.g., Ayurveda, indigenous medicines, massage), which may be a combination of more than one or even all of these categories.

One of Health Canada's main concerns is about 'consumers' using biomedicine and TCAM at the same time, and the potential adverse interactions between the two approaches, especially plant-based medicine and pharmaceuticals (Health Canada 2003a). It envisages a crucial role for government in developing regulation of TCAM practices in order to ensure consumer safety. This includes government input into implementing and standardising TCAM in biomedical curricula, and to this end, Health Canada has worked in collaboration with a Canadian university to create a 'curriculum-related research initiative to facilitate the physician's role with respect to complementary and alternative medicine' (Health Canada 2003a). This initiative was part of the complementary and alternative medicine in undergraduate medical education (CAM in UME) project which aimed to facilitate integration and standardise how TCAM is taught in biomedical education.

In another Health Canada web-based document, it states that the increased visibility and public use of TCAM is posing a challenge to biomedical dominance and the social authority that has been afforded to physicians and that physicians should oversee TCAM (Health Canada 2003b). Many TCAM practices are unregulated in Canada, and Health Canada views this lack of regulation as an ethical issue. From this perspective, the regulation and inclusion of TCAM in biomedical education may be interpreted as a way to control this challenge to biomedicine's social authority, as well as a means of constraining TCAM practices themselves (Coburn et al. 1983). However, Health Canada does go on to state that:

[t]he history of osteopathy and chiropractic reveals that the process of recognising and regulating an alternative practice can be highly charged politically. The process does not leave the alternative practice unchanged... (Health Canada 2003a: 11)

This quote illustrates the subtle, and not so subtle, forces at play in the reinterpretation and perhaps even eventual erasure of non-biomedically rooted healthcare practices and knowledges that may occur with increased regulation and integration. Health Canada has stated that the co-option of TCAM by biomedicine could:

stifle the evolution and knowledge acquisition of an alternative health care system that may eventually prove more robust and effective than the present conventional medical system, which limits itself to the philosophy of biological reductionism. (Health Canada 2003a: 12)

However, Health Canada's own emphasis on the categorisation, standardisation, and regulation of TCAM using a biomedical model remains.

Summary and Discussion

The World Bank, WHO, and Health Canada are governing institutions that exercise power through policy recommendations and policymaking (Prah and Yach 2009). As illustrated in the previous sections, central themes and keywords emerging from the World Bank, WHO, and Health Canada sample documents suggest a biomedicalisation of non-biomedically oriented health beliefs and practices, and the further entrenchment of biomedical hegemony, which may be further facilitated through the integration of TCAM in biomedical education. Analysing World Bank, WHO, and Health Canada TCAM-related documents for language, central themes, and keywords helped contextualise the nature of TCAM's integration into public health systems and its existence in biomedical education. It is also suggestive of the level of influence these institutions have on the 'everyday world' (Wedel et al. 2005) in Canada 'through' these institutions (Wedel et al. 2005), thus connecting questions about differing medical belief systems within a broader context that includes issues of dominance and biomedical hegemony (see Khan 2006; Nichter and Lock 2002).

The main difference between these three institutions involves their scope and jurisdiction. In 1978, the World Bank endorsed selective primary healthcare, which focuses on low-cost technical health interventions rather than addressing global social inequities (Cueto 2004), and the WHO followed suit soon after (Banerji 1984; Rifkin and Walt 1986; Stuckler and Segal 2011; Yalamala 2013). Likewise, Health Canada tends to be caught between maintaining a public system and privatisation as per other economically liberal nations, such as the US (Armstrong and Armstrong 2009). As Navarro and Shi have argued (2001), unlike the social democratic Western nations, in Canada and the US, the 'market reigns supreme' (p. 19), and this paradigm fits very well with the approaches of the World Bank and the WHO, with their profit motive in mind (Armada et al. 2001).

A key thematic continuity between the World Bank, WHO, and Health Canada is the focus on safety through surveillance to the exclusion of other important concerns. The materials we reviewed from Health Canada in particular repeatedly refer back to the importance of including TCAM in biomedical education so that doctors can oversee patient TCAM use. They also emphasise how doctors need to learn how to advise their patients on the safe and effective use of TCAM. In a preliminary examination of some TCAM-related curriculum documents taken from the CAM in UME project, for example, the website includes a 'Quackwatch' screening guide (CAM in UME project, 2013), which divides up TCAM practitioner behaviour into 'Red Flag' and 'Yellow Flag' categories. These categories cite specific behaviours physicians should be on the lookout for so they can advise patients against these therapies. Neglected in these discussions are many possible behaviours and practices that may be ethically questionable for any health practitioner, such as accepting gifts from pharmaceutical companies, overprescribing medication (Haque et al. 2013), the many adverse medical events that occur each day in healthcare (Illich 1976; Wazana 2000), financial benefit from industry (Barnes 2017), and ghostwriting (Sismondo 2009). Instead, the focus is only on TCAM practitioners as potential charlatans. Physicians are portrayed as somehow above unethical behaviour, implying that public safety is ensured against charlatanism by modern science (Haque et al. 2013). Interestingly, a more recent search for the CAM in UME project turned up empty. The only information we could find about it was located on a new association website called the Canadian Integrative Medicine Association (CIMA). On the CIMA website they state that the CAM in UME project 'is a wealth of knowledge and resources regarding CAM and integrative medicine', yet when you click on the link it is empty. CIMA's focus is on postgraduate medical training and fellowships related to TCAM and integrative medicine, most of which are in the US. CIMA membership and access to the various resources is only open to medical doctors.

Our analysis reveals thematic continuities between the World Bank, the WHO, and Health Canada. This is suggestive of how these institutions may be influencing why and how TCAM is being integrated into healthcare and biomedical education in Canada. Our analysis suggests that efforts to standardise, regulate, and biomedicalise TCAM, which may be further facilitated through its integration into biomedical education, are reflective of the pervasive nature of biomedical hegemony. While it has been argued that biomedical dominance is not forever assured (Moore and McLean 2010), we suggest that the easy adaptability of biomedicine to market interests makes it hard to resist, and relatedly, knowledge that doesn't conform or measure up to biomedical benchmarks is at risk of being reinterpreted and lost. In light of this, it is important to continue to investigate the ways that TCAM is 'integrated' into public healthcare, who decides what is included, what is left behind, and what is lost in this process.

Similar to processes that occurred during the colonial era, the 'integration' of TCAM practices into biomedical settings, such as medical curricula, may be viewed as part of an entrenched pattern of indigenous knowledge and worldview expropriation, homogenisation, and in some cases even erasure. From this perspective, 'integration' may actually lead to the contortion of practices towards a logic that places profit and the expanding neoliberal market (Navarro 2007; McKenna 2010, 2012) above people and health. Further, it circumscribes and constrains other ways of understanding health and healing from actually being 'integrated' into medicine. Medicine is about more than it is being reduced to by biomedicine (McKenna 2010). Allowing biomedical hegemony to become further entrenched takes with it any chance of an expanded health system or systems and the possibility of non-biomedical health practices and knowledges maintaining their differing strengths, strengths that could instead serve to improve healthcare in areas where biomedicine is weak (such as chronic diseases and subclinical illness).

Tsing (2000) suggests that the circulation of knowledge and culture, and their artifacts, such as healthcare practices, are components of globalisation; however, she also highlights how merely focusing on their circulation and contact doesn't take into account the ways that agency, and power, influence the direction of movement and quality of circulation, and we would add the outcome of that circulation. The networks of knowledge(s) between TCAM and biomedicine that may occur through integration are influenced by factors internal and external, internally through the actual structures of knowledge themselves, and externally through capitalism, hegemony, power, agency, and their impact on the day-to-day knowledge transmission in this context.

In closing, we would like to draw the reader's attention to Fournier's experiences when working as a massage therapist. Throughout this study she was teaching at a massage therapy school in Canada. Perhaps because of being so immersed in this study and critically analysing biomedicine, each time she taught she came face to face with the ways that massage therapy is becoming contorted through its increased regulation and surveillance. Touch, palpation, and intuition are forms of knowledge that are integral to massage but also forms of knowledge that are increasingly being viewed as illegitimate and overlooked in favour of so-called hard or real science in contemporary Canadian massage therapy curricula. For example, many biomedical forms of measuring and assessing have overshadowed other ways of understanding and approaching treatment, such as simple touch and palpation. Teaching massage therapy within the context of a formal institution, Fournier was constrained in her approach by the push to emphasise the visible and measurable components of practice. She was constrained by a curriculum contorted by biomedical hegemony.

The implications of the integration of TCAM with biomedicine include both the influence on TCAM practices and the potential for improvements in healthcare. Latour's argument that we tend to conceive of hybrids, such as knowledge and practices in medicine, as deriving from two 'pure forms' and that we tend to try and 'split mixtures apart' (1993: 78) that are actually more fluid is crucial here. If differing forms of medicine are involved in processes of contact and exchange, given that biomedicine is already an assemblage or mixture of knowledge(s), then perhaps the process of contact and exchange with TCAM might lead to knowledge assemblages and innovations that are even harder to gauge and predict. What may be more traceable are the socio-economic and political factors at play in their contact and why and how powerful governing institutions such as the World Bank and WHO, and national governing institutions such as Health Canada, are integrating TCAM into the public healthcare system, including how doctors are trained. This has significant implications for the very survival of the practices in question and the potential for improvements in public healthcare.

Notes

1. The terms CAM and TCAM are used interchangeably at times. The WHO and World Bank use TCAM or T&CM while in medical education the term CAM is more common.
2. We use the Constitutional language with the 's' at the end of the word. Adding the 's' to the word was fought for to resist assimilating the concept of a singular 'Aboriginal people' in Canada and to recognise diversity.

References

Adams, V. (2002). Randomized controlled crime: Postcolonial sciences in alternative medicine research. *Social Studies of Science, 32*(5), 650–690.
Adams, V., Schrempf, M., & Craig, S. R. (Eds.). (2013). *Medicine between science and religion: Explorations on Tibetan grounds*. Oxford: Berghahn Books.

Adler, S. (2008). Integrative medicine and culture: Toward an anthropology of CAM. *Medical Anthropology Quarterly, 16*(4), 412–414.

Aikenhead, G., & Ogawa, M. (2007). Indigenous knowledge and science revisited. *Cultural Studies of Science Education, 2*(3), 539–620.

Armada, F., Muntaner, C., & Navarro, V. (2001). Health and social security reforms in Latin America: The convergence of the World Health Organization, the World Bank, and transnational corporations. *International Journal of Health Services, 31*(4), 729–768.

Armstrong, P., & Armstrong, H. (2009). Contradictions at work: Struggles for control in Canadian health care. In C. Leys & L. Panitch (Eds.), *Morbid symptoms: Health under capitalism* (pp. 1–29). Wales: The Merlin Press.

Arnold, D. (1988). *Imperial medicine and Indigenous societies*. Manchester: Manchester University Press.

Attaran, A., Attaran, K., Barnes, I., Bate, R., Binka, F., d'Alessandro, U., et al. (2006). The World Bank: False financial and statistical accounts and medical malpractice in malaria treatment. *The Lancet, 368*(9531), 247–252.

Baer, H. (2004). U.S. health policy on alternative medicine: A case study in the co-optation of a popular movement. In A. Castro & M. Singer (Eds.), *Unhealthy health policy: A critical anthropological examination* (pp. 317–329). Plymouth: Alta Mira Press.

Baer, H., & Coulter, I. (2008). Taking stock of integrative medicine: Broadening biomedicine or co-option of complementary and alternative medicine? *Health Sociology Review, 17*(4), 331–341.

Baer, H., Singer, M., & Susser, I. (2003). *Medical anthropology and the world system: A critical perspective* (2nd ed.). Westport, CT: Praeger.

Banerji, D. (1984). Primary health care: Selective or comprehensive. *World Health Forum, 5*(4), 312–315.

Barimah, K., & van Teijlingen, E. R. (2008). The use of traditional medicine by Ghanaians in Canada. *BMC Complementary and Alternative Medicine, 8*(30), 1–10.

Barnes, B. (2017). Financial conflicts of interest in continuing medical education: Implications and accountability. *JAMA, 317*(17), 1741–1742.

Baronov, D. (2008). Biomedicine: An ontological dissection. *Theoretical Medicine and Bioethics, 29*(4), 235–254.

Barry, C. A. (2006). The role of evidence in alternative medicine: Contrasting biomedical and anthropological approaches. *Social Science and Medicine, 62*(11), 2646–2657.

Berg, B. L. (2009). *Qualitative research methods for the social sciences* (7th ed.). Boston: Pearson Publishing.

Bernard, H. R. (2006). *Research methods in anthropology* (4th ed.). London: Rowman & Littlefield Publishers.

Betancourt, M. T., Roberts, K. C., Bennett, T.-L., Driscoll, E. R., Jayaram, G., & Pelletier, L. (2014). Monitoring chronic diseases in Canada: The chronic disease indicator framework. *Chronic Diseases and Injuries in Canada, 34*(1), 1–30.

Biehl, J., & Petryna, A. (Eds.). (2013). *When people come first: Critical studies in global health*. Princeton: Princeton University Press.

Bodecker, G., & Kronenberg, F. (2002). A public health agenda for traditional, complementary, and alternative medicine. *American Journal of Public Health, 92*(10), 1582–1591.

Boomgaard, P. (2003). Dutch medicine in Asia, 1600–1900. In D. Arnold (Ed.), *Warm climates and Western medicine: The emergence of tropical medicine 1500–1900* (pp. 42–65). Amsterdam: Rodopi.

Brown, T., & Bell, B. (2008). Imperial or postcolonial governance: Dissecting the genealogy of a global public health strategy. *Social Science and Medicine, 67*(10), 1571–1579.

Coburn, D., Torrance, G. M., & Kaufert, J. M. (1983). Medical dominance in Canada an historical perspective: The rise and fall of medicine? *International Journal of Health Services, 13*(3), 407–432.

Complementary and alternative medicine in undergraduate medical education project. (2013). Retrieved May 2015, from http://www.caminume.ca/.

Cueto, M. (2004). The origins of primary health care and selective primary health care. *American Journal of Public Health, 94*(11), 1864–1874.

Esmail, N. (2017). *Complementary and alternative medicine: Use and public attitudes 1997, 2006, and 2016*. Fraser Institute. Retrieved June 1, 2017, from http://www.fraserinstitute.org.

Evans, S. (2008). Changing the knowledge base in Western herbal medicine. *Social Science & Medicine, 67*(12), 2098–2106.

Fournier, C. (2016). Book review – Naraindas, H., Quack, J., & Sax, W. S. (Eds.) Asymmetrical conversations: Contestations, circumventions, and the blurring of therapeutic boundaries. *The Journal of the Royal Anthropological Institute, 22*(2), 439–441.

Gale, N. (2014). The sociology of traditional, complementary and alternative medicine. *Social Compass, 8*(6), 805–822.

Gautam, V., Raman, R. M., & Kumar, A. (2003). *Exploring Indian healthcare: Export of Ayurveda and Siddha products and services.* Mumbai: Quest Publications.

Gordon, D. R. (1988). Tenacious assumptions in Western medicine. In M. Lock & D. Gordon (Eds.), *Biomedicine examined* (pp. 19–56). Dordrecht: Kluwer Academic Publishers.

Haque O. S., De Freitas, J., Bursztajn, H.T., Cosgrove, A., Gopal, A., Robindra P., et al. (2013). *The ethics of pharmaceutical industry influence in medicine.* UNESCO Report.

Harding, S. (1998). *Is science multicultural? Postcolonialisms, feminisms, and epistemologies.* Indianapolis: Indiana University Press.

Harding, S. (Ed.). (2011). *The postcolonial science and technology studies reader.* London: Duke University Press.

Harris, S. (2010). Non-native plants and their medicinal uses. In E. Hsu & S. Harris (Eds.), *Plants, health and healing: On the interface of ethnobotany and medical anthropology* (pp. 83–130). Oxford: Berghan Books.

Health Canada. (2003a). *Taking stock: Policy issues related to CAHC.* Health Policy Bulletin, 7 November.

Health Canada. (2003b). *Complementary and alternative health care: The other mainstream.* Health Policy Research November 7, 2003. Retrieved December 2013, from http://www.hc-sc.gc.ca/sr-sr/alt_formats/hpb-dgps/pdf/pubs/hpr-rps/bull/2003-7-complement/2003-7-complement-eng.pdf.

Health Canada. (2003c). *Developing a national vision for complementary and alternative medicine in undergraduate medical education.* Report on an invitational workshop held September 27–28, 2003. Retrieved December 2013, from http://www.phac-aspc.gc.ca/publicat/pcahc-pacps/pdf/comp_intro.pdf.

Hollenberg, D., & Muzzin, L. (2010). Epistemological challenges to integrative medicine: An anti-colonial perspective on the combination of complementary/alternative medicine with biomedicine. *Health Sociology Review, 19*(1), 34–56.

Horden, P., & Hsu, E. (2013). *The body in balance: Humeral medicines in practice.* Oxford: Berghahn Books.

Hsu, E., & Harris, S. (Eds.). (2010). *Plants, health and healing: On the interface of ethnobotany and medical anthropology.* New York and Oxford: Berghahn Books.

Illich, I. (1976). *Medical nemesis: The expropriation of health.* New York: Pantheon Books.

Jacklin, K. M., & Warry, W. (2004). The Indian health transfer policy in Canada: Toward self determination or cost containment. In A. Castro & M. Singer (Eds.), *Unhealthy health policy: A critical anthropological examination* (pp. 215–234). Plymouth: Alta Mira Press.

Kelton, P. (2007). *Epidemics and enslavement: Biological catastrophe in the native southeast, 1492–1715.* Lincoln and London: University of Nebraska Press.

Khan, S. (2006). Systems of medicine and nationalist discourse in India: Towards 'new horizon' in medical anthropology and history. *Social Science & Medicine, 62*(11), 2786–2797.

Kincheloe, J. (2006). Critical ontology and Indigenous ways of being: Forging a postcolonial curriculum. In Y. Kanu (Ed.), *Curriculum as cultural practice: Postcolonial imaginations* (pp. 181–197). Toronto: University of Toronto Press.

King, N. (2002). Security, disease, commerce: Ideologies of postcolonial global health. *Social Science & Medicine, 32*(5–6), 763–789.

Krippendorff, K. (2013). *Content analysis: An introduction to its methodology* (2nd ed.). London: SAGE.

Latour, B. (1993). *We have never been modern.* Cambridge, MA: Harvard University Press.

Leslie, C., & Young, A. (1992). *Paths to Asian medical knowledge: Comparative studies of health systems and medical care.* Berkeley: University of California Press.

Leys, C. (2009). Health care under capitalism. In C. Leys & L. Panitch (Eds.), *Morbid symptoms: Health under capitalism* (pp. 1–29). Wales: The Merlin Press.

Maar, M. A., & Shawande, M. (2010, January). Traditional Anishinabe healing in a clinical setting: The development of an Aboriginal interdisciplinary approach to community-based Aboriginal mental health care. *Journal de la santé autochtone, 6*, 18–27.

Manitowabe, D., & Shawande, M. (2013). Negotiating the clinical integration of traditional Aboriginal medicine at Noojmowin Tej. *Canadian Journal of Native Studies, 1*, 97–128.

Martin, E. (2001). *The woman in the body: A cultural analysis of reproduction.* Boston: Beacon Press.

Martin-Hill, D. (2003, March). Traditional medicine in contemporary contexts: Protecting and respecting indigenous knowledge and medicine. *National Aboriginal Health Organization, 19*, 3–35.

Massey, A., & Kirk, R. (2015). Bridging indigenous and western sciences: Research methodologies for traditional, complementary, and alternative medicine systems. *SAGE Open, 5*(3), 1–15. https://doi.org/10.1177/2158244015597726

McKenna, B. (2010). Take back medical education: The primary care 'shuffle'. *Medical Anthropology: Cross-Cultural Perspectives in Illness and Health, 29*(1), 6–14.

McKenna, B. (2012). Medical education under siege: Critical pedagogy, primary care, and the making of 'slave doctors'. *International Journal of Critical Pedagogy, 4*(1), 95–117.

Mehta, L. (2001). The World Bank and its emerging knowledge empire. *Human Organization, 60*(2), 189–196.

Mgbeoji, I. (2006). *Global biopiracy: Patients, plants and Indigenous knowledge.* Ithaca: Cornell University Press.

Moore, R., & McLean, S. (Eds.). (2010). *Folk healing and health care practices in Britain and Ireland: Stethoscopes, wands and crystals.* New York and Oxford: Berghahn Books.

Morgan, M. W., Zamora, N. E., & Hindmarsh, M. F. (2007). An inconvenient truth: A sustainable healthcare system requires chronic disease prevention and management transformation. *Healthcare Papers, 7*(4), 6–23.

Nabipour, I., Burger, A., Moharreri, M. R., & Azizi, F. (2009). Avicenna, the first to describe thyroid-related orbitopath. *Thyroid, 19*(1), 7–8.

Nanda, M. (2001). A 'broken people' defend science: Reconstructing the Deweyan Buddha of India's Dalits. *Social Epistemology: A Journal of Knowledge, Culture and Policy, 15*(4), 335–365.

Navarro, V. (1976). *Medicine under capitalism.* New York: Prodist.

Navarro, V. (2007). Neoliberalism as a class ideology, or the political causes of growth inequalities. In V. Navarro (Ed.), *Neoliberalism, globalization and inequalities: Consequences for health and quality of life* (pp. 9–27). New York: Baywood Publishing.

Navarro, V., & Shi, L. (2001). The political context of social inequalities and health. *International Journal of Health Services, 31*(1), 1–21.

Nayak, J. (2012). Ayurveda research: Ontological challenges. *Journal of Ayurveda & Integrative Medicine, 3*(1), 17–20.

Nichter, M., & Lock, M. (2002). *New horizons in medical anthropology: Essays in honour of Charles Leslie.* London: Routledge.

Oakley R. (forthcoming). The wrong names': Non-status aboriginality and well being. In A. S. Grøsneth (Lillehammer) & J. Skinner (Roehamptom) (Eds.),

Mobilities of wellbeing, suffering and misfortune: Knowledge beyond evidence and causality. Carolina Academic Press.

Oakley, R., & Grøsneth, A. S. (Eds.). (2007). Ethnographic humanism: Migrant experiences in the quest for well-being. *Special Edition of Anthropology in Action Health, 14*, 1–11.

Oakley, R., Yalamala, R., & Kasi, E. (2013). Social exclusion in India: Critical ethnographic discourse from the margins. *Annuaire Roumain d'Anthropologie, 50*, 1–86.

Patwardhan, B., Vaidya, A., & Chorghade, A. (2004). Ayurveda and natural products drug discovery. *Current Science, 86*(6), 789–799.

Patwardhan, B., Warude, D., Pushpangadan, P., & Bhatt, N. (2005). Ayurveda and traditional Chinese medicine: A comparative overview. *Evidence-based Complementary and Alternative Medicine, 2*(4), 465–473.

Prah, R. J., & Yach, D. (2009). *The global role of the World Health Organization.* Retrieved May 2015, from http://www.ghgj.org/Ruger%20and%20Yach_The%20Global%20Role%20of%20WHO.pdf.

Quah, S. R. (2003). Traditional healing systems and the ethos of science. *Social Science & Medicine, 57*(10), 1997–2012.

Quan, H., Lai, D., Johnson, D., Verhoef, M., & Musto, R. (2008). Complementary and alternative medicine use among Chinese and white Canadians. *Canadian Family Physician, 54*(11), 563–569.

Rifkin, S. B., & Walt, G. (1986). Why health improves: Defining the issues concerning 'comprehensive primary health care' and 'selective primary health care'. *Social Science Medicine, 23*(6), 559–566.

Robbins, J., & Dewar, J. (2011). Traditional Indigenous approaches to healing and the modern welfare of traditional knowledge, spirituality and lands: A critical reflection on practices and policies taken from the Canadian Indigenous example. *The International Policy Journal, 2*(4), 1–17.

Ruger, J. P. (2005). The changing role of the World Bank in Global health. *American Journal of Public Health, 95*(1), 60–70.

Ruger, J. P. (2007). Global health governance and the World Bank. *The Lancet, 370*(9597), 1471–1474.

Sax, W., & Nair, H. (2014). A healing practice in Rwanda. In H. Naraindas, J. Quack, & W. Sax (Eds.), *Asymmetrical conversations: Contestations, circumventions, and the blurring of therapeutic boundaries* (pp. 200–237). Oxford: Berghahn Books.

Scheper-Hughes, N. (1992). *Death without weeping.* Berkeley: University of California Press.

Sefa-Dei, J. S., Hall, B. L., & Goldin-Rosenberg, D. (Eds.). (2000). *Indigenous knowledges in global contexts: Multiple readings of our world.* Toronto: University of Toronto Press.

Semali, L., & Kincheloe, J. L. (Eds.). (1999). *What is Indigenous knowledge? Voices from the academy.* New York: Taylor and Francis.

Shiva, N. (2000). Cultural diversity and the politics of knowledge. In J. S. Sefa-Dei, B. L. Hall, & D. Goldin-Rosenberg (Eds.), *Indigenous knowledges in global contexts: Multiple readings of our world* (pp. xii–xix). Toronto: University of Toronto Press.

Shore, C., & Wright, S. (Eds.). (2003). *Anthropology of policy: Perspectives on governance and power.* London: Routledge.

Silnicki, A. (2013). *Why won't premiers defend public health care?* Canadian Perspectives, Autumn, 22–23. Retrieved March 2017, from http://canadians.org/sites/default/files/publications/premiers-healthcare.pdf.

Siraisi, N. (1987). *Avicenna in renaissance Italy: The Canon and medical teaching in Italian universities after 1500.* Princeton: University Press.

Sismondo, S. (2009). Ghosts in the machine: Publication planning in the medical sciences. *Social Studies of Science, 39*(2), 171–198.

Smith, T. L. (1999). *Decolonizing methodologies: Research and Indigenous peoples.* London: Zed Books.

Statistics Canada. (2017). Retrieved June 1, 2017, from http://www23.statcan.gc.ca/imdb/p3VD.pl?Function=getVD&TVD=139116&CVD=13.

Stuckler, D., & Segal, K. (Eds.). (2011). *Sick societies: Responding to the global challenge of chronic disease.* Oxford: Oxford University Press.

Sundar Rajan, K. (2007). *Biocapital: The constitution of postgenomic life.* Durham: Duke University Press.

Timmerman, K. (2003). Intellectual property rights and traditional medicine: Policy dilemmas at the interface. *Social Science and Medicine, 57*(4), 745–756.

Tovey, P., Easthope, G., & Adams, J. (Eds.). (2004). *Mainstreaming complementary and alternative medicine: Studies in social context.* London: Routledge.

Towghi, F. (2004). Shifting policies towards traditional midwives: Implications for reproductive health care in Pakistan. In A. Castro & M. Singer (Eds.), *Unhealthy health policy: A critical anthropological examination* (pp. 317–329). Plymouth: Alta Mira Press.

Tsing, A. (2000). The global situation. *Cultural Anthropology, 15*(3), 327–360.

Ventola, C. L. (2010). Current issues regarding complementary and alternative medicine (CAM) in the United States. *Pharmacy and Therapeutics, 35*(8), 461–468.

Wazana, A. (2000). Physicians and the pharmaceutical industry: Is a gift ever just a gift? *JAMA, 283*(3), 373–380.

Wedel, J., Shore, C., Feldman, G., & Lathrop, S. (2005). Toward an anthropology of public policy. *The Annals of the American Academy of Political and Social Science, 600,* 29–51.

WHO. (2002). *WHO traditional medicine strategy 2002–2005.* Retrieved June 2013, from http://www.who.int/medicines/publications/traditionalpolicy/en/.

WHO. (2004). *WHO guidelines on developing consumer information on proper use of TCAM.* Retrieved June 2014, from http://apps.who.int/medicinedocs/en/d/Js5525e/.

WHO. (2010). *Benchmarks for training in traditional/complementary and alternative medicine: Benchmarks for training in traditional Chinese medicine.* Retrieved June 2016, from http://apps.who.int/medicinedocs/documents/s17556en/s17556en.pdf.

WHO. (2013a). *TCAM and policy and public health perspectives.* Retrieved June 2016, from http://www.who.int/bulletin/volumes/86/1/07-046458/en/.

WHO. (2013b). *Traditional medicine strategy 2014–2013.* Retrieved October 2016, from http://apps.who.int/iris/bitstream/10665/92455/1/9789241506090_eng.pdf.

World Bank. (2004a). *Conditions for effective collaboration between modern and traditional medicine.* Retrieved June 2013, from https://openknowledge.worldbank.org/handle/10986/10772.

World Bank. (2004b). *Conditions for effective collaboration between modern and traditional medicine.* Retrieved June 2013, from https://openknowledge.worldbank.org/handle/10986/10772.

World Bank. (2004c). *Local pathways to global development: Marking five years of the World Bank knowledge for development program.* Retrieved June 2013, from http://www.worldbank.org/afr/ik/ikcomplete.pdf.

World Bank. (2013b). *Traditional medicine; and the World Bank.* Retrieved June 2013, from http://go.worldbank.org/433PVWTQL0.

Xue, C. C. (2008). Traditional, complementary and alternative medicine: Policy and public health perspectives. *WHO Bulletin, 86*(1), 1–80.

Yalamala, R. (2013). Beyond the institutionalized approach to research ethics: Anthropology and systems of health exclusion. *Annuaire Roumain d' Anthropologie, 50,* 65–78.

Zargaran, A., Zarshenas, M., Mehdizadeh, A., & Mohagheghzadeh, A. (2013). Management of tremor in medieval Persia. *Journal of the History of the Neurosciences, 22,* 53–61.

Zhan, M. (2001). Does it take a miracle? Negotiating knowledges, identities, and communities of traditional Chinese medicine. *Cultural Anthropology, 16*(4), 453–480.

Zhang, E. (2007). Switching between traditional Chinese medicine and viagra: Cosmopolitanism and medical pluralism today. *Medical Anthropology, 26*(1), 53–96.

10

Epistemic Hybridity: TCM's Knowledge Production in Canadian Contexts

Ana Ning

Introduction

Recent scholarly analyses of complementary and alternative medicine's (CAM) global developments have interrogated taken-for-granted dichotomies between CAM and biomedicine as distinct health modalities, with separate ideological and pragmatic underpinnings. Rather than viewing CAM as a monolithic 'Other' versus a hegemonic biomedicine, many point to their significant overlap in the ways they legitimate, standardise, integrate, and globalise their knowledges and practices in diverse settings (Fries 2008; Gale 2014; Givati and Hatton 2015; Hampshire and Owusu 2013; Ning 2013). Ideologies such as holism, vitalism, naturalism, humanism, and spiritualism, long perceived to be unique features of CAM, in contrast to biomedicine's dualism, reductionism, materialism, scientism, and individualism, have been problematised as Western binary oppositions (Givati 2015; Fries 2013; Ning 2013; Zhan 2014).

The consequences of the interaction between CAM and biomedicine in Western industrialised societies have been the subject of intense

A. Ning (✉)
King's University College, Western University, Oakville, ON, Canada

© The Author(s) 2018
C. Brosnan et al. (eds.), *Complementary and Alternative Medicine*, Health, Technology and Society, https://doi.org/10.1007/978-3-319-73939-7_10

247

scholarly debate around the issues of integrative medicine, integrative health care[1], and CAM co-optation by biomedicine (Baer 2008; Baer and Coulter 2008; Coulter et al. 2008; Boon et al. 2004; Hollenberg 2006; Hollenberg and Muzzin 2010; Tataryn and Verhoef 2001). Increasingly, scholars argue that CAM and biomedicine are co-constituted in a complex nexus of negotiated power enabled by transnational cultural flows (Coulter et al. 2008; Fries 2008; Gale 2014; Hampshire and Owusu 2013; Quah 2008). Given the extent of engagement between diverse healing modalities at both informal and formal levels[2] worldwide, 'hybridity' becomes a more spatially informed analysis of the co-constitution between CAM and biomedicine (Coulter et al. 2008; Fries 2008; Gale 2014; Hampshire and Owusu 2013). 'Hybridity' (Appadurai 1996) helps illuminate the myriad ways in which CAM and biomedical knowledges and practices flow from original settings to new locations, facilitated by globalisation.

Although 'hybridity' has been used in CAM analyses to critically examine the integration of CAM and biomedicine in different regions (Fries 2008; Gale 2014; Khan 2006; Obadia 2007), I will use *epistemic hybridity* as a heuristic tool to show how the knowledge production of a particular type of CAM—Traditional Chinese Medicine (TCM)—takes shape and shifts in very complex and sometimes contradictory ways within local contexts. By focusing on TCM as encompassing incompatibilities and intersections with Western science, my chapter endeavours to move beyond a larger theoretical debate that situates TCM's increasing global appeal within the structure/agency binary: *either* as a broader social phenomenon consistent with a global move towards 'scientific evidence' (Baer 2008; Coulter 2004; Fries 2008, 2013; Iedema and Veljanova 2013) *or* as a counter-hegemonic movement that reveals TCM proponents' conscious efforts to actively legitimise a unique tradition within biomedically dominant arenas (Barnes 2005; Dew et al. 2008; Saks 2003; Kelner and Wellman 1997, 2014).

Drawing upon ethnographic field research[3] with TCM practitioners in British Columbia (BC) and Ontario, Canada, regarding constructions of TCM evidence of safety and effectiveness, I aim to demonstrate how TCM evidence is produced and applied in context, thus suggesting possible ways to address Gale's (2014) 'big question'—how and whether

CAM therapies work. The TCM practitioners' narratives that appear later in this chapter will uncover highly hybridised TCM knowledges and practices in which 'epistemic disunity' (Knorr Cetina 1999), that is, different theoretical and methodological approaches, occurs within TCM itself and not only in relation to other health practices. In so doing, my chapter contributes to a larger social science debate about identifying multiple legitimate 'evidence bases' to evaluate different health modalities that include diverse ways of knowing and doing, rather than the current emphasis on a single biomedical epistemology.

Rethinking Therapeutic Evidence

The question of appropriate evidence bases, in which bio-scientific standards to evaluate the safety and efficacy of any therapeutic modality are privileged, is a major controversy in the integration of CAM practices into the public healthcare domain (Barry 2006; Daly 2005; De Bruyn 2001; Dean 2004; Denny 1999; Rappolt 1997; Villanueva-Russell 2005). The concept of evidence itself is highly contested: different stakeholders define and interpret evidence differently for their own purposes of recognising, legitimising, and regulating health professions. To date, limited ethnographic research has been conducted that clarifies what constitutes 'sufficient evidence' to assess complex, multifactorial, synergistic, and interactive health systems such as TCM in order to support its integration, although significant qualitative research addresses TCM effectiveness in transnational encounters (Barnes 2005; Baer 2008; Farquhar 1994; Kelner and Wellman 2014; Zhan 2009, 2014).

In this chapter, I explore contemporary constructions of TCM evidence as a complex undertaking in which practitioners, knowledge, experiences, and science intersect in interesting and sometimes contradictory ways. To understand how TCM evidence is produced and used in context against rigid boundaries, I draw upon an emerging social science literature (Barry 2006; Broom and Tovey 2007; Brosnan 2016; Gale 2011, 2014; Ziguras 2004; Zhan 2009, 2014) that considers the relevance of multiple epistemic frameworks to evaluate diverse therapeutic outcomes. This analytical approach sheds light on broader definitions of 'evidence' in which bioscience and traditional knowledge can coexist within a knowledge-making culture such as TCM. In particular, Brosnan (2016) and Zhan (2014) highlight the importance of both areas of knowledge in shaping TCM as a 'living tradition' (Scheid and Lei 2014), whereby the tension between aligning with the biomedical approach to produce mainstream forms of evidence and being committed to traditional healing principles to emphasise its unique systemic logic renders its knowledge-making process fluid—neither strictly 'experiential' nor 'scientific'. Taking this theoretical orientation as a point of departure, my chapter seeks to rethink another unexamined dichotomy underlying contemporary representations of TCM's knowledge production that situate TCM's increasing global move towards *either* scientific evidence to achieve legitimacy alongside biomedicine *or* to actively carve out a space within biomedically dominant arenas as a unique systemic tradition premised upon distinct principles.

Historically, TCM's cited experiential basis revolves around its theory, philosophy, and approach to illness. TCM is known for emphasising the unique constitution of each individual, the integration of body, mind, and spirit, the flow of energy or vital force (*qi*) as a source of healing, and disease as having multiple dimensions beyond the purely biological (Scheid 2002; Unschuld 1992). Central to the concept of vital force is the idea that the human body has the ability to self-heal and the task of TCM practitioners is to assist this process, a perspective that is seen as fundamentally different from biomedicine (Vincent et al. 1998). TCM is usually viewed within a paradigm with a holistic theory of disease known as a 'whole medical system'. A fundamental aspect of TCM's understanding of bodily dysfunctions and source of disease is the idea of a general imbalance whereby *qi* energy becomes blocked within one's body system and it must be 'unblocked' to restore the flow of energy, thus ensuring a healthy body system.

Currently, to maintain the integrity of this type of systemic logic which is also apparent in other CAM systems, many leading CAM researchers in Canada are pursuing 'whole-systems' research as a new mode of research inquiry (Verhoef et al. 2005; Ijaz et al. 2016; Torri and Hornosty 2017). Their ultimate goal through 'whole-systems' research is to challenge biomedical dominance by actively seeking to validate unique CAM methods to evaluate therapeutic evidence.

Further, many scholars have found that TCM has undergone a process of biomedicalisation, whereby its practitioners have adopted the biomedical model and rejected the more holistic aspects of traditional practice. This biomedicalisation of TCM is a result of pressure to gain recognition, legitimacy, and regulation in local and global contexts where the 'gold standard' for establishing scientific evidence of therapeutic efficacy and safety is mainly randomised controlled clinical trials (RCTs) (Barry 2006; Brosnan 2016; Ernst 2000; McClean 2003; Ning 2008; Saks 1992).

Rather than viewing the knowledge-making of TCM as a stable or dichotomous endeavour, oscillating between 'traditional' and 'scientific' paradigms, I believe it is more fruitful to situate the often ambiguous processes of TCM knowledge production and translation in terms of *epistemic hybridity*. My theorising of *epistemic hybridity* adds to Brosnan's (2016) and Zhan's (2009, 2014) research by showing that the empirical bases of TCM evidence—experiential, historical, observational, oral—inform TCM practitioners' identities and practices, yet they also negotiate the dominant biomedical evidence.

In particular, I want to call attention to more encompassing types of evidence that TCM practitioners rely upon in TCM interventions that facilitate a complex synergy between patients, healers, and their shared healing experiences. These intersubjective experiences constitute sufficient 'evidence' for TCM practitioners to continue undertaking personally meaningful practices that are often discounted by biomedical practitioners due to limited 'scientific' bases. Here, I want to emphasise that to better understand TCM's therapeutic effects, we must take into consideration broader factors beyond individual bodies' functioning. As such, TCM practitioners' reliance upon multiple evidence frameworks strictly mirrors neither a sense of historical continuity with 'traditional' Chinese medical knowledge nor concerted efforts to fit TCM within currently dominant bio-scientific lenses. Rather, by denoting incompatibilities and intersections between TCM and Western science in the production of therapeutic evidence, I am highlighting the coexistence of diverse 'sciences' that are equally valid, thus questioning the presumed naturalness and primacy of Western science as the most acceptable method of knowledge production. As Knorr Cetina (1999) already noted, even the body of knowledge that characterises 'Western science' is not homogeneous but is comprised of separate knowledge-making cultures.

This chapter aims to explore the following research questions:

1. What constitutes legitimate types of TCM evidence of therapeutic effectiveness and safety?
2. How do TCM practitioners integrate experiential and scientific evidence in their regular practices?
3. What constitutes 'sufficient evidence' to validate successful treatments in the absence of scientific evidence?

Methodology

This chapter is based on ethnographic field research with TCM practitioners in BC and Ontario, Canada, regarding constructions of TCM evidence of safety and effectiveness. Given ethical concerns raised by the Research Ethics Review Committee (RERC) at my university about potential conflicts of interest associated with eliciting permission from TCM practitioners' patients to observe actual clinical interactions, I received ethics approval to only conduct field research with TCM practitioners. The RERC was concerned that patients could feel compelled to give consent to participate in my research once they knew their health providers were part of it. Thus, upon informed consent, my ethnographic data collection began with participant observation and field note taking of initial conversations with five TCM practitioners at their offices across Ontario. During these meetings, they showed me how acupuncture worked as a TCM treatment by targeting specific body meridians outlined on medical mannequins. I also had the opportunity to observe and discuss with them about the various TCM herbal remedies that were packaged in pill form within sealed bottles resembling pharmaceuticals, and which were sold in their offices.

Additionally, I conducted in-depth, open-ended interviews with a total of 15 TCM practitioners in each province, who were recruited from personal and professional connections as well as via snowball sampling. Prior to meeting and interviewing the practitioners individually in their homes, offices, or public venues (restaurants, coffee shops), I sent them a detailed copy of my research protocol, including its ethical clearance from my university, as well as a tentative list of research questions in three main areas: background training and experience, individual descriptions and meanings of 'evidence', and types of scientific and non-scientific evidence used in TCM practices.

All of the practitioners in my research were ethnically Chinese, ranged in age from early 40s to late 50s, were originally trained in mainland China and had been in Canada between 10 and 25 years. They were selected for their extensive knowledge of and experience in TCM so that they could address complex questions about TCM evidence. Such questions may not have been possible to elicit from locally trained TCM practitioners whose training remains more limited in both scope and practice in comparison to those trained overseas. In Canada, TCM training is limited to private, non-degree, and non-university accredited institutions, offering two-, three-, or four-year diplomas in acupuncture or TCM, although some acupuncture courses are taught as elective courses at the university level. The first Canadian and the only publicly funded TCM training programme in an accredited community college was implemented in Toronto, Ontario, in the fall of 2016, offering a three-year diploma in TCM.

Because some of the participants are very well known in their respective TCM communities, their names have been changed to protect their identity. The stories that follow are mainly compiled from information gathered over several recorded interviews lasting one to several hours. The latter were transcribed verbatim and analysed for thematic content using NVivo, a qualitative software programme.

Engaging with Narratives of TCM Practitioners' Lived Experiences: Stories of Triumph and Ambivalence About TCM Evidence

All 30 participants interviewed were clinically trained in both TCM and biomedicine, being qualified to practise both modalities in mainland China prior to immigrating to Canada. In countries like China and

India, indigenous healing systems have long co-existed with biomedicine, sharing legitimacy and popularity. In China, TCM still provides significant healthcare for much of the population, especially in rural areas.

In their homeland, 17 of my participants had exclusively practised TCM, and the remaining 13 had primarily practised biomedicine as their main specialisations. In Canada, they can only practise TCM as they could not obtain medical licensing as foreign-trained physicians due to language and accreditation barriers. This situation has presented both opportunities as well as challenges. For example, Martha is a TCM practitioner with nearly 30 years of experience practising TCM in both her home and host countries. After graduating from a five-year programme in TCM, she found employment in a prestigious department of internal medicine at a local TCM university where she held teaching, research, and clinical responsibilities for four years prior to immigrating to Canada in the mid-1980s. In Canada, she furthered her studies in reproductive biology, earning a master's in science which enabled her to work as a researcher on gene therapy. She later left this position to develop her own school of TCM in Toronto, offering the first comprehensive TCM programme of its kind in Ontario. Despite many successful patient testimonials about her TCM treatments, she doesn't feel her skills are recognised in Canada because TCM is perceived as an alternative treatment rather than being fully integrated into the public healthcare system. She claims to have faced much criticism, scepticism, and disrespect about her work from biomedical practitioners who questioned the legitimacy of her treatment outcomes due to the absence of appropriate evidence bases. In the following section, she expresses candidly her second-class treatment as a TCM practitioner in Canada for being unable to demonstrate scientific evidence in her successful fertility treatments:

> Last week I gave a talk at a fertility clinic in downtown Toronto. I shared many successful stories of patient testimonials about their TCM treatments for fertility issues. I have several patients who got pregnant after many years of trying conventional methods, and they were more surprised when they found out they got pregnant the second time! They didn't think they could get pregnant so fast the second time! The fertility specialists however, were very sceptical about TCM. They kept asking me, 'Where's your proof?

Where are your articles? Where's your hard evidence? Where are your clinical trials?' Regardless of patient testimonials, and detailed philosophical explanations of *yin/yang*, they still dismissed me by claiming that my results were a mere coincidence, they were individual cases, and basically their question was 'where are your evidence bases?' I know there's some proof regarding acupuncture for fertility, which has been published in some articles, but I didn't want to argue with them ... Everything is evidence based, double-blinded clinical trials; you can't change people's mentality. I have a lot of patient testimonials—why not consider this as evidence? Even in biomedical journals, there are single case reports, why not TCM? It's unfair, these double standards, we're treated as second class.

Similar to many CAM studies (Coulter 2004; Hare 1993; Kelner and Wellman 1997; Siapush 1999; Thorpe 2008; Zhan 2009), my research has found that TCM practitioners working in Canadian settings are usually the last resort for treating challenging, chronic conditions unsuccessfully treated by biomedicine. Zhan (2009) has noted that TCM practitioners in North America are often sought out as 'miracle-making', which can backfire on them as shown in Martha's example, being dismissed by biomedical counterparts for merely providing coincidental results that cannot be substantiated by 'scientific evidence'. However, since TCM in Canada is not covered by public or most private health insurance plans, the TCM practitioners' credibility and economic survival in local settings mainly depend on word of mouth referrals from successfully treated patients.

Sam and Teresa are a husband and wife team of TCM practitioners who run their own TCM clinic in downtown Vancouver, BC, which they opened after immigrating to Canada about 16 years ago. Both were trained as (biomedical) physicians and TCM practitioners in China, but they specialised in TCM. By the time they arrived in BC in the early 2000s, TCM had become a regulated health profession, which meant that they were required to pass written and practical tests before practising TCM in that province. Both Sam and Teresa noted that being allowed to practise TCM only has proved beneficial because it enabled them to improve their skills, concentrating on one modality of care to treat mostly chronic cases. In their view, focusing on challenging health conditions has made it possible for them to develop a deeper appreciation for

TCM. As Teresa put it, 'we saw how Chinese medicine is better than Western medicine … Chinese medicine has a perfect foundation'. They cite numerous success stories in their current practice, which earned them more patient referrals, increasing their sense of pride and confidence in their work as TCM practitioners. Here is Sam's account of a major success story:

> We have a recent case, a 58-year-old woman with terminal lung cancer. She has a big tumor that spread to the liver, below the bronchial area, and spread to the bones. Western medicine doctors told her she had 2 or 3 months to live. It was also terminal for us. We told her we can do something, but it's not guaranteed. We gave her some herbs, acupuncture, and she's doing much better. The tumor is shrinking, there's no water in her lungs. She's taking other lung cancer medication, but 4 other patients like her who were taking the same medication, have all died…

Echoing other TCM practitioners interviewed, Sam acknowledged that different foundational principles underlie TCM and biomedicine, resulting in different approaches to diagnosis and treatment:

> Our theories have different foundations. TCM is more inductive. Before we have organs, there's *qi*, which you can't see. When it becomes a real problem, then we can see. Western medicine focuses mostly on what you see … For example, when your kidney functions are good, because 90% of functions are left, that's considered okay, you have only 10% damage. From 90% to 10%, it's a long time, your kidneys may be good for 5 to 10 years, so let's wait until it's really bad. In Chinese medicine, before blood test says you have a problem, Chinese medicine can see it. We fix it before it's too late. We can provide early detection and treatment before the problem appears…

As communicated earlier in this chapter, Sam suggests a major 'epistemic disunity' (Knorr Cetina 1999), that is, theoretical and methodological differences between TCM and biomedicine that lead to their respective use of different types of evidence to establish a clinical diagnosis and treatment programme. In his viewpoint, TCM has the preventative value of contributing to early detection of chronic health issues prior to biomedical standardised tests. The latter may detect conditions at an advanced stage, which can constrain effective treatment. Later in this chapter, Wayne expands on these differences in terms of TCM's capability to detect and address early 'functional' disorders before they manifest into chronic, potentially untreatable 'structural' disorders.

Similar to Sam and Teresa, Wayne was primarily trained as a clinician in TCM in China, who also trained as a researcher in molecular biology and physiology. He came to Canada in the early 1990s to pursue a post-doctoral fellowship in molecular biology and eventually settled in Toronto, working as a researcher at a Toronto public hospital. Unlike other TCM practitioners interviewed, Wayne combines both TCM and biomedicine in his research work that focuses on identifying active ingredients in Chinese herbs to treat cystic fibrosis. Here, he shares observations gained in over 20 years of research in Toronto that reveals incompatibilities and intersections between biomedical and TCM types of evidence for evaluating therapeutic efficacy:

> TCM is most effective as a prevention method … Structural disorders like cancer for example, always come after functional disorders. When the body goes wrong, the first reaction is your functional disorder. This cannot show in standardised tests like urine, blood, medical imaging, however it can be told by patients' feelings, patients feeling uncomfortable, tired, frustrated, and doctors usually don't pay enough attention to this unless they find something solid, or what they call hard evidence. I would say, medical data can be half soft data, something you can describe but cannot show such as through patients' feelings, pulse diagnosis, looking at a person's vitality, all these are very important. Hard data, you can see through the number of blood pressure, x-ray, etc. Soft data are very critical, they contain more information for TCM practice, but hard to standardise. You can tell how a functional disorder develops in an earlier stage, providing earlier detection than biomedicine. Take diabetes for example. It is diagnosed by biomedicine only when the sugar level is high. TCM can make an earlier diagnosis based on someone's taste, appetite, feeling of thirst, and can provide treatment before the disease appears…

Wayne's insights and familiarity with TCM and biomedicine demonstrate his ability to comfortably navigate both medical worlds, appreciating what each approach can offer, unlike Sam and Teresa who are clearly partial to TCM. Nonetheless, these three practitioners' narratives imply that TCM's higher effectiveness is based on its unique foundation.

My previous research (Ning 1997, 2008, 2013), which showed that many TCM practitioners assert the legitimacy of their TCM practices by biomedicalising their practices, has not fully held in my latest findings. In the current Canadian settings, my interviews with TCM practitioners reveal more nuanced narratives about the evidence bases of their regular practices. The TCM practitioners in Canada use multiple types of legitimate evidence to justify their therapeutic practices in ways that often suggest the higher effectiveness of TCM over biomedicine. Brosnan (2016) has found similar ambivalences in her research with TCM academics in Australian universities. She describes how TCM academics follow a biomedical approach of RCT research to sustain TCM as an academic discipline and to enhance its legitimacy by producing mainstream forms of evidence. Yet, during their teaching activities, they engage with broader constructions of TCM evidence that includes both traditional knowledge and bioscience.

Epistemic Hybridity: TCM Practitioners' Constructions of Legitimate Types of TCM Evidence

In responses to my question—what constitutes appropriate TCM evidence to validate effectiveness and safety of their therapeutic practices?—many TCM practitioners resort to what Hobsbawm and Ranger (1983) have called the 'invention' of tradition. In particular, they emphasise the validity of unique experiential or 'soft' types of evidence that are inherent to the original philosophy of TCM and which they claim are equally compelling or even more reliable than the scientific or 'hard' evidence underlying biomedicine. In their perspective, TCM has its own epistemology, which may not befit the biomedical standards of evaluation based on RCTs. As Martha explains:

You have to understand, TCM did not come from test tubes, labs, molecular biology, chemistry, cell research—it was empirical, experimental, based on daily lives. It was the way people found out about medicine when they were searching for food, finding ways to fight against natural disasters, finding ways to fight against diseases, then TCM was discovered. TCM is empirical—do you believe in that or not? When people searched for food, they came across food that gave diarrhoea, yet some thought it might stimulate bowel movement in others. When it was too cold, you could take spicy food. When you press in certain points, it alleviates headaches, toothache—that's how meridians were discovered.

By declaring TCM's reliance on experiential, 'soft' evidence as a reflection of its unique philosophy and practice, some TCM practitioners specifically highlighted the positive attributes of what biomedical practitioners discount as 'non-scientific' evidence. One of them—Joanne, trained in both TCM and biomedicine in China—uses primarily acupuncture in her Vancouver-based practice. Acupuncture is compatible with most of her Canadian patients' preference to avoid potential hazardous interactions with biomedical interventions. It is generally believed to have no side effects if practised competently and is also one of the few TCM components that has successfully undergone RCTs for various conditions (Ernst 2000; Huang and Chen 2008; Isoyama et al. 2012; Rubin et al. 2012). Hence, Western audiences seem more inclined to use it. As Joanne maintains,

Not everything can show—spirit, energy ... [l]ike religion, you cannot show which one is good or better. But you can show that people are getting better. Isn't this enough evidence? We cannot show how energy moves, but we can show more people coming to see a TCM doctor. Most people have to pay; if it wasn't effective, they wouldn't come back. Even if they don't have any pain or other problems, many of my patients still want to do acupuncture once a month just to feel good.

The notion of what is visible/invisible is a recurring theme in the TCM practitioners' constructions of TCM knowledge-making to affirm differences between TCM and biomedical conceptualisations of the empirical world. In Teresa's words:

Chinese medicine has a perfect foundation, diagnosis and perfect treatment, but you can't see the energy when you do pulse readings, or apply
acupuncture needles, it is hard to learn to feel it [energy]. Authentic TCM
knowledge can only be learned with a few masters who pass their knowledge within certain families, and it's not passed through academic institutions. Today, only 30% of medical graduates in China practise TCM
because their knowledge is incomplete…

By emphasising TCM's focus on elusive energy, and what constitutes
'authentic' knowledge-making, I contend that Teresa is asserting the
validity of a 'tradition'—the use of empiricism and the art of training
with a master to legitimise a health profession with deeper historical roots
than biomedicine. 'Tradition' creates a sense of authenticity and ownership for TCM practitioners attempting to make 'objective' knowledge
claims. Understanding tradition as (re)invented (Hobsbawm and Ranger
1983) does not invalidate its authenticity or the right of a group or culture to claim it; rather it draws analytical attention to the processes of its
production and use (MacDonald 2008). Indeed, Zhan (2014) has argued
that the knowledge-making of TCM as 'experiential' served important
political interests in China in the 1950s to produce a 'TCM with two
fists', paired with biomedicine.

While the TCM practitioners in my research allude to differing notions
of the empirical in TCM and biomedical knowledge-making, a closer
examination of TCM's and biomedicine's foundations demonstrates that
the boundaries between them are more fluid than commonly thought.
Biomedicine and TCM are foundationally empirical. That is, they use
observation to explain or predict nature's phenomena. TCM uses experience to verify knowledge without constructing an ordered scientific system (Scheid 2002; Unschuld 1985). Biomedicine tends to discount the
'invisible' or elusive aspects of TCM that cannot be 'objectively' measured by scientific methods. However, Brown (1998), in studying the
shamanic beliefs of indigenous groups in Northeast Peru offers a different
insight into the intersecting worlds of traditional medicine and biomedicine. His study demonstrates that the indigenous groups accept that only
a shaman can see and remove 'spirit darts' as causes of disease during
healing rituals and that a similar logic underlies the reality of biomedicine

and of our trust in it, since many of us believe in viruses or bacteria that cause diseases, even though we cannot see them through the naked eye. Asked why TCM knowledge production is concentrated in the hands of a few masters who transmit it only within particular families rather than making it more publicly available, Teresa used an interesting analogy: 'As people say it, 1% of the population controls 90% of the wealth in the world...'. Indeed, most of the TCM practitioners interviewed confirmed that they must attend frequent professional development workshops offered by reputable TCM masters in order to continually upgrade their skills. Access to such exclusive knowledge is very costly, not only in Canadian settings when invited masters from mainland China provide guest lectures and demonstrations but also when the TCM practitioners must frequently travel back to mainland China to attend equally expensive workshops.

As can be seen through these ethnographic examples, 'epistemic disunity' (Knorr Cetina 1999) occurs within TCM itself and not only in relation to other health modalities. The TCM practitioners themselves are (re)producing hierarchies between 'authentic' TCM knowledge that is monopolised by limited individual masters and incomplete TCM knowledge that is produced in formal university settings where they undertook their training in China. As such, they are positing a hierarchy of value between more comprehensive TCM knowledge that is produced and transmitted by experienced masters and partial TCM knowledge that is produced in academic institutions. Thus, 'epistemic disunity' manifests intra-professionally (within TCM) and not only inter-professionally (between TCM and other health professions like biomedicine), beyond the confines of scientific evidence.

Interestingly, TCM's popularity in China is declining during the country's twenty-first-century economic boom, as cosmopolitan consumers now interpret it as a 'traditional' practice, less desirable than the 'modern' Western biomedicine (Karchmer 2010). The latter's association with the more prestigious symbols of science and technology is valorised over the traditional Chinese diagnostic practices, which rely strongly on sensorial experiences like touching, feeling, observing, smelling, and listening to patients' bodies. The current Chinese government is adopting Western biomedical standards for evaluating the safety, efficacy, and educational standards of all medical practice, thus overturning the long-standing prestigious place of TCM in Chinese history (Brosnan 2016; Karchmer 2010; Qiu 2007).

In effect, James and Marilyn, another husband and wife TCM team, specialising in the treatment of fertility issues in their two private TCM clinics in Vancouver and Richmond, BC, are sceptical about TCM's reliance on 'non-scientific' evidence. Both were primarily trained in biomedicine in China and subsequently obtained master's degrees in clinical immunology and molecular biology overseas.[4] Because they were unable to find research work in Canada due to language barriers and limited local experience, friends encouraged them to practise TCM without a licence, given that it was an unregulated profession in BC in the mid-1990s. James began refreshing his limited TCM training by working in a local Chinese herbal store and by observing his friends practising TCM. Meanwhile, Marilyn returned to China to sharpen her TCM skills and after four years in Canada, they opened their first TCM clinic in Vancouver. Despite their successful use of TCM in the treatment of male and female infertility in their Canadian clinics, James argues that the exclusive use of TCM in health care is insufficient because of its lack of 'scientific' evidence:

> Purely Chinese medical diagnosis is insufficient because it's not scientific. Sixty percent of my mind follows the Western medical model. When a patient comes with a problem, I still want to know the Western diagnosis. I ask them, did you see your family physician, what kind of lab work have you done? All this is very helpful. Even in purely TCM hospitals in China, they still use CT scans, ultrasounds, to diagnose problems. There's a lot of intersection in China. There, TCM relies on Western diagnostic tools to establish the best diagnosis.

Asked what constitutes 'enough evidence' of effectiveness in their TCM practices in the absence of scientific evidence, Marilyn responded:

> Patients' feelings—for example, if pain has improved after two or three [TCM] treatments. In the case of infertility, it is easy to demonstrate how our treatments are effective. …We check if sexual activity has improved … let's say, previously a patient only had sex once a week, but after treatments,

it increased to three times a week. We also do a pulse reading to check the *qi* rating, look at the colour of tongue, use acupuncture points to improve irregular menstrual periods.

Although James points to TCM's lack of scientific validity in diagnosis and treatment, both he and Marilyn have successfully used TCM to treat fertility issues. Just as conventional biomedical practitioners' scepticism of alternative health practices is shaped by the cultural lens of their bio-scientific training (Helman 2002), as Canadian TCM practitioners, and Chinese biomedical physicians, James' and Marilyn's practice of TCM is also influenced by Western scientific discourse. This tension between legitimising health practices through Western science ('hard evidence') or traditional medicine ('soft evidence') is continually played out in many TCM practitioners' interpretations of their work, especially as they engage with biomedically minded individuals who question their evidence bases for the purposes of evaluating their legitimacy within the mainstream health care system. However, in their everyday practices, this tension does not necessarily undermine their own confidence in treating patients, as they are often sought out to address chronic conditions unsuccessfully treated by biomedicine.

Beyond the Boundaries of Experiential and Scientific Evidence

While there appears to be justification for the biomedicalisation of contemporary TCM in local and global settings—namely, legal recognition and adherence to dominant scientific evidence bases (Brosnan 2016; Saks 1992; Scheid 2002; Ning 2008, 2013)—the conversations in this chapter paint a more complex picture. As these conversations illustrate, the reinterpretation of tradition to demonstrate TCM's effectiveness is juxtaposed with rejection and accommodation of biomedicine to explain the successful outcomes of TCM. Thus, *epistemic hybridity* more accurately describes the complex processes of TCM knowledge production and translation in which TCM practitioners negotiate the feasibility of multiple types of legitimate evidence.

Despite the strong direction by the current Chinese government and TCM practitioners like James and Marilyn to fit TCM into biomedical standards to ensure a rigorous approach in medical care, most TCM practitioners in my study agreed that a combination of experiential types of evidence that are inherent to the foundational knowledge of TCM and biomedical evidence bases provide the most compelling evidence to validate treatment outcomes. These findings confirm previous research that traditional knowledge and bioscience constitute TCM as a 'living tradition'— it retains a recognisable form, all the while adapting to advances in science (Brosnan 2016; Scheid and Lei 2014; Zhan 2014).

Martha, despite being a strong advocate of TCM's unique philosophy and experiential basis, agrees that combining biomedicine and TCM provides the most reliable methods to achieve proper diagnosis and treatment for any condition but especially for women's health issues:

Western diagnosis is very important, especially through regular physicals, scans. TCM is essential not to diagnose diseases, but to differentiate syndromes, to find the nature of the conditions, whether they are caused by heat, cold, dampness, dryness, and then which organ or meridian is obstructing the flow of energy … Differentiation is very important because individuals are different, constitutions are different, signs and symptoms are manifested differently … I wouldn't say that certain conditions are better treated by TCM alone, because people are different, there are many options, but some conditions can be better addressed with TCM because it's natural, less invasive, and these can be menstrual problems, menopause and fertility issues.

In turn, Wayne, who is comfortable navigating between the TCM and biomedical worlds, acknowledges the strengths and limitations of biomedical evidence bases and shares how TCM can effectively address genetic conditions like cystic fibrosis:

Evidence exists at different levels…. For example, what works at a molecular level may not work at a cellular level. What works at a cellular level, may not repeat in an animal level. And what works at an animal level, may not work at a human level. From a TCM perspective, we look at disease from different angles … TCM can compensate for a defective gene like in cystic fibrosis, by adjusting the body holistically. Western medicine discovered the defective gene in 1989, and after 25 years of research, there is still no cure ... patients are only offered antibiotics and physio. We can compensate for the defective gene by using existing TCM treatments for asthma ... By using acupuncture, herbal treatments, we can improve symptoms, and patients become more comfortable, their asthma is not as severe, their life span is prolonged. The usual life span for a CF patient is 20 years, but now we have patients who are 50 and still alive. We can't say we have the cure for the disease because of the defective gene, but we can help patients become a carrier of a mutant gene.[5] This is very good evidence that TCM is effective.

In biomedical reports of unsuccessful acupuncture treatments for several conditions like cardiovascular disease, chronic pain, infertility, among other issues, they often omit factors that extend beyond the singular applications of acupuncture prior to biomedical interventions (El-Toukhy and Khalaf 2009; Madaschi et al. 2010; Pastore et al. 2011). TCM, like many other CAM treatments, does not consider a therapeutic effect such as successful conception to rest on a single remedy (e.g., herb) or technique (e.g., acupuncture) but in an energetic system that comprises the patient, the prescribed treatment, the healer, and the treatment setting (Barry 2006: 2647). By engaging with synergistic evidence, observing, and adjusting to the entire healing situation, the TCM practitioners in this study account for broader factors beyond the physical body (e.g., lifestyle, vital energies, diet, environment) to address their patients' ailments. Since many also incorporate biomedical evidence bases into their regular practices, *epistemic hybridity* unveils their reliance upon more encompassing types of evidence, hence, illustrating the production and co-constitution of multiple *sciences* to validate treatment outcomes.

Conclusion

In conclusion, TCM practitioners in Canadian contexts construct evidence of effectiveness and safety of their practices by what I call *epistemic hybridity*. That is, in describing how and why TCM works, they refer to multiple epistemic frameworks of evidence. On the one hand, by integrating experiential and bio-scientific evidence as reliable sources of therapeutic effectiveness, TCM practitioners go beyond common boundaries that distinguish between TCM as experiential and biomedicine as scientific. *Epistemic hybridity* also sheds light on the production of TCM knowledge that entails incompatibilities and intersections with Western science, thus challenging a commonly held assumption that TCM's global expansion is essentially either driven by its production of scientific evidence *or* by active efforts to preserve its traditional knowledge.

On the other hand, the TCM practitioners' narratives presented here illustrate that theoretical and methodological differences exist within TCM itself and not only in relation to other practices. By declaring that 'authentic' TCM knowledge is mainly found among individual TCM masters rather than in academic settings, and by valorising broader definitions of evidence, the TCM practitioners also establish new hierarchies within TCM knowledge-making beyond the 'experiential/science' binary. In particular, a hierarchy of value is established between more comprehensive forms of knowledge that are concentrated in the hands of a few experienced masters and the partial knowledge that is allegedly produced in formal institutions. In addition to this, a hierarchy of value arises from privileging both traditional knowledge *and* bioscience as more appropriate forms of evidence in their therapeutic practices, rather than following closely a traditional *or* scientific approach.

In light of the more encompassing types of evidence that TCM practitioners count on to validate their treatment experiences beyond the confines of bio-scientific evidence bases, this chapter illuminates the relevance of multiple types of evidence that co-constitute diverse, yet equally valid, *sciences*. In the accounts of TCM practitioners, TCM knowledge systems are equally valid with their own internal logic that makes sense to those who partake in them. As such, my chapter calls for a more expanded conceptual framework to evaluate the evidence bases of any health modality that includes diverse ways of knowing and doing, rather than the current emphasis on a single biomedical epistemology.

Notes

1. In Canada, 'integrative healthcare' is a more recent and increasingly preferred term to describe a non-hierarchical, collaborative interaction between CAM and biomedicine that respects each other's unique epistemologies (theories and methods). In contrast, 'integrative medicine' presupposes a hierarchical relationship between diverse health practices, in which biomedicine co-opts other modalities (Boon et al. 2004).

2. Informal integration of CAM and biomedicine is visible in the diversity of health beliefs and practices within and across different societies—as part of the cultural traditions of certain groups, personal choice, or affordability—regardless of the dominant form of healthcare. At a formal level, different levels of integration of CAM modalities with biomedical care are also apparent worldwide. For example, Traditional Chinese Medicine (TCM) and East Indian Ayurvedic Medicine have long co-existed with biomedicine in the provision of mainstream health care, in their respective countries of origin. Even in Western countries like Italy, Germany, France, and England, where biomedicine is the dominant modality of health care, it is not ideologically bound against other health traditions such as humoralism and homeopathy (Hogle 1999; Payer 1990; Whitaker 2003).

3. My research entailed an initial 12 months of fieldwork in two distinct phases (August 2010–December 2011 and January–August 2012) with five TCM practitioners in British Columbia (BC) and five in Ontario (ON). Additionally, from June 2014 to August 2016, I engaged in field research with ten TCM practitioners in BC and ten in Ontario.

4. James received masters of science degrees in clinical immunology and molecular biology and Marilyn received her master's degree in molecular biology.

5. According to biomedicine, cystic fibrosis (CF) is caused by two copies of a mutated gene that a patient has inherited from both parents. In principle, a CF carrier does not have the disease but can pass it on to their offspring, if their partner is also a CF carrier. By citing the benefits of TCM treatment for CF, Wayne is suggesting that CF patients can potentially live long enough to be carriers of the disease, although they may not be cured from it.

References

Appadurai, A. (1996). *Modernity at large: Cultural dimensions of globalization.* Minneapolis: University of Minnesota Press.

Baer, H. (2008). The emergence of integrative medicine in Australia: The growing interest of biomedicine and nursing in complementary medicine in southern developed society. *Medical Anthropology Quarterly, 22*(1), 52–66.

Baer, H., & Coulter, I. (2008). Taking stock of integrative medicine: Broadening biomedicine or co-optation of complementary and alternative medicine? *Health and Sociology Review, 14*(4), 331–341.

Barnes, L. (2005). American acupuncture and efficacy: Meanings and their points of insertion. *Medical Anthropology Quarterly, 19*(3), 239–266.

Barry, C. (2006). The role of evidence in alternative medicine: Contrasting biomedical anthropological approaches. *Social Science and Medicine, 62*(11), 2646–2657.

Boon, H., Verhoef, M., O'Hara, D., Findlay, B., & Majid, N. (2004). Integrative healthcare: Arriving at a working definition. *Alternative Therapies, 10*(5), 48–56.

Broom, A., & Tovey, P. (2007). Therapeutic pluralism? Evidence, power and legitimacy in UK cancer services. *Sociology of Health and Illness, 29*(4), 551–569.

Brosnan, C. (2016). Epistemic cultures in complementary medicine: Knowledge-making in university departments of osteopathy and Chinese medicine. *Health Sociology Review, 25*(2), 171–186.

Brown, M. (1998). Dark side of the shaman. In P. Brown (Ed.), *Understanding and applying medical anthropology* (pp. 170–173). Mountain View, CA: Mayfield Publishing Company.

Coulter, I. (2004). Integration and paradigm clash: The practical difficulties of integrative medicine. In P. Tovey, J. Adams, & G. Easthope (Eds.), *The mainstreaming of complementary and alternative medicine: Studies in social context* (pp. 103–122). London: Routledge.

Coulter, I., Hilton, L., Ryan, G., Ellison, M., & Rhodes, H. (2008). Trials and tribulations on the road to implementing integrative medicine in a hospital setting. *Health Sociology Review, 17*(4), 368–384.

Daly, J. (2005). *Evidence-based medicine and the search for a science of clinical care.* Berkeley: University of California Press.

De Bruyn, T. (2001). Taking stock: Policy issues associated with complementary and alternative health care. In *Perspectives on complementary and alternative health care: A collection of papers prepared for Health Canada* (pp. 17–29). Ottawa: Health Canada.

Dean, K. (2004). The role of methods in maintaining orthodox beliefs in health research. *Social Science and Medicine, 58*(4), 675–685.

Denny, K. (1999). Evidence-based medicine and medical authority. *Journal of Medical Humanities, 20*(4), 247–263.

Dew, K., Plumridge, E., Stubbe, M., Dowell, T., Macdonald, L., & Major, G. (2008). "You just got to eat healthy": The topic of CAM in the general practice consultation. *Health Sociology Review, 17*(4), 396–409.

El-Toukhy, T., & Khalaf, Y. (2009). The impact of acupuncture on assisted reproductive technology outcome. *Current Opinion in Obstetrics and Gynaecology, 21*(3), 240–246.

Ernst, E. (Ed.). (2000). *Herbal medicine: A concise overview for professionals.* Oxford: Butterworth-Heineman.

Farquhar, J. (1994). *Knowing practice: The clinical encounter in Chinese medicine.* Boulder, CO: Westview Press.

Fries, C. (2008). Governing the health of the hybrid self: Integrative medicine, neoliberalism, and the shifting biopolitics of subjectivity. *Health Sociology Review, 17*(4), 353–367.

Fries, C. (2013). Self-care and complementary and alternative medicine as care for the self: An embodied basis for distinction. *Health Sociology Review, 22*(1), 37–51.

Gale, N. (2011). From body-talk to body-stories: Body work in complementary and alternative medicine. *Sociology of Health & Illness, 33*(2), 237–251.

Gale, N. (2014). The sociology of traditional, complementary and alternative medicine. *Sociology Compass, 8*(6), 805–822.

Givati, A. (2015). Performing "pragmatic holism": Professionalisation and the holistic discourse of non-medically qualified acupuncturists and homeopaths in the United Kingdom. *Health, 19*(1), 34–50.

Givati, A., & Hatton, K. (2015). Traditional acupuncturists and higher education in Britain: The dual, paradoxical impact of biomedical alignment on the holistic view. *Social Science and Medicine, 131*, 173–180.

Hampshire, K., & Owusu, S. (2013). Grandfathers, Google, and dreams: Medical pluralism, globalization and new healing encounters in Ghana. *Medical Anthropology, 32*(3), 247–265.

Hare, M. (1993). The emergence of an urban U.S. Chinese medicine. *Medical Anthropology Quarterly, 7*(1), 30–49.

Helman, C. (2002). *Culture, health and illness* (5th ed.). Oxford: Butterworth and Heineman.

Hobsbawm, E., & Ranger, T. (1983). *The invention of tradition.* Cambridge: Cambridge University Press.

Hogle, L. (1999). *Recovering the nation's body: Cultural memory, medicine and the politics of redemption.* New Jersey: Rutgers University Press.

Hollenberg, D. (2006). Uncharted ground: Patterns of professional interaction among complementary/alternative and biomedical practitioners in integrative health care settings. *Social Science and Medicine, 62*(3), 731–744.

Hollenberg, D., & Muzzin, L. (2010). Epistemological challenges to integrative medicine: An anti-colonial perspective on the combination of complementary/alternative medicine with biomedicine. *Health Sociology Review, 19*(1), 34–56.

Huang, S., & Chen, A. (2008). Traditional Chinese medicine and infertility. *Current Opinion in Obstetrics and Gynaecology, 20*(3), 211–215.

Iedema, R., & Veljanova, I. (2013). Lifestyle science: Self-healing, co-production and DIY. *Health Sociology Review, 22*(1), 2–7.

Ijaz, N., Boon, H., Muzzin, L., & Welsh, S. (2016). State risk discourse and the regulatory preservation of traditional medicine knowledge: The case of acupuncture in Ontario, Canada. *Social Science and Medicine, 170,* 97–105.

Isoyama, D., Cordts, E., van Niewegen, A., Carvalho, W., Matsumura, S., & Barbosa, C. (2012). Effect of acupuncture on symptoms of anxiety in women undergoing in vitro fertilization: A prospective randomized controlled study. *Acupuncture in Medicine, 30*(2), 85–88.

Karchmer, E. (2010). Chinese medicine in action: On the postcoloniality of medical practice in China. *Medical Anthropology, 29*(3), 226–252.

Kelner, M., & Wellman, B. (1997). Health care and consumer choice: Medical and alternative therapies. *Social Science and Medicine, 45*(2), 203–212.

Kelner, M., & Wellman, B. (2000). Introduction: Complementary and alternative medicine: Challenge and change. In M. Kelner, B. Wellman, B. Pescosolido, & M. Saks (Eds.), *Complementary and alternative medicine: Challenge and change.* Australia: Harwood Academic Publishers.

Kelner, M., & Wellman, B. (2014). Introduction: Complementary and alternative medicine: Challenge and change. In M. Kelner, B. Wellman, B. Pescosolido, & M. Saks (Eds.), *Complementary and alternative medicine: Challenge and change* (pp. 1–24). New York: Routledge.

Khan, S. (2006). Systems of medicine and nationalist discourse in India: Towards "new horizons" in medical anthropology and history. *Social Science and Medicine, 62*(11), 2786–2797.

Knorr Cetina, K. (1999). *Epistemic cultures: How the sciences make knowledge.* Cambridge, MA: Harvard University Press.

MacDonald, M. (2008). *At work in the field of birth: Midwifery narratives of nature, tradition and home.* Nashville: Vanderbilt University Press.

Madaschi, C., Braga, D., Figueira, R., Iacorelli, A., & Borges, E., Jr. (2010). Effect of acupuncture on assisted reproductive treatment outcomes. *Acupuncture in Medicine, 28*(4), 180–184.

McClean, S. (2003). Doctoring the spirit: Exploring the use and meaning of mimicry and parody at a healing Centre in the North of England. *Health, 7*(4), 483–500.

Ning, A. (1997). Regulating health professions and Chinese medicine in Ontario. In R. Andersen, J. T. H. Connor, & J. K. Crellin (Eds.), *Alternative health care in Canada: Nineteenth and twentieth-century perspectives* (pp. 231–241). Toronto: Canadian Scholars' Press.

Ning, A. (2008). Paradoxes of integrative health care: The question of legitimate evidence bases. *International Journal of Diversity in Organizations, Communities and Nations, 7*(6), 237–248.

Ning, A. (2013). How "alternative" is CAM? Rethinking conventional dichotomies between biomedicine and complementary/alternative medicine. *Health, 17*(2), 135–158.

Obadia, L. (2007). The economies of health in Western Buddhism: A case study of a Tibetan Buddhist group in France. In D. Wood (Ed.), *Economics of health and wellness: Anthropological perspectives* (Vol. 26, pp. 227–259).

Pastore, L., Williams, C., Jenkins, J., & Patrie, J. (2011). True and sham acupuncture produced similar frequency of ovulation and improved lh to fsh ratio in women with polycystic ovary syndrome. *The Journal of Clinical Endocrinology and Metabolism, 96*(10), 3143–3150.

Payer, L. (1990). Borderline cases: How medical practices reflects national culture. *The Sciences, 30*(4), 38–42.

Qiu, J. (2007). China plans to modernize traditional medicine. *Nature, 446,* 590–591.

Quah, S. (2008). In pursuit of health: Pragmatic acculturation in everyday life. *Health Sociology Review, 17*(4), 419–422.

Rappolt, S. (1997). Clinical guidelines and the fate of medical autonomy in Ontario. *Social Science and Medicine, 44*(7), 977–987.

Rubin, L., Opsahl, M., & Ackerman, D. (2012). Acupuncture improves in vitro fertilization live birth outcomes: A retrospective chart review. *BMC Complementary and Alternative Medicine, 12*(Suppl. 1), 71.

Saks, M. (1992). The paradox of incorporation: Acupuncture and the medical profession in modern Britain. In M. Saks (Ed.), *Alternative medicine in Britain* (pp. 183–200). Oxford: Clarendon Press.

Saks, M. (2003). *Orthodox and alternative medicine: Politics, professionalization and health care.* London: Sage.

Scheid, V. (2002). *Chinese medicine in contemporary China: Plurality and synthesis*. Durham, NC and London: Duke University Press.

Scheid, V., & Lei, S. H. L. (2014). Introduction. *East Asian Science, Technology and Society: An International Journal, 1*, 1–7.

Siapush, M. (1999). Why do people favour alternative medicine? *Australian and New Zealand Journal of Public Health, 23*(3), 266–271.

Tataryn, D., & Verhoef, M. (2001). Combining conventional, complementary and alternative health care: A vision of integration. In *Perspectives on complementary and alternative health care: A collection of papers prepared for health Canada* (pp. 87–109). Ottawa: Health Canada.

Thorpe, R. (2008). Integrating biomedical and CAM approaches: The experiences of people living with HIV/AIDS. *Health Sociology Review, 17*(4), 410–418.

Torri, C., & Hornosty, J. (2017). *Complementary, alternative, & traditional medicine: Prospects and challenges for women's reproductive health*. Toronto: Women's Press/Canadian Scholars.

Unschuld, P. (1985). *Medicine in China: A history of ideas*. Berkeley, CA: University of California Press.

Unschuld, P. (1992). Epistemological issues and changing legitimation: Traditional Chinese medicine in the 20th century. In C. Leslie & A. Young (Eds.), *Paths to Asian medical knowledge* (pp. 44–62). Berkeley, CA: University of California Press.

Verhoef, M., Lewith, G., Ritenbaugh, C., Boon, H., Fleishman, S., & Leis, A. (2005). Complementary and alternative medicine whole systems research: Beyond identification of inadequacies of the RCT. *Complementary Therapies in Medicine, 13*(3), 206–212.

Villanueva-Russell, Y. (2005). Evidence-based medicine and its implications for the profession of chiropractic. *Social Science and Medicine, 60*(3), 545–561.

Vincent, C., Furrnham, A., & Richardson, P. (1998). *Complementary medicine: A research perspective*. New York: John Wiley & Sons.

Whitaker, E. (2003). The idea of health: History, medical pluralism, and the management of the body in Emilia-Romagna, Italy. *Medical Anthropology Quarterly, 17*(3), 348–375.

Zhan, M. (2009). *Other-worldly: Making Chinese medicine through transnational frames*. Durham, NC: Duke University Press.

Zhan, M. (2014). The empirical as conceptual: Transdisciplinary engagements with an "Experiential Medicine". *Science, Technology, & Human Values, 39*(2), 236–263.

Ziguras, C. (2004). *Self-care: Embodiment, personal autonomy and the shaping of health consciousness*. New York, NY: Routledge.

11

Shaping of 'Embodied Expertise' in Alternative Medicine

Inge Kryger Pedersen and Charlotte Andreas Baarts

Introduction

The most recent representative National Health Interview Survey in Denmark (2013) estimates that 53.2 per cent of respondents are current or previous users of alternative medicine; 27.0 per cent have used such services within the preceding year, compared with 10.0 per cent in 1987 (Ekholm et al. 2015). Defined as treatment not usually offered within the ordinary health service and without public support or control, alternative medicine is offered on a fee-for-service basis by non-authorised practitioners with varying training and certification and is widespread in the Scandinavian welfare states and elsewhere. The overall question we tackle here is how to explain the widespread use of alternative medicine. This is a puzzle that we and other scholars have tried to solve. Explanations for the popularity of alternative medicine typically fall into two camps: societal or user-oriented (c.f., Pedersen 2012; Baarts and Pedersen 2009; Ziguras 2004). Another explanation relates to the development of

I. K. Pedersen (✉) • C. A. Baarts
Department of Sociology, University of Copenhagen,
Copenhagen, Denmark

© The Author(s) 2018
C. Brosnan et al. (eds.), *Complementary and Alternative Medicine*, Health,
Technology and Society, https://doi.org/10.1007/978-3-319-73939-7_11

diseases, in particular the increase in chronic diseases. Biomedical institutions have not been able to solve the problems of chronically ill patients and this impasse might have stimulated an increasing interest in what the expertise of alternative practitioners may have to offer. Indeed, in most studies of alternative medicine, practitioners and users address chronic ill health (e.g., Lee-Treweek 2002; Connor 2004; Sointu 2013). In this chapter, we will bypass such explanations and focus on the arrangements and conditions available in the practitioner-user encounter that allow for individuals' ailments to become the objects of alternative practitioners' labour.

In the absence of a consensus among scientific or health professionals on the basis for decision-making in alternative treatments, the distinction between lay and expert is sometimes blurred (Johannessen 2007; Gale 2011; Nissen 2013). The capacity of the therapies to stimulate collaboration between practitioners and users has contributed to multifaceted treatments, and users have themselves become the 'experts' in heterogeneous, context-specific dimensions of knowledge (Cant and Sharma 1999; Pedersen 2017). In a previous article we examined how users describe and construct practitioners' expertise in alternative treatments (Pedersen and Baarts 2010). Whereas that chapter explored how users ascribed legitimacy to the therapies and practitioners, in this chapter we revisit the empirical material in order to address which features develop embodied expertise in clinical encounters between practitioners and users. As such, this chapter focuses neither on the practitioners nor the users as so-called experts in their own fields of knowledge. Instead, we acknowledge the analytical shift suggested by the American sociologist Gil Eyal (2013) from investigating experts to researching expertise.

While Eyal has studied expertise as 'networks' that 'link together objects, actors, techniques, devices, and institutional and spatial arrangements' (Eyal 2013: 864), we aim to describe the relationships that comprise embodied expertise. Relationships include here what unites or differentiates human forces, such as client-practitioner encounters, as well as human and non-human forces, for example, practitioners and tools or spatial arrangements. Later we will demonstrate how 'embodied expertise' in alternative treatments is constructed. We first discuss the conceptual framework—the notion of embodied expertise and how it relates to alternative treatments. The next section 'Research material and methods' presents methodological considerations and describes the production of empirical material gathered from clinics of alternative medicine. We have organised the analysis of embodied expertise through discussions of three dimensions that have evolved from the empirical material: skills, knowledge, and spatiality. Demonstrating these dimensions by way of three relationships: (1) expert and lay, (2) experience and evidence-based knowledge, and (3) clinic and home, we show how embodied expertise of alternative medicine includes the practitioner's skills in a broader sense than certified knowledge; it does so by including experience-based knowledge and practice, as well as other actors, indeed the users, and objects that might not fall under biomedical knowledge.

Embodied Expertise

As Eyal has noted, 'expertise' derives from the Latin root *experiri*—that is, 'to try' and means know-how (Eyal 2013: 869). 'Profession' derives from the word for the vows or 'public declarations taken upon entering a religious order'; 'experts' make jurisdictional claims over a task 'by "professing" their disinterest, skill, and credibility', whereas 'expertise' covers 'the sheer *capacity* to accomplish this task better and faster' (Ibid.). Eyal argues that the latter definition of expertise, as presented by Collins and Evans (2002, 2007), for example, is 'unsatisfactory' because to evaluate skills and capacities involves the sociologist in playing the normative role when 'assigning differential worth to competing claims and performances' (Eyal 2013: 870). Therefore, he continues, it is not sufficient to focus on actors and their skills but necessary also to consider tools and devices, as well as their makers. Eyal also suggests that contributions by others, namely laypeople and 'the mechanisms by which their cooperation has been secured', should be included in a 'complex make-up of expertise' (Ibid.: 871). Thus, instead of focusing on a group of experts, he considers a network of relations 'that produces, reproduces, and disseminates expert statements or performances' (Ibid.: 875), which raises the question of what mechanisms secure the co-operation of the actors involved.

Eyal argues for contrasting and replacing the sociology of professions with that of expertise. Although we are not convinced by his argument (see also Abbott 1988 and 2005 for an ecological approach to analyses of professions), Eyal's notion of embodied expertise proves convenient for covering multifaceted practices within alternative medicine that are not solved or addressed by professions as such but open up contributions made by different actors for extending the capacity to solve or address tasks and problems. Eyal certainly distinguishes between understanding expertise and understanding treatment practices as a profession's monopoly and highlights expertise as practices that are co-produced. The understanding of expertise is 'extended via generosity and dialogue' (Ibid.: 876) different from professions' monopoly and autonomy, which may serve to weaken and prevent relations of expertise being extended.

According to Eyal (2013: 872) two important questions are central to an analysis of embodied expertise: (1) jurisdiction, that is, who has control and to what extent over a set of tasks and (2) expertise or what arrangements must be in place for a task to be accomplished. Through his work on the first question Abbott has contributed analyses and conceptual tools to allow insights into historical processes that show how jurisdictions become available and are formed (1988, 2005). Eyal has included the second question in a 'genealogy' of the autism epidemic and historical tracing of how a form of expertise is made. Although this chapter draws on these two questions, we will not focus on the historical processes of developing jurisdiction or expertise within alternative medicine, which is a multifaceted field. Neither can we outline here the conditions and arrangements that have been necessary for the popularity of alternative medicine to evolve. However, we touch upon the latter question when we approach alternative treatments in the Danish welfare state at the beginning of the twenty-first century.

In this chapter, we investigate how alternative treatments can be characterised by relational connections between practitioners and other experts, users, tools, concepts, and institutional and spatial arrangements. We attend to the relationships among relevant actors within the field of alternative medicine, such as users, practitioners, and medical doctors. Other relational connections include variations in understandings of validity or legitimate knowledge, emerging from, for example, therapeutic processes or evidence-based knowledge or from variations in spatial arrangements. The analytical object entails what constitutes formations of relational connections, that is: (1) What are the roles of the practitioners and users? (2) Which kind of knowledge is developed and involved in the practitioner-client encounter? (3) Which spatial arrangements are brought into play in clinics of alternative medicine? These empirical questions are addressed in the analysis and discussion section within three sets of relationships: (1) between expert and lay; (2) between experience and evidence-based knowledge; and (3) between clinic and home. In so doing, we will demonstrate how embodied expertise is composed of actors and arrangements and involves the co-construction of validity in the relationships.

Research Material and Methods

We refer to the science-based Western medical system as 'biomedicine', viewing biomedicine as 'a comparable cultural system' (Barry 2006: 2646). Instead of complementary and alternative medicine—CAM—we prefer the term 'alternative medicine' to highlight the philosophies that often underpin these systems of medicine. As Barry has put it, 'complementary' is 'often used in a relational sense to biomedicine and implies that the two systems are compatible' (Ibid.). The definition of alternative medicine in our introduction was used both in Danish law and in the National Health Interview Surveys in Denmark while we were doing our empirical studies. We have drawn on this definition when selecting clinics to be included in the study, and it allows for addressing alternative practitioners in a broader sense than as a 'profession' or as 'experts'.

We followed 46 users of acupuncture, reflexology, or mindfulness meditation, conducted three in-depth interviews with each participant (138 interviews), and observed 92 of the interviewees' treatment sessions. Our study was designed to reflect the wide variety in:

- the nature of the treatment (indirect touch [acupuncture], direct touch [reflexology], and cognitive techniques [mindfulness meditation]);
- the immediate reason for seeking alternative treatment (a broad spectrum of illnesses, ailments, problems, and challenges); and
- the age, gender, education, and employment of the participants.

The study was conducted from 2006 to 2007 in Copenhagen and adjoining municipalities and was reported to and acknowledged by the Regional Committee on Health Research Ethics and The Danish Data Protection Agency. Users attending reflexology, acupuncture, or mindfulness meditation were individually followed over six treatments and interviewed after the second, fourth, and sixth treatments. The interviews were supplemented by observations of the second and fourth treatments, aimed at gaining insight into the actual practice of the treatment, the users' reactions as treatment was carried out, and the kinds of advice and guidance given. In addition, users and practitioners were asked to keep diaries between treatments, and during the second interview, the interviewees filled in a questionnaire about their gender, age, family, education, and employment, as well as reasons for seeking alternative treatment. These additional sources are only used as background information in this chapter, where we focus on practitioner-user interactions and therapeutic situations, drawing predominantly on the interview data.

Recruitment was carried out with the help of representatives from the three treatments, each of whom suggested four or five registered practitioners within the Copenhagen area. Thus, the research team contacted 14 practitioners with varying training and certification but no state authorisation, and all agreed to participate. To ensure that the selection of users was appropriate, the representatives and practitioners co-operated with our research group in identifying certain selection criteria, such as users should be Danish-speaking adults who had sought out treatment on their own initiative. One concern was to ensure sufficient variation in the study population by involving a minimum of 15 users from each treatment. Moreover, the users should not have consulted other alternative practitioners within the last year, since as far as possible the experiences they reported should relate only to the particular treatment observed by the researchers during the study. At the first treatment, the reflexologists and acupuncturists each asked 15 users and the mindfulness meditation practitioners 16 users—in sum 46—if they agreed to participate. The users selected paid for their own treatments and differed in their immediate reason for seeking alternative treatment (illnesses, problems, or challenges), as well as age, gender, education, and employment. Participants were between 22 and 81 years. Thirty-two of the 46 were women

(70 per cent). The participants' age, gender, and education corresponded closely to those of participants in the Danish National Health Survey's population (2005) who stated that they had used alternative medicine within the preceding year. Women, persons aged 25–64, and those with 3–4 years of higher education predominated among the alternative medicine users in the survey population (Ekholm and Kjøller 2007).

The observations and most of the interviews took place at the practitioners' clinics. The interviews were semi-structured and followed on our prior observation of the treatment sessions. In particular, we encouraged users to comment on their bodily reactions and practitioners' handling of specific situations. All interviews were audio recorded, transcribed, and then coded in dimensions and categories with NVivo software. To protect privacy, we have not mentioned participant names. Insights from the studies were condensed based on ethnographic principles (Spradley 1979) and phenomenological analysis (Hycner 1999) to generate more generalised themes (Charmaz 2000). The accounts were analysed by both authors based on the agreed themes that emerged from the interviews. Interviewees' accounts selected for this chapter illustrate the theme of 'expertise' primarily mentioned by participants when asked about bodily experiences connected with specific treatments. The analytical approach to the accounts followed Michael (1996: 108) by focusing on the users' self-ascriptions of ignorance or lack of knowledge about the practice and 'outcomes' of alternative medicine. Through the selected accounts we aim to demonstrate how users articulate their experiences, justifications, and explanations.

How Embodied Expertise Is Shaped in Clinics of Alternative Medicine

In this section, we examine different markers for alternative medicine that define a kind of territory for treatment practice. The analysis is based on data from clinical settings with a focus on the informal arena that is the 'workplace', shaped by action and practice (Abbott 1988: 66–68), rather than on formal arenas that are public and legal (see instead Mizrachi and Shuval 2005). As Mizrachi and Shuval have noted, the territory of biomedicine is demarcated by its 'scientific infrastructure: laboratory experiments, a list of scientific methods used to establish causal relations and predictive power, on-going research, and the scientific ethos of skepticism' (2005: 1652), whereas alternative medicine often is portrayed as based on anecdotal evidence (Ibid., see also Saks 2001; Wahlberg 2007). Alternative medicine is, as Mizrachi and Shuval put it, 'placed outside the realm of diagnosis and treatment of "disease" (…) and focuses primarily on the patients' experience of "illness"' (2005: 1653). Yet session-based alternative medicine offers treatments by practitioners. In the first of three subsections that follows, *Between expert and lay*, we focus on which practitioner skills are appreciated by users in the alternative treatment process, also on tools, exchange, co-operation, dialogue, and concrete forms of reasoning. *Between experience and evidence-based knowledge* then addresses ambiguities observed among users when they evaluate their treatment course. Finally, *Between clinic and home* describes spatial arrangements that underline different ways of inviting users into clinics and shaping embodied expertise.

Between Expert and Lay

As the editors of this book note in their Introduction, alternative medicine is 'a contested space where legitimate science and knowledge are negotiated and given meanings' (p. 8). This is evident in our study where we observed and, together with practitioners and users, participated in different kinds of negotiations not only about legitimacy of knowledge and effects (cf. Baarts 2009) but also the meaning of attending alternative treatments. We understand these negotiations to reflect how constructions of embodied expertise in the clinics emerge through encounters between practitioners and users, as well as in interviews with us researchers. Such negotiations are necessary to users and practitioners because alternative treatments are not officially approved and state subsidised in Denmark, calling for other ways of legitimising their validity.

The absence of official recognition and the fact that sensations are not considered valid outcomes of treatments raise a question about who can be acknowledged as the expert in alternative medicine. In this context the practitioner who is trained in a specific treatment approach, and the user who is supposed to be actively involved in the treatment process and can describe bodily sensations as kinds of 'effects', may both be considered experts. Medical doctors and scholars may be the experts when assessing and testing the treatment effects, as may be politicians who refer to and decide on the basis of (lack of) evidence-based knowledge about such effects. What differentiates these experts from one another is the platform on which they ground their expert knowledge.

Practitioners of alternative medicine are sometimes certified and formally trained professionals and as such are not members of the lay public (Pedersen and Baarts 2010: 1072–1074; Brosnan 2015; Givati and Hatton 2015). A medical doctor who offers alternative therapies might formally be considered an expert when biomedicine is the high-status medical care and established form of treatment, as in Denmark and most Western countries. Despite the hegemony of biomedicine in the Danish healthcare system, formal training within the various fields of alternative medicine is also seen, at least within those fields and by some users, as a valid basis for constructing expertise. As one of the reflexology users says when suggesting formal training as the key to legitimacy: 'they [the practitioners] have a training in reflexology. Well, it should be brought together and organised in some way or another. And then there should be people in the approved system to approve it, right'.

In biomedical contexts, users of alternative medicine are sometimes reduced to 'passive victims' (Mizrachi and Shuval 2005: 1659; see also Beyerstein 2001). However, many social studies researchers describe users as active consumers. They attend alternative treatments on the 'grey' market and, at least in Denmark, pay out of their own pockets, whereas biomedical treatments are officially subsidised. When choosing among the many non-authorised treatments in the private market, users draw on widely different media, connections, networks, and resources. Under these circumstances the practical skills and educational status of the practitioner serve as signposts for users' judgements and choices. A reflexology user says: 'But I'm also very accepting of authority, as I can remember I also said to you the first time, that … [laughs] … I wouldn't have any doubts about it if one could get a referral from one's doctor…' An acupuncture user adds:

it suits me very well, as I said, that I know [the acupuncturist] also has a background as a trained medical doctor. That really suits me. I'm completely sure I know what she's doing and I feel I'm in competent professional hands. I feel really good about that. So that's really fine for me. I also feel that earlier on I would have asked somewhat more about what the things do. I don't have as many questions about things now. I have more faith that it works and can feel that it works. And that's fine for me. So I have confidence that she knows what she's up to in what she does.

In this sense users construct expertise not necessarily only as a form of 'doing', but also as a form of 'being', based on the practitioner's formal training or certification in a health-related field. Moreover, embodied expertise is constructed on the grounds of what users feel when receiving treatments. Users' ascriptions of expertise to the practitioner in the treatment process, however, show their desire or appreciation for him or her to focus on their experience of illness or ailments, pain and suffering, their feelings, well-being, efforts to improve their body's 'self-healing', as well as quality of life. In this study, particularly those users with chronic or terminal diseases approve of alternative medicine when seeking emotional support, whereas personal attention may not be offered to the same degree within conventional medical care (see also Mizrachi and Shuval 2005: 1653). Thus, all users appreciate practitioners offering personal attention and giving more time per patient than is possible in the public healthcare system.

Most of the alternative treatments involve more talking and touching than is often typical of biomedical treatments. These seem to be reassuring processes and several users in our study precisely appreciate their practitioner's voice and hands. A woman with abdominal muscle pains says:

I'm slightly uneasy in the sense that I don't know her [the reflexologist] that well—this is the second time I've been here. And [I'm] also a bit uneasy thinking: What's actually going to happen today? What does she actually do? Can I take it? This chair starts creaking at the slightest provocation! Things like that. But you also get used to that! But it's generally just certain small things. Your hearing is also incredibly vulnerable when you're lying on one of these beds. And she has a fantastically good voice. It's so firm and simple, and she also has fantastic hands, I mean, she's so good at it! (…) What I meant to say really was that I find my body relaxes.

Despite her uncertainty, the user still exclaims: 'she's so good at it!' This construction of competence is grounded in the user's judgement about the practitioner's 'fantastic hands' and her 'good voice' (see also Pedersen and Baarts 2010: 1070). These 'small things' make the user relax and act confidently. Other studies (e.g., Ong and Banks 2003; Lee-Treweek 2002) emphasise too the importance of practitioners' communication skills—in particular listening rather than talking and taking part in conversation (Pedersen 2014), as well as giving time to users—as shaping embodied expertise in alternative treatments.

Interviewees in our study sometimes turned to alternative medicine owing to a reluctance to ingest pharmaceuticals or undergo surgeries. Yet many people use an alternative practitioner while still receiving care from a medical doctor (e.g., Druss and Rosenheck 1999; Cant and Sharma 1999; Ni et al. 2002). In Denmark, The National Health Surveys indicate that more users than non-users of alternative medicine use conventional medicine (Ekholm and Kjøller 2007). Contrary to prevailing assumptions, the reasons for the growing interest in alternative medicine should not primarily be sought in a rejection of conventional medical treatment (e.g., Boon et al. 1999; Fadlon 2004). Scholars (e.g., Boon et al. 1999; Foote-Ardah 2004) have emphasised that the use of alternative medicine represents a health strategy through which individuals struggle to gain control over their situation. Moreover, as we have argued elsewhere, users' decisions to undergo alternative therapies also reflect new and more conscientious ways of living and imagining one's life and oneself in the future, all of which can be considered 'derivative benefits' of alternative treatments (Baarts and Pedersen 2009).

Users may also acknowledge their own responsibility for a successful alternative treatment, as one user expresses about the reflexologist: 'I have faith in what she's doing, and what points she's activating, that's her [business]. But I say to myself that the other thing [that's my business]—because there's a fair bit of psychological work to do as well!'. In this sense embodied expertise not only is constructed on behalf of the practitioner's competences and knowledge but also on the beliefs and attitudes of the user. To optimise treatment, users might also serve as their own experts, for example, by combining conventional and alternative medicine. This suggests a blurred division between laypersons and experts in the development of embodied expertise in alternative treatments.

Between Experience and Evidence-Based Knowledge

The institutional framing wherein practitioners are not officially authorised by the Danish healthcare system—and therefore 'alternative'—
reflects the age-old gap between conventional and alternative medicine
(Baarts 2009). Many trained alternative practitioners are organised in
associations eager to be accorded the same legitimacy as established biomedical professions. However, at least formally, biomedical discourse has
succeeded in securing its dominant position and has retained epistemological hegemony and institutional control. In the informal arena of the
clinics, users seem interested in concrete outcomes rather than abstract
knowledge and solutions. The users in our study did not incorporate
scientific judgements when framing their experiences of treatments.
They appreciated alternative practitioners not taking a 'one-size-fits-all'
approach to care.

Some users were sceptical at the beginning of the course, and many
wondered whether the treatments would work. After six treatment sessions, all but one user said about their bodily experiences that 'something'
was happening. As we have noted elsewhere (Baarts and Pedersen 2009;
Pedersen and Baarts 2010: 1070), these users became convinced of
positive benefits from alternative medicine, even when they were not
relieved of their symptoms or ailments. One of the reflexology users
explains:

> I had hoped that it [the pain] would disappear. That's why I came. But
> although it hasn't, I've at least got something else out of it. I didn't know it
> would be so nice. I would like to continue with reflexology once a month,
> but I don't expect to get rid of the pain problem.

The users experienced a diverse array of bodily sensations when undergoing treatments. A reflexology user says:

> These [reflexology treatments] have given me what I came for. Because I
> wanted to find out what kinds of tensions I'm walking around with, [ten-
> sions] that I've created in my body. I don't want to have these any more. And
> I've obtained an enormous understanding of what kinds of tensions these are.

A user participating in mindfulness meditation says: 'When I pause [am mindful] during an argument, I calm down, so I can get control over the nervous bodily sensations such as palpitations, sweat, and cold fingers'. The users consider such bodily sensations to be effects of the alternative treatments resulting in increased awareness and a sense of mastery. Although these sensations are real to the users, they originate in the encounters with the practitioners and alternative treatments. As such, these experiences develop from ongoing processes through which both users and practitioners construct embodied expertise based on their mutual encounters.

Regardless of the outcome, most users reported that they had achieved increased well-being through their treatment course. In interviews and diaries, they search for criteria other than evidence-based knowledge on which to build their belief in what they generally term 'successful outcomes'. The users were mainly pragmatic in their construction of practitioners' expertise, based on the commitments and predispositions available in the specific encounter, although most of those participating in our study valued formal training among the practitioners (Pedersen and Baarts 2010). For example, a woman suffering from cancer says: 'I definitely think it's obvious that the combination of having a professional medical angle—I'm not saying necessarily only a doctor—but having the security that people [alternative practitioners] have a knowledge of the physical … I mean how the skeleton is constructed, all those things'.

Differences in understandings of validity and acknowledgement of different forms of knowledge also can be traced to users who seek out alternative medicine. The ambiguities among users in our study did not directly reflect political or scientific controversies such as paradigmatic differences about validity but rather doubts concerning personal beliefs or convictions, which were either challenged or supported in their encounters with the practitioner. From the perspective of alternative medicine, the critique of the biomedical model has included its very restrictive view on therapeutic processes and measurement of effectiveness on reductionist notions (Broom and Tovey 2008: 30). Biomedicine has been viewed as strictly disease-centred, failing to acknowledge the implications of therapeutic processes on treatment and curing of patients. Although slogans such as 'the patient in focus' (*patienten i centrum*) have been part of healthcare discourse for decades in the Danish system, the biomedical model has not succeeded in changing the increasing popularity of alternative medicine. From a biomedical perspective, randomised controlled trials are often the most proper means of producing knowledge about 'effects', and alternative medicine, which represents other forms of knowledge production and treatment practices, has succeeded little in becoming an established form of knowledge. However, alternative medicine seems to have succeeded in being user-centred.

Between Clinic and Home

Alternative therapies' sites of treatment include private clinics and homes. Pedersen et al. have shown, by drawing on the present and two more studies, how the material setting is important in establishing trust in the practitioner-client encounter (2016: 51–52). Identifying with and valuing certain kinds and styles of decorations, furnishing, remedies, posters, and environment might differ among practitioners and users. The contextual and material settings frame the therapeutic practices: 'Clothing and interior decorations establish the practitioner in specific ways and draw on different sources of legitimacy, thereby "catering for" potentially different types of clients' (Pedersen et al. 2016: 51). Many users live with different kinds of ailments, many in worlds of pain, and are sensitive to the layout of clinics. One of this chapter's authors has in another paper described how users' homes also sometimes frame alternative treatments (Pedersen 2014: 52–54), depending, for example, on the user's condition. The feeling that space is populated with emotional experiences was noticed by some interviewees. Without being asked, some users described how they sensed the environs of the clinics, which made them relaxed and sure of the practitioner's capacity. Later in the chapter, one of the interviewees also comments on how incense-burning practitioners do not convey 'professionalism' to her.

The clinics in our study represented a continuum. Some were in modern buildings with dentist-like white paint and sparsely decorated with anatomical drawings of the human body; here, the practitioner dressed in a white coat and white clogs and used electronic equipment. In contrast, other clinics had colourful walls, seashells, flowery pictures, and meditative music in the background, with the practitioner dressed in colourful loose clothing, signalling a different basis for authority than in conventional medicine (Pedersen et al. 2016: 51).

Some users expressed a preference for clinics that were not 'too alternative' (see also Pedersen and Baarts 2010: 1072), including in their décor. For example, a user of reflexology emphasised that she felt comfortable and safe with a 'biomedical clinic look' that to her denoted efficiency and competence:

> I like it when the practitioner isn't the type that burns incense! In this clinic, it's kind of businesslike. That's what appeals to me (…) [The reflexologist] doesn't believe I need salvation, but acts professionally. And I appreciate professionalism. Here is a computer with a program designed for users. I like those kinds of things.

Some users however liked a more relaxed treatment setting, and another reflexology user found it relaxing and cosy if the clinic's decor did not mimic a conventional medical clinic and was modelled on a 'cosier' ('hyggelig') style with domestic touches. He said:

> you are drawn out of your everyday life and you come to these pleasant rooms. There's a pleasant atmosphere (…). A couch is in the middle of the room. You can see it's a practitioner's room. A poster is up there (…) with different kinds of breathings and so on, but it's not very clinical. It also seems cosy, like a cosy courtyard here in [the city], such a relaxed atmosphere, she's good at cooling you down.

The diverse material objects in the clinics, such as ointments and potions, occasional music, decorative objects, and dress code of the practitioners, were part and parcel of the therapeutic process itself. These material objects form an aspect of the treatment situation and reflect a kind of relational landscape, in this context an emotional and embodied one. The cultural geography perspective has indeed drawn attention to the material dimension of emotions (Davidson and Milligan 2004; Thrift 2004). For example, Lupton has noted that emotions 'take place within and around the body as it moves through space and interacts with other bodies and with objects' (2013: 639). We consider that the examples from our study illustrate research benefitting from an engagement with place and space to understand how the people-place relationship matters to attribution of 'professional' capacity.

Whereas evidence-based medicine seeks to ensure that clinical practice decisions are not contingent on practitioners' personal opinion and individual experience, alternative treatments are in general context-dependent and link knowledge to decision-making, mostly in collaboration with the user. Moreover, alternative practitioners and users seem to contend with how spatial surroundings shape bodies and vice versa. Scholars within the field of alternative medicine have suggested that more patient-centred and subjective understandings of validity should be recognised, including notions of well-being, healing, and achieving 'balance', thus, that patient needs may not easily be solved within the framework imposed by the biomedical model (Paterson et al. 2009). This field—and the sociological study of it—might be strengthened by eventually drawing on spatial tools of analysis currently being developed as spatial sociology emerges as a 'new field' (e.g., see the monograph issue of *Current Sociology*, Patel 2017).

Conclusion and Perspectives

Whereas evidence-based medicine and standardisation are crucial in helping to determine the effectiveness of caring and healing practice within biomedicine, alternative medicine is less rule-bound, non-authorised, and with no standard system of control or training of practitioners. Alternative medicine offers very limited scientific evidence but still acts as a popular health provider alongside the state in most countries. Based on qualitative research within three of the most popular forms of session-based alternative medicine in Denmark, this chapter has focused on dimensions of embodied expertise in alternative medicine and how these contribute to explaining its popularity.

Embodied expertise has been a neglected area in healthcare research of alternative medicine compared with, for example, studies of effects and effectiveness or patients' dissatisfaction with conventional healthcare. Drawing on a concept of expertise different from 'expert' and 'profession', the empirical findings in this chapter point to elements such as practitioners' and users' involvement, including listening and using all senses in treatments. As such, embodied expertise draws not only on (therapeutic) conversation and knowledge of anatomical and physiological data but also on contextual issues in the encounter between the practitioner and the user in clinics. Thus, we have explored embodied expertise by bringing into play various criteria other than the practitioner's skills. Drawing on our empirical material, we have suggested three pairs of relationships as markers for constructing embodied expertise in session-based alternative medicine. These markers refer to skills, knowledge and spatiality, and respectively concern the relationships between: (1) lay and expert; (2) experience and evidence-based medicine; and (3) home and clinic:

1. The boundaries between lay and expert are blurred. Co-operation between practitioner and user contributes to the construction of embodied expertise. Users are involved as responsible participants in their own healing, pain relief, self-development, or any other treatment goal.
2. Compared with the biomedical paradigm, alternative practitioners' expertise remains weak. No evidence-based knowledge exists for the effectiveness of the treatments discussed here. Nevertheless, users still find support for their construction of embodied expertise by relying on elements from biomedicine, such as when the alternative practitioner also holds a medical degree. Yet the success of alternative therapies is not due to their scientific or technical superiority but to social and bodily innovativeness.
3. The material setting as a framework for the therapeutic practice has been illustrated by clinics' décor, users' reflections, and the wish to be treated in private homes. These elements also demonstrate how forms of embodied expertise are constructed in alternative treatment clinics through spatial arrangements.

Although alternative practitioners' expertise cannot be legitimised when it comes to evidence-based knowledge and organisational power, their embodied expertise is powerful in securing and facilitating users' co-operation in treatment approaches. Mechanisms that secure the co-operation of users are activated by assumptions such as that the user knows more about his or her own dysfunctions or ailments than the practitioner, and the user might also know better on what to do about it. When users become experts on their own health, the lack of legitimacy of the alternative practitioner is less important.

The analysis has indicated that users of alternative medicine need 'care' and assistance in making choices and are not 'ordinary' consumers. They might need experts other than those who provide purely professional, technological, or scientific answers to their problems. The users do not need a 'cure' if their condition is chronic, but they may need to be 'capable' at home, in the workplace, and with friends and family. Common to alternative treatments is that they individualise the user, tailoring a unique treatment course to each user's deficits, strengths, and sensitivities. Different from the standard issue, the 'one-size-fits-all' mechanism, alternative medicine does not promote a common agenda for users. The goal of treatment is co-produced with the individual user, and the practitioners as users are taught to view themselves and their bodies as self-healing. This may facilitate hope for users that healing is possible, perhaps also contributing to the popularity of alternative medicine. Finally, the target of treatment is not so much the particular disease as the skills to be acquired and the concrete behaviours to be modified to provide pain relief, self-development, well-being, quality of life, or tools and practices for living with a chronic disease.

Surveys tell us that not only in Denmark but in many Western countries alternative medicine has become a mainstream health commodity since the 1970s. Its popularity, along with public health concerns about health promotion and prevention of chronic diseases, has led to political interest, albeit scattered, in alternative treatments as a medical system. Paradoxically, as health policy has encouraged patients to assume a more prominent role in care, many people have taken on this role by opting for alternative medicine. However, the burden of care does not seem to have shifted from the subsidised public healthcare system to active, self-managing citizens. Users of alternative medicine do not necessarily portray conventional treatment as something to be avoided. Rather, in exploring various expert systems and technologies for curing disease and enhancing health, they are 'hunting' for different solutions to, and perhaps also meaning in, a range of problems.

Although in recent decades anthropologists, sociologists, and scholars within cognate social sciences and humanities have contributed increasing studies of alternative medicine, we need more knowledge about how the growing power of patients as consumers, and people seeking care, is playing a role in legitimising alternative medicine. Moreover, the effectiveness of alternative treatments and the role of alternative practitioners are issues of scientific complexity and conflicting interests. They are also issues of uncertainty, in which the risks perceived by various actors are affected by different claims about the truth of alternative treatments (e.g., Coward 1989; Sered and Agigian 2008; Pedersen 2013). For these reasons we scholars should be careful not to focus exclusively on the informal arena or the clinics—although we still need more systematical knowledge about this informal arena to study external linkages such as professional knowledge and networks and health policy(making). Here approaches such as Abbott's (1988, 2005) and Eyal's (2013) are important and should be developed, alongside the Science and Technology Studies-informed approaches to knowledge production included in this volume.

References

Abbott, A. (1988). *The system of professions: An essay on the division of expert labor.* Chicago: University of Chicago Press.

Abbott, A. (2005). Linked ecologies: States and universities as environments for professions. *Sociological Theory, 23*(3), 245–274.

Baarts, C. (2009). Stuck in the middle: Research ethics caught between science and politics. *Qualitative Research, 9*(4), 1–17.

Baarts, C., & Pedersen, I. K. (2009). Derivative benefits: Exploring the body through complementary and alternative medicine. *Sociology of Health & Illness, 31*(5), 719–733.

Barry, C. A. (2006). The role of evidence in alternative medicine: Contrasting biomedical and anthropological approaches. *Social Science & Medicine, 62*(11), 2646–2657.

Beyerstein, B. L. (2001). Alternative medicine and common errors of reasoning. *Academic Medicine, 76*(3), 230–237.

Boon, H., Brown, J. B., Gavin, A., Kennard, M. A., & Stewart, M. (1999). Breast cancer survivors' perceptions of complementary/alternative medicine (CAM): Making the decision to use or not to use. *Qualitative Health Research, 9*(5), 639–653.

Broom, A., & Tovey, P. (2008). *Therapeutic pluralism: Exploring the experiences of cancer patients and professionals.* London: Routledge.

Brosnan, C. (2015). "Quackery" in the academy? Professional knowledge, autonomy and the debate over complementary medicine degrees. *Sociology, 49*(6), 1047–1064.

Cant, S., & Sharma, U. (1999). *A new medical pluralism? Alternative medicine, doctors, patients and the state.* London: UCL Press.

Charmaz, K. (2000). Grounded theory: Objectivist and constructivist methods. In N. K. Denzin & Y. S. Lincoln (Eds.), *Handbook of qualitative research* (pp. 509–535). Thousand Oaks, CA: Sage.

Collins, H. M., & Evans, R. (2002). The third wave of science studies: Studies of expertise and experience. *Social Studies of Science, 32*(2), 235–296.

Collins, H. M., & Evans, R. (2007). *Rethinking expertise.* Chicago: University of Chicago Press.

Connor, L. H. (2004). Relief, risk and renewal: Mixed therapy regimens in an Australian suburb. *Social Science & Medicine, 59*(8), 1695–1705.

Coward, R. (1989). *The whole truth: The myth of alternative health.* London: Faber.

Davidson, J., & Milligan, C. (2004). Embodying emotion sensing space: Introducing emotional geographies. *Social & Cultural Geography, 5*(4), 523–532.

Druss, B. G., & Rosenheck, R. A. (1999). Association between use of unconventional therapies and conventional medical services. *JAMA, 282*(7), 651–656.

Ekholm, O., Christensen, A. I., Davidsen, M., & Juel, K. (2015). *Alternativ behandling. Resultater fra Sundheds- og sygelighedsundersøgelsen.* Copenhagen: SIF, Syddansk Universitet.

Ekholm, O., & Kjøller, M. (2007). Brugen af alternativ behandling i Danmark: resultater fra den nationalt repræsentative Sundheds- og sygelighedsundersøgelse 2005. *Tidsskrift for Forskning i Sygdom og Samfund, 6,* 15–24.

Eyal, G. (2013). For a sociology of expertise: The social origins of the autism epidemic. *American Journal of Sociology, 118*(4), 863–907.

Fadlon, J. (2004). Meridians, chakras and psycho-neuro-immunology: The dematerializing body and the domestication of alternative medicine. *Body & Society, 10*(4), 69–86.

Foote-Ardah, C. E. (2004). Sociocultural barriers to the use of complementary and alternative medicine for HIV. *Qualitative Health Research, 14*(5), 593–611.

Gale, N. K. (2011). From body-talk to body-stories: Body work in complementary and alternative medicine. *Sociology of Health & Illness, 33*(2), 237–251.

Givati, A., & Hatton, K. (2015). Traditional acupuncturists and higher education in Britain: The dual, paradoxical impact of biomedical alignment on the holistic view. *Social Science & Medicine, 131*, 173–180.

Hycner, R. H. (1999). Some guidelines for the phenomenological analysis of interview data. In A. Bryman & R. Burgess (Eds.), *Qualitative research* (Vol. III, pp. 143–164). London: Sage Publications.

Johannessen, H. (2007). Body praxis and the networks of powers. *Anthropology & Medicine, 13*(3), 267–278.

Lee-Treweek, G. (2002). Trust in complementary medicine: The case of cranial osteopathy. *The Sociological Review, 50*(1), 48–68.

Lupton, D. (2013). Risk and emotion: Towards an alternative theoretical perspective. *Health, Risk & Society, 15*(8), 634–647.

Michael, M. (1996). Ignoring science: Discourses of ignorance in the public understanding of science. In A. Irwin & B. Wynne (Eds.), *Misunderstanding science? The public reconstruction of science and technology* (pp. 107–125). Cambridge: Cambridge University Press.

Mizrachi, N., & Shuval, J. T. (2005). Between formal and enacted policy: Changing the contours of boundaries. *Social Science & Medicine, 60*(7), 1649–1660.

Ni, H., Simile, C., & Hardy, A. M. (2002). Utilization of complementary and alternative medicine by United States adults: Results from the 1999 national health interview survey. *Medical Care, 40*(4), 335–358.

Nissen, N. (2013). Women's bodies and women's lives in western herbal medicine in the UK. *Medical Anthropology: Cross-Cultural Studies in Health and Illness, 32*(1), 75–91.

Ong, C. K., & Banks, B. (2003). *Complementary and alternative medicine: The consumer perspective*. London: The Prince of Wales's Foundation for Integrated Health.

Patel, S. (Ed.). (2017). Spatial sociology: Relational space after the turn. *Current Sociology*, Monograph 2, 65(4).

Paterson, C., Baarts, C., Launsø, L., & Verhoef, M. (2009). Evaluating complex health interventions: A critical analysis of the 'outcomes' concept. *BMC Complementary and Alternative Medicine, 9*(1), 1–11.

Pedersen, I. K. (2012). *Kampen med kroppen. Alternativ behandling i et bruger- og samfundsperspektiv* [The Body in Borderland: Alternative Medicine in a Societal and Users' Perspective]. Aarhus: Aarhus Universitetsforlag.

Pedersen, I. K. (2013). 'It can do no harm': Body maintenance and modification in alternative medicine acknowledged as a non-risk health regimen. *Social Science & Medicine, 90*, 56–62.

Pedersen, I. K. (2014). Lytninger i alternativ behandling – en fænomenologisk analyse [Listenings in session-based alternative medicine: A phenomenological analysis]. *Tidsskriftet Antropologi, 69*, 45–63.

Pedersen, I. K. (2017, October 14). Striving for self-improvement: Alternative medicine considered as technologies of enhancement. *Social Theory & Health*. https://doi.org/10.1057/s41285-017-0052-3.

Pedersen, I. K., & Baarts, C. (2010). 'Fantastic hands' – But no evidence: The construction of expertise by users of CAM. *Social Science & Medicine, 71*(6), 1068–1075.

Pedersen, I. K., Hansen, V. H., & Grünenberg, K. (2016). The emergence of trust in clinics of alternative medicine. *Sociology of Health & Illness, 38*(1), 43–57.

Saks, M. (2001). Alternative medicine and the health care division of labour: Present trends and future prospects. *Current Sociology, 49*(3), 119–134.

Sered, S., & Agigian, A. (2008). Holistic sickening: Breast cancer and the discursive worlds of complementary and alternative practitioners. *Sociology of Health and Illness, 30*(4), 616–631.

Sointu, E. (2013). Complementary and alternative medicines, embodied subjectivity and experiences of healing. *Health, 17*(5), 530–545.

Spradley, J. P. (1979). *The ethnographic interview*. Orlando: Harcourt Brace Jovanovich College Publishers.

Thrift, N. (2004). Intensities of feeling: Towards a spatial politics of affect. *Geografiska Annaler, 86*(1), 57–78.

Wahlberg, A. (2007). A quackery with a difference: New medical pluralism and the problem of "dangerous practitioners" in the United Kingdom. *Social Science & Medicine, 65*(11), 2307–2326.

Ziguras, C. (2004). *Self-care: Embodiment, personal autonomy and the shaping of health consciousness*. London: Routledge.

12

Institutionalising the Medical Evaluation of CAM: Dietary and Herbal Supplements as a Peculiar Example of (Differential) Legitimisations of CAM in the USA

Geoffroy Carpier and Patrice Cohen

In our socio-anthropological research focusing on the federal institutionalisation of Complementary and Alternative Medicine (CAM) in the USA, we found that 'dietary and herbal supplements' (D/HS)[1] represented and still represent today a very relevant example of different and specific configurations of the medical evaluation of CAM. These products have benefitted from various processes of institutionalisation at the federal level since the 1990s and now face multiple scientific challenges in their evaluation.

In 1994, in order to 'protect the right of access of consumers to safe dietary supplements',[2] the Congress enacted the Dietary Supplement Health and Education Act (DSHEA) legally defining dietary supplements as:

a product … intended to supplement the diet that bears or contains one or more of the following dietary ingredients: (A) a vitamin; (B) a mineral;

G. Carpier (✉) • P. Cohen
Université de Rouen, Mont Saint Aignan, France

© The Author(s) 2018
C. Brosnan et al. (eds.), *Complementary and Alternative Medicine*, Health, Technology and Society, https://doi.org/10.1007/978-3-319-73939-7_12

(C) an herb or other botanical; (D) an amino acid; (E) a dietary supplement for use by man to supplement the diet by increasing the total dietary intake; or (F) a concentrate, metabolite, constituent, extract, or combination of any ingredient described in clause (A), (B), (C), (D), or (E). (sect. 3, DSHEA 1994)

Under this law, the Food and Drug Administration (FDA) regulates dietary supplements as 'food', exempting them a priori from the requirement of new drug approvals. Their medical evaluation has been the result of an original institutionalisation since the 1990s implemented through the creation of three federal entities in charge of medical research on CAM as part of the Department of Health and Human Services: the Office of Dietary Supplements (ODS, since 1995), the National Center for Complementary and Integrative Health (NCCIH, formerly the Office of Alternative Medicine from 1992 to 1998, and then the National Center for Complementary and Alternative Medicine, NCCAM, from 1998 to 2014), and the Office of Cancer CAM (OCCAM, since 1998) at the National Cancer Institute (NCI), all part of the National Institutes of Health (NIH). In the early 2000s, in collaboration with ODS, the National Institute of Standards and Technology (NIST) from the Department of Commerce joined this institutionalisation (Fig. 12.1).

Subsequent to surveys since the 1990s revealing the prevalent use of such D/HS among American CAM users,[3] these products have been part of the natural product branch of CAM as officially defined by these institutions in the USA.[4] The definition and categorisation of D/HS as CAM by those federal entities brought with it specific configurations of medical research on those products.

Based on an ethnographic approach[5] to studying this institutionalisation of CAM in the USA through these federal entities (2014–2017), this chapter explores various processes in the medical evaluation of D/HS, oriented towards various diseases (including cancer). Because D/HS are categorised as CAM by them, we have considered the emic terminology of CAM as many historical, social, and political characteristics of the legitimisations at stake (Jütte 2001). We focused our investigation

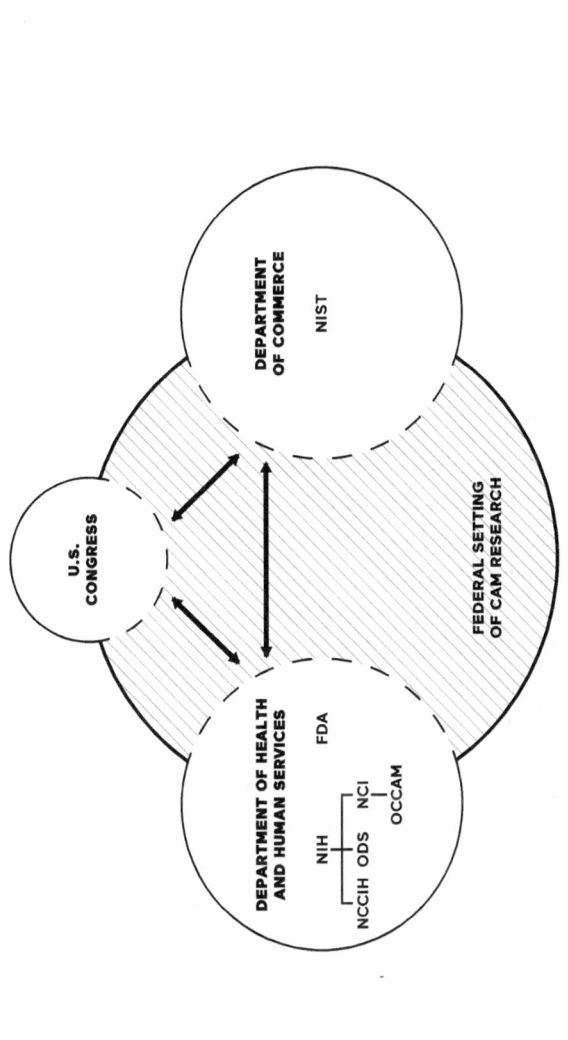

Fig. 12.1 Main federal institutions participating in the federal setting of CAM research

NIH: NATIONAL INSTITUTES OF HEALTH

NCCIH: NATIONAL CENTER FOR COMPLEMENTARY & INTEGRATIVE HEALTH

OCCAM: OFFICE OF CANCER COMPLEMENTARY & ALTERNATIVE MEDICINE

FDA: FOOD AND DRUG ADMINISTRATION

ODS: OFFICE OF DIETARY SUPPLEMENTS

NIST: NATIONAL INSTITUTE OF STANDARDS & TECHNOLOGY

NCI: NATIONAL CANCER INSTITUTE

on both non-State and State institutions in medical research on CAM. We have studied how negotiations are built up among institutional and individual agents all together enshrined in specific time and space contexts. In fact, this mixed social space of medical research on CAM is occupied by a plurality of individual and institutional agents (and their network of interactions) that we met with during the course of our research, for the most part, including, federal institutions that we mentioned earlier, non-federal institutions (such as clinical centres, universities, research laboratories, patient associations), researchers from various medical disciplines (such as biochemistry, oncology, pharmacology, family medicine), patient advocates, medical practitioners, and CAM practitioners. A specific investigation on different sources[6] is used here to make more explicit the context of ethnographic interviews and observations.[7] For the sake of clarity, we will refer to archival and fieldwork sources ((s)) as follow in the endnotes: (name, date) (s).

Considering some specific cases of very well-known D/HS, it is mostly through specific scientific controversies that we will outline the construction of different medical evaluations of CAM efficacy, safety, standardisation, and integration. We will borrow analytical tools from different sociological traditions, between constructivism and interactionism, such as the sociology of institutions (Offerlé and Lagroye 2011; Fuselier and Marquis 2009; Dubet 2002) and the interactionist school (Strauss 1978; Baszanger 1986). Those negotiations about what are the most relevant protocols in addressing CAM efficacy and safety reveal competitions over the places assigned to CAM in the broader health system around terms such as 'alternative', 'complementary', and 'integrative'. Section 1 outlines how D/HS are defined by and caught in different institutional articulations between the FDA, NIH, and other institutions, around ideas of safety and efficacy, via analysis of controversies surrounding Ephedra. Through the specific case of a controversial D/HS for cancer, Section 2 shows how D/HS represented challenges for CAM research concerning the definition of D/HS and for the structure within which research on D/HS is framed, and Section 3 shows how both examples revolve around the development of new research standards.

Efficacy and Safety of Dietary and Herbal Supplements: The Controversial Case of Ephedra

The DSHEA (1994) establishes a particular legal status for D/HS. In contrast with the new conventional drugs, their constraining legislative measures framing market approvals are not built upon the same basis. The FDA requires conventional drugs to have proven both their efficacy and their safety before being released on the market, notably by implementing randomised control trials (RCTs) (Bothwell and Podolsky 2016; Meldrum 2000).[8] D/HS are governed by a hybrid regime sliding almost in between food and drugs (Chen 2009: 79–91). D/HS manufacturers are only required by the FDA to evaluate the identity, composition, and strength of their D/HS. Such requirements are not aimed at demonstrating D/HS efficacy and safety. In fact, like food, the proof of their efficacy is not required, and the proof of their safety is not produced a priori, as for conventional drugs, but a posteriori, after their release on the market.[9] Specific legal regulations provide a framework around what manufacturers can and cannot write on the label and on other advertising presenting their specific D/HS on the market. Thus, any therapeutic claim of a potential curative, preventive, or diagnostic benefit for a specific disease on the label will make a D/HS fall into conventional drug regulations, putting it at risk of being considered by the FDA as a non-approved drug.[10] Manufacturers may provide general health information related to the D/HS they release on the market, such as addressing a nutrient deficiency, promoting or supporting health, or a specific body function. This hybrid regime, as we will see further, sums up the regulatory ambiguity into which D/HS falls, and to which federal and non-federal agents answer.

Facing the lenient regulation of D/HS by the FDA, different agents from our studied social space came to fill the regulatory void left by the DSHEA, which was sometimes considered by them as unduly permissive. The case of Ephedra[11] as a D/HS provides an illustrative example of two major questions regarding D/HS: their safety and efficacy. It then allows an understanding of the institutional controversies on this scientific debate—considered as a 'war', a 'scandal', or an 'important issue' by NIH agents and non-NIH researchers working on D/HS.

Chronology of the Ephedra Case: From Medical Concerns to the Ban of a D/HS

On 21 December 2000, in response to the enthusiasm towards the use of this plant or plant extracts by patients seeking weight loss, two medical doctors commissioned by the FDA and NIH analysed data collected by the FDA since 1999 and demonstrated that the use of Ephedra could be associated with risks of cardiovascular complications. Their publication in the *New England Journal of Medicine*[12] sparked controversies regarding this D/HS. In April 2001, the Office of Inspector General from the Department of Health and Human Services voiced criticism about the FDA's inefficacy to regulate D/HS on the market; their agents published a report[13] decrying the inexpediency of the FDA's MedWatch Program concerning D/HS—a program allowing both practitioners and patients to report 'adverse effects' of medications. On 5 September 2001, the controversy regarding D/HS regulation by the so-called Snake Oil Protection Act (DSHEA)[14] translated to public health policy concerns. In response, the non-profit patient advocacy organisation, Public Citizens' Health Research Group, initiated a petition calling for the FDA to ban D/HS containing ephedrine alkaloids.[15] In February 2003, the polemic dramatically hit the news when the Baltimore Orioles player, Steve Blecher, died during a baseball game. The cause of his death was partly attributed by the medical examiner to the use of Ephedra.[16]

The NCCAM's Advisory Council archives indicate that on 17 March 2003, at the request of the Department of Health and Human Services, two bodies of the NIH—NCCAM and ODS—had already begun tackling the issue by funding a meta-analysis of available data at the time. During this meeting, NCCAM and ODS members as well as the attending audience, pondered over the necessity of conducting more research including 'case-control studies' and 'clinical trials'. Implicitly reiterating the NCCAM's public mission to inform patients and practitioners, the director stated:

> The real question [about Ephedra] is whether the products people are taking are dangerous or not…. [The] bar to prove scientifically that something is unsafe is very high.[17]

On 26 March 2003, an article in the *Journal of the American Medical Association (JAMA)* was then asking federal institutions for further regulation of D/HS in the wake of the scandal aroused by Ephedra.[18] Less than a month later (18 April), one of the Public Citizen founders, medical doctor, researcher, and patient advocate, Sydney Wolfe,[19] renewed in the journal *Science* the call for banning the release of D/HS containing ephedrine alkaloids on the market. At the same time, he criticised the juridical gap left by the FDA regarding D/HS.

It was not until 2004 that the FDA definitively prohibited the sale of D/HS containing ephedrine-like alkaloids.[20] The same year, the FDA Center for Drug Evaluation and Research published non-binding recommendations[21] for manufacturers regarding a new drug category, those derived from botanicals, in order to ensure quality and safety processes. Nonetheless, the legal status of D/HS and the status of recommendations of those latter regulations still give a panoply of possibilities to D/HS manufacturers: either following the pre-market legal route for new drug approvals or, as they all do, stepping onto the less constraining framework of D/HS.

Filling the Void of the DSHEA and Addressing Controversies: Regulatory Versus Research Science

Keeping in mind the aforementioned facts, two logics are actually pitching against each other at the federal level. This controversy around Ephedra is well known by NIH agents, researchers, and clinicians working on D/HS. They often mention it when they explain the articulations between the drug regulatory institution and the work in medical research at NIH. Two scientific logics will then be at stake here, namely: the FDA rationale—an administrative and legal logic, the one from the denominated 'regulatory science', spearhead of the FDA (for more details about 'regulatory science', see Jasanoff 1990)[22] and the other defended by NIH agents as 'research science'—informing both professionals and patients about the efficacy, use, and safety of CAM modalities and their mission of promoting and conducting research on CAM.

Agents involved in a 'research science' paradigm criticise the role of the FDA as overly permissive where D/HS are concerned:

So Ephedra, you can still find that in Chinese pharmacies because Ephedra is still a drug that's used in TCM [Traditional Chinese Medicine] practice, but the FDA turns a blind eye to that stuff. (A researcher in biochemistry specialised in botanicals who worked with NIH, February 2017)

They just use regulatory discretion. You won't find that written down anywhere, but you can walk into a Chinese pharmacy, everywhere, and find products that we would consider toxic and that we would not like to see as an OTC [over-the-counter] product. (A researcher in pharmacognosy who previously worked for the FDA, January 2017)

The Ephedra scandal spurred NCCAM to position itself in relation to the drug regulatory institution, disarmed in the face of the DSHEA not allowing it to regulate D/HS in a stricter way.[23] The NCCAM seized upon those questions of D/HS regulation evading the FDA's control, namely the efficacy and safety of D/HS as public health concerns, applying the federal model of drug approvals in effect, although they were supposedly not required to do so:

Apart from the legalities, sellers of dietary supplements have no obligation to provide data on effectiveness and little obligation to pursue safety issues (although toxicities of which they become aware must be reported). [NCCAM Director said] that all NCCAM's studies on natural products have met FDA standards for Investigational New Drug (IND) applications and that NCCAM uniformly encourages this. [FDA member] said that NIH studies are not required to have INDs.[24]

In the aftermath of its creation in 1994, NCCAM aimed at 'speed[ing] the discovery, development, and validation of potent treatments that may be added to the complementary wheel of alternatives currently available to patients and practitioners' and at giving a strong scientific basis to the 'foundation for the development of a whole new system of medicine'.[25] To those founding promises is articulated the necessity of evaluating D/HS according to the regime of proof applicable to conventional drugs.

Carving out its place and crafting its role in the legitimisation of CAM, by articulating research policies and public health policies, has been a major concern for the institution dedicated to researching CAM—shaping D/HS as a CAM category which, even a posteriori, has to be accountable or amenable to conventional pharmaceutical drug models, adhering to dominant standards of proof-making on their efficacy and establishing evidence of their safety.

In Conclusion: Reading Institutional Processes Through the Ephedra Case

Public health issues were at the core of the original mandate of CAM research in the early 1990s: studying CAM modalities as they relate to the management of chronic health conditions (allergies, cancer, pain, depression, hypertension, etc.).[26] The federal institution dedicated to medical research on CAM justifies its missions through the construction of public health concerns, particularly the general public appeal of the use of a specific D/HS, such as Ephedra; but in the wake of controversies, NCCAM negotiated collaborations within NIH (with ODS) and within the Department of Health and Human Services (with the FDA) to fill the legal void regarding D/HS. Entering a 'struggle for territory' (Meimon 2011) or an interactive institutional 'bricolage' (Castel and Friedberg 2010), NCCAM had to transact and demarcate its own territory of competence and action: controlling D/HS through 'research science' rather than 'regulatory science'.

Recent Evolutions in Research Policies: Contributions from the PC-SPES Investigations

In the wake of another controversy regarding research and what a journalist called the 'gaps in regulation' of D/HS,[27] it was within the realm of cancer research that major reconfigurations of research conditions emerged. Facing new challenges, federal institutions thus designed new programs, supposedly to give a framework to D/HS. Orientating research on common bases was apparently at stake. A precise characterisation of D/HS compounds, an overhaul of experimental protocols to implement, and the peculiar place granted to D/HS as CAM have been the major issues discussed in research policies. In this section, we will illustrate these new trends through the specific case of PC-SPES, a dietary supplement oriented towards Americans with hormone-refractory prostate cancers.

The PC-SPES Case: A Turning Point of NCCAM Research Policies Concerning D/HS 'Integrity'

As an NIH researcher interviewed in July 2016 explained, 'PC stands for Prostate Cancer and SPES is Latin for hope'. With this suggestive name, this product became popular in the mid-1990s among individuals who were living with particular hormone-sensitive prostate cancers and could not find satisfying conventional therapeutic treatments. PC-SPES was a blend of eight herbs imported from Asia and manufactured by a Californian company, BotanicLab. According to the NCI, each herb has been reported by the manufacturer to have anti-inflammatory, antioxidant, or anticarcinogenic properties. Regulated as a D/HS by the FDA, the packaging then indicated that PC-SPES was designed to improve 'prostate health'. According to an NCCAM Press Release, surveys revealing that the majority of patients undergoing treatment for cancer used CAM modalities, along with the popularity of PC-SPES, urged NCCAM to fund research projects on PC-SPES in the early 2000s.[28]

In February 2001, the NCCAM Advisory Council indicated that the Johns Hopkins University's CAM Cancer Centre, which was funded by NIH, was recruiting 100 men affected by prostate cancer for a 'double-blind RCT' comparing PC-SPES to Estradiol. Those studies on cancer CAM were still a research priority for NCCAM at the time, and in 2002, their budget validation before Congress confirmed the ongoing importance of cancer research, including research on PC-SPES.[29] NCCAM was about to be confronted with a new dilemma. This new research funding was strongly supported by previous research funded in part by NCI demonstrating the anticarcinogenic potential of PC-SPES for certain types of prostate cancer.[30] Nonetheless, in 2002, a research team from the State of California Department of Health, commissioned to analyse its composition, determined that PC-SPES contained not only plant extracts but was contaminated or adulterated with several conventional drugs such as Warfarin, Indometacin, Alprazolam, and also Diethylstilbestrol.

Subsequently, NCCAM initiated a change in research efforts in this field by addressing issues related to D/HS integrity, specifically a characterisation and standardisation to fit within research settings. The issue raised by PC-SPES adulteration led NCCAM to grasp D/HS quality issues: its authenticity and its interactions with conventional drugs. In fact, in January 2004, the NCCAM Advisory Council's observation had drastically shifted. Noticing the lack of standardised and well-characterised D/HS in clinical trials, NCCAM recalibrated its research efforts towards pre-clinical and early-phase clinical studies, setting aside RCTs. In the words of its Advisory Council (2004), this change revolved around the idea of producing sufficient standardisation of D/HS in order to ultimately design better clinical trials. The PC-SPES issues were the starting point of this shift.[31] Soon thereafter, NCCAM would put an end to all research on PC-SPES in order to halt what most agents called either a 'fiasco', a 'controversy', or a 'scandal', despite the supposed therapeutic promises of this D/HS.[32] Those adulterations of D/HS by conventional drugs became a focal point even though they were not newcomers on the D/HS marketplace (Foster 2011).[33]

In interviews, several federal and non-federal agents with chemistry, pharmacognosy, and biology research backgrounds argued that the addition of pharmaceutical compounds into the blend could have occurred at different moments in the production line in order to either enhance the therapeutic potential of PC-SPES or to alleviate undesirable side effects of the blend such as thrombosis. PC-SPES composition was highly inconsistent and variable from one batch to another. Those reasons led institutions and agents to negotiate research efforts on D/HS.

Restructuring Institutional Research Efforts on D/HS at NIH: Aims of a New Balanced Research Portfolio

These debates mobilised the scientific communities, leading NCCAM to position itself regarding new research policy on D/HS, around different points. The first one deals with the characterisation and regulation of the biological profile of the research object. PC-SPES led agents to elaborate solutions in pharmacognosy related to D/HS 'integrity' within research settings—that is, producing or getting access to D/HS that are not contaminated and that are sufficiently stable in their composition from one batch to another. It is illustrated by the new policies that NCCAM presented before Congress in 2003. Prior to new clinical studies, an unadulterated version of PC-SPES had to be 'fully characterised and standardised'.[34]

The second point relates to the place assigned to CAM modalities within the American health system. Research efforts on D/HS headed then towards the study of their interactions with the therapeutic orthodoxy, negotiating the manner by which to consider multimodal recourses to CAM as 'complementary' rather than 'alternative'. Those research efforts focused on D/HS in interaction with conventional drugs, effectively prioritising the therapeutic effects of conventional drugs and considering D/HS as products supposed to support the former:

> Drugs and herbal products or other natural supplements … could have a broad array of interactions with conventional drugs. Herbals can enhance drug activity and evoke greater drug toxicity, or they can speed the metabolism of drugs and diminish their therapeutic benefits.[35]

The third point focuses on protocols of D/HS evaluation. The aftermath of PC-SPES centred on the manner of producing scientific knowledge regarding D/HS. It was about embracing 'all levels of complexity' related to D/HS,[36] which, in the words of NCCAM, implied the necessity of re-routing the chain of research from RCTs to more basic science research. Shifting from clinical settings to lab investigations on D/HS alone, thus setting aside human subjects and ethical concerns, knowledge production on these products at NCCAM started focusing on determining their biological mechanisms of action. To do so, this NIH centre decided to promote the use of cutting-edge approaches such as DNA microarray and proteomics to establish D/HS profiles at the molecular, cellular, and biochemical levels. To resume clinical trials in the future, basic research including mechanistic studies on D/HS as complementary to conventional drugs had to be done.[37]

In Conclusion: What PC-SPES Has Provided to Institutional Research Policies

Through those reconfigurations of research policies, NCCAM sought its legitimate place among other NIH institutes. NCCAM first embraced the federal dominant model of proof-making, RCTs, described by Marks (1997) as a 'negotiated order'. The decision of carrying out the gold standard in medicine to assess the efficacy and safety of CAM modalities—randomised clinical trials—will be 'as much a scientific as it is an economic and political one' (Petryna 2009). But facing new research challenges, such as complex and non-standardised controversial research objects, this NIH centre played a major role in the field of medical research on CAM by reinventing its research policies while still aligning them with high evidence-based standards. It allowed this centre to defend and re-assert its legitimate place at NIH and more generally in the arena of medical research. NCCAM became a major institution in the field of medical research on CAM, stimulating and orienting research efforts, funding projects, and instituting D/HS as CAM and as complementary, rather than alternative, to conventional care.

Crafting New Research Standards for the Evaluation of D/HS

Those evolutions in research policies on D/HS led to new research protocols and new research standards, allowing researchers to better 'characterise' those products, to better include them within new protocols in the search for scientific evidence, and to administer their 'integration' within complementary strategies of care, notably where cancer is concerned.

Characterising and Proving: The Issues of Integrity, Standardisation, and Reproducibility

Both federal and non-federal researchers on D/HS indicate that, regarding a lot of previous studies, protocols lacked scientific rigour for diverse reasons. The nature of these products (those on the market, with an unclear and highly variable composition), the large panel of different analytical methods used both by researchers and manufacturers, and the lack of recording and assessing of different steps within the experimental protocol (batch-to-batch consistency, temperature, storing conditions, reaction time, etc.) are reasons researchers give for the need for better articulations between research programs. The necessity of research reproducibility represented an appeal to the production of a 'common language for talking about CAM'[38]: the making of shared, recognised, and validated practices by NIH cutting-edge research settings. The stakes of D/HS 'integrity', 'authenticity', and also 'quality' will translate through the elaboration of standard methods and standardised compounds. Their underlying mission will consist of reinventing the chain of D/HS supply for research, by an instituted federal standardisation of studied compounds, thus making D/HS as a CAM 'amenable' to scientific research.[39]

In the early 2000s, several initiatives emerged at NIH to coordinate research on D/HS considering the risks of D/HS adulterations. In 2002, ODS created the Dietary Supplement Analytical Methods and Reference Materials (AMRM) Program on Congress' demand to address and solve the problematic aforementioned issues regarding D/HS. Under the auspices of this program, this NIH Office collaborated with the NIST to elaborate stable D/HS compounds for research, including reference material data banks determining their concentration for certain plants within the D/HS under study, echoing the galenic composition of conventional drugs. Notably, Ephedra was one of the first D/HS to follow this process of compliance and standardisation. Around 2006, in the interests of aligning research policies on D/HS with the 2004 FDA recommendations,[40] a working group was set up at NCCAM to ponder programmatic solutions. From this working group emerged the NCCAM's Product Integrity Policy, which requires any research to produce proof of non-adulteration and to indicate the precise composition of the studied D/HS. The history of the creation and articulation of those programs directly answers concerns raised by both Ephedra and PC-SPES, as a federal researcher in chemistry working on D/HS familiar with those programs told us (December 2016):

the original language said 'primarily for botanicals' because that seemed to be the issue. But it's the reason of those programs, it's to create standard methods of analysis and give researchers, manufacturers and regulators the tools giving you the right answer and techniques.

Characterising and standardising D/HS were the necessary steps for the construction of proof and for future clinical trials. In 2004, in an article published in the *JAMA*, the former director of NCCAM, Stephen Strauss, described the scientific research priorities of his institution as based upon the necessity of 'randomized, placebo-controlled clinical trials for assessing the efficacy of CAM treatments whenever feasible and ethically justifiable'.[41,42] Following these paradigms of evidence-based medicine (EBM), this policy is confronted by the fact that CAM does not necessarily fit within RCT settings. In an article published in 2015, the director of extramural research in charge of the NCCIH portfolio on D/HS takes stock of the research work from 2002 to 2012: regarding 17 research studies presented here, dealing with D/HS, proofs of efficacy are considered as weak or even not established.[43] Subsequent to those programmatic solutions at NIH and NIST, both NIH and non-NIH researchers consider that D/HS represents challenges for research inasmuch as they are recognised as highly complex botanical entities, derived from plants, calling for various approaches. Taking into consideration the complexity of D/HS, particularly when they are labelled as 'natural products' and mixtures or 'polyherb blends',[44] raises challenges for the identification of botanical mechanisms of action determining every polychemical element,[45] as federal researchers explain:

Hyperferin is the known active compound of St John's Wort but there are hundreds of compounds in St John's Wort that are probably working together, and you know if you look at nutrition generally. (A researcher in pharmacology working on D/HS and cancer, funded by NIH, November 2016)

Criticising the Conventional Models of Evaluation: Paths to Defend Specificities of CAM in Research Settings

Many researchers and clinicians working on CAM or integrative medicine and/or cancer are critical of the FDA's use of the pharmaceutical model of drug evaluation and development and the burdens this creates for D/HS research. In particular, critiques emerge from researchers working on D/HS associated with products used in Traditional Chinese Medicine (TCM). For example, a researcher in pharmacology specialising in pre-clinical cancer studies and focusing on a herbal blend from TCM describes the pharmacological model as incompatible with TCM paradigms:

> The current paradigm of mainstream pharmaceutical discovery uses a reductionist approach.... Therefore, a new paradigm for future medicine is a multipletarget and polychemical medicine instead of a onechemical medicine with a systembiology approach in mind.[46]

This polychemical approach of D/HS derived from TCM revolves around an intention of 'hybridation [hybridisation]' (Micollier 2011) between biomedical and TCM paradigms within the scope of cancer. It is then—as another researcher in pharmacology working on D/HS from TCM told us in December 2016—a question of developing a new medicine based on a regime of proof whereby 'West meets East' and 'East meets West', and it will consist of moving from a single-molecular model to a polychemical one, linked to D/HS as 'polyherb blends', within developmental avenues of new cancer therapies.

Other critiques around the current biomedical regime of proof were also frequently found in our research, usually made by agents with both medical practice backgrounds (such as family medicine, oncology, and integrative medicine) and research backgrounds (such as epidemiology and clinical research). These involve a critical reassessment of the proof hierarchy produced by EBM[47] as putting too much emphasis on RCTs in the face of both clinical knowledge and clinical experiences, whereas research on CAM has, since the 1990s, accounted for the appeal of therapeutic modalities to patients.[48] Usually echoing classic critiques of RCTs as inadequate in accounting for CAM's complexity (Hess 1999), they solicit a re-evaluation of EBM and its research protocols, understood as onerous, long, and difficult to set in place. Those critiques of EBM tend to invert the hierarchy of proof by focusing primarily on the various clinical practices of integrative medicine itself, usually defined by researchers and clinicians as 'collaborative' between the medical team and the patient, or 'patient-centred'. In fact, new studies in integrative medicine are thus focusing on effectiveness—an efficacy defined by clinicians and researchers in integrative medicine as centred on clinical experiences and patient outcomes. In 2007, a large network of (mostly academic) clinical centres in integrative medicine (some members of which were interviewed) organised the PRIMIER project: Patients Receiving Integrative Medicine Interventions Effectiveness Registry. In reaction to the marginalisation of clinical and patient experiences within the EBM hierarchy, this network of pioneer clinical institutions in integrative medicine is gathering data on different clinical practices through 'Patient-Reported Outcomes' which are 'basically a patient's feedback on their feelings or functions as they are dealing with chronic diseases or conditions [...] such as the importance of fatigue to cancer'.[49] One agent from a similar network, a director of one of the ten or so leading university clinical programs in integrative medicine in the USA, indicated that RCT and research mechanisms tending to reach a minimal bias threshold do not allow researchers and clinicians to evaluate multimodal approaches of integrative medicine, combining both conventional and CAM modalities (including D/HS), which would better account for patient-centred clinical data:

[talking about impediments in gaining funding for research on D/HS within the scope of integrative medicine] This doesn't get a chance to get funded, they said: 'you have too many CAM modalities!' (a clinician and researcher in integrative medicine, February 2017)

Depending on their professional specialisation and institutional affiliations, agents are thus re-negotiating plural modalities of research on D/HS considered as more capable of rigorously reflecting the complexity of both the use and the mechanisms of action of D/HS. They are contributing to the production of multiple definitions of CAM efficacy: a clinical evaluation that is usually multimodal and patient-centred, a polychemical and synergistic approach towards D/HS within the development of new treatments, a pluri-paradigmatic approach, and a mechanistic research approach by bioactive compounds on different modalities of D/HS action.

Integrating? The Place of Disease and Treatment in CAM Research

Nowadays, NCCIH justifies its public health mission (protecting patients and informing them about CAM use) towards D/HS by the necessity of ensuring the safety of the products. Research on Ephedra and PC-SPES among others will also lead institutions to position themselves regarding the place of D/HS vis-à-vis conventional treatments. In 2015, the director of extramural research and research policies on D/HS at NCCIH expressed that:

> NCCIH would consider research focused on disease treatment a low priority…. Surveys consistently show that for those people who take dietary supplements, their primary reason for doing so is not for disease management but for general health promotion.[50]

This risk-management policy oriented towards conventional treatments is also articulated with a less probabilistic discourse regarding conventional drug-D/HS interactions than research results on CAM efficacy, as our analysis of NCCIH institutional archives tends to show. St John's Wort (*bot. Hypericum perforatum*), one of the plants most commonly used as D/HS in the USA, is an emblematic example of it. When research on its efficacy for mental health conditions either failed or revealed inconsistencies or conflicts in research results, several studies published by NCI led to strict precautionary recommendations (contraindications). This D/HS is associated with modifications of the efficacy and absorption mechanisms of drugs prescribed for cancer (Irinotecan: antineoplastic medication to treat colon and rectal cancer) and HIV (Indinavir: prothease inhibitor).[51]

The uncertainties of research results on CAM efficacy have a different status to the more affirmative and clear-cut risks expressed for drug-CAM interactions. Those differential discourses are criticised by stakeholders that we interviewed and in documents we analysed as instituting CAM as hierarchically beneath conventional drugs and their 'real' efficacy. Some agents we interviewed are regretting the discourse of their colleagues not working on CAM, as a researcher in epidemiology and CAM reported to us (March 2016): '[According to them] "There is medicine that works and medicines that don't work"'. She then explained that, for them, there is no such thing as 'complementary' or 'alternative' when it 'works', implying that conventional medicine works per se by virtue of the proof of its efficacy, such as conventional drugs according to the standards of EBM. Some agents, usually medical doctors, working in integrative settings that we have interviewed (March 2017) criticise this difference of research result and the place it implies for CAM modalities within conventional care settings. They consider that benefits of conventional medicine and CAM therapies are 'both real', and they are 'both central to the optimal health of somebody' as a clinician and researcher in integrative medicine said. Critiques are formulated on how research results on D/HS are differentially used depending on the research scope (efficacy vs. drug-CAM interactions), as illustrated by another researcher and clinician in integrative medicine (July 2016):

> There are certainties spoken when it comes to any problem and then you can have 35 trials on that D/HS that 'may provide' [a therapeutic benefit] … And yet, people point to the negative ones.

The pejorative connotation of the term 'alternative' meets general consensus among all agents. The renunciation of treatment as a D/HS research priority then echoes challenges, controversies, and discussions raised by PC-SPES and Ephedra on the mission of research on CAM efficacy and safety in articulation with research standards in conventional drug development. This is following a well-known and long history of 'alternative' cancer treatments which have sometimes been discredited, such as Laetrile in the 1970s (Markle and Petersen 1980), the Gerson therapy since the 1930s (Hess 2002: 76–96), and the antineoplastons of

Stanislaw Burzinsky since the 1970s (Smith 1992).[52] These are still vivid in the memory of these agents. These agents thus define what they consider the 'zone of comfort' for CAM research: the management of symptoms rather than the treatment of a disease, and an approach considering CAM as adjuncts to conventional treatments. This is translated into a programmatic manner at NCCIH which henceforth focuses its research efforts on the non-pharmacological management of pain, investing opioid use and over-prescription as a major public health issue in the USA. Both federal and non-federal researchers and clinicians, for instance, allude to the regime of CAM integration to which research should answer, that being CAM as complementary to conventional treatments. It will then be about observing a position of compromise or concession towards conventional medicine within research:

[Questioning the complementary and/or alternative aspects of CAM as symptom management instead of treatment in research settings] You're not putting yourself in a confrontational position. (A researcher in pharmacology and D/HS, December 2016)

[Talking about cancer and D/HS] You can't use the word cancer 'out loud' in conjunction with the word DS because DS are not allowed to cure or treat or medicate a disease. (A researcher in biochemistry working on D/HS, November 2016)

Despite this dominant symptom-based approach, practical and discursive negotiations about the research object at stake among some researchers working on D/HS seem to play around it by implicitly designating a specific disease by its related symptoms, and at the same time by acknowledging that the frontier between disease treatment and symptom management is not strictly sharp:

[about research on D/HS] I cannot look at disease outcomes, I can look at symptom-management. If I'm gonna look at a disease outcome, I have to file this as an investigational new drug, even if it's not a drug. I mean, we are actually investigating a herbal formula that has [herb A], [herb B], that may help manage [cause of the disease], and I'd like to do it for [this disease] but I can't because they would consider that a drug, because [this disease] is a disease, but for pre-[this disease] or symptoms of [this disease], and not mentioning the actual disease, I can … You know you're always dancing this dance. (A clinician and researcher in integrative medicine working on D/HS, February 2017)[53]

In Conclusion: Contrasting Institutional Research and Interactive Positioning of Agents

Those reconfigurations at different levels could then explain the making of obstacles to research done by an office of NCI devoted to the study of cancer CAM. The pioneer OCCAM-NCI program since 1998, the Best Case Series (BCS), has focused on clinical cases of alternative cancer treatments outside complementarity with conventional therapeutics. Those BCS are based upon data gathered in clinical settings by clinicians or researchers and provided by them to this office. They could be considered as research initiators, prior to RCT, within the EBM hierarchy. Clinicians or researchers can send to OCCAM-NCI a case report that will be examined by OCCAM members.[54] They must prove that patients have been treated with one or more CAM modalities in the absence of conventional treatment, that those patients are affected by cancer, and that a decrease in the tumour size can be observed on radiography.[55] But since the creation of OCCAM at NCI, no BCS has led to further investigation. Facing a mixed social space of CAM research tending to define CAM aside from nosology and as adjuncts validated by EBM standards and integrated within conventional care settings, impediments to further the BCS towards RCT will then answer to political and social reconfigurations of CAM research rather than scientific and functional reasons.

While NCCAM/NCCIH stimulates research on D/HS aligned with high scientific evidence-based standards, by instituting a common language to research CAM complexities, other agents in this space negotiate the place assigned to CAM modalities alongside the research protocols to prove their efficacy. Different and sometimes competing and pluri-paradigmatic approaches articulate with the federal standardisation of what is a CAM modality amenable to scientific research. They question the EBM and pharmaceutical standards of proof by creating and implementing research protocols amenable to a more rigorous understanding of CAM modalities within the American health system. Institutions play an important role in this balance of negotiations but ultimately agents take distance from them through critiques, compromises, and innovations in the definition of the place assigned to CAM.

Discussion

Understanding the Transactional Shifts in the Making of Proof Around CAM: A Plurality of Agents and Networks

Our ongoing analysis in this chapter could be understood as socio-historically evolving and at the intersection of different histories: the history of federal institutions, the history of CAM, the history of integrative medicine, the history of medical and CAM research, the history of pharmacology and chemistry, the history of cancer, and the history of social movements in health, to name a few. Consideration of both Ephedra and PC-SPES as peculiar and structuring examples of CAM research reconfigurations sheds light on the fact that this ongoing construction of legitimisations towards CAM relies on a plurality of individual and institutional agents (and a plurality of disciplines), such as federal institutions (from Congress to NIH), laboratories, universities and academic clinical centres, private clinics, patient associations, D/HS manufacturers, academic societies, and national and international consortia.

The study of those institutional constructions of legitimisations towards CAM in the USA allows us to identify at least two processes: the competition between different paradigms for the evaluation of CAM and the ever-changing distribution of both individual and institutional agents on different networks of interaction involved in these constructions, fostering transactions, alliances, competition, disregard, and distinctions among them. They all compete at different levels on the regime of proof that should be assigned to the evaluation of CAM efficacy and safety.

They reveal sophisticated negotiations on research protocols, on the definition of the research object and on the translationality of CAM research, differentially distributed among agents.

Research policies on CAM from NIH institutions—illustrated by the focus on D/HS—are caught up in, and by, different institutional games and are answering to diverse societal stakes regarding health. And ultimately, interactions between plural agents and the constitution of various social sub-spaces within CAM research are embodied by complex arrangements and re-adjustments of CAM evaluation, translating into both practical and discursive reconfigurations revealing this co-construction of the place assigned to CAM within the American health system. Those manifold and entangled interactions occur at different levels, strategically and tactically, within the particularities of the medical arena and the larger scientific field.

Those analytical elements invite us to take into consideration the constitution of various networks of interactions and knowledge production participating in legitimisations towards CAM within this mixed social space, also caught in an ongoing move towards the globalisation of interactions, dissemination and conduct of research as evidenced by the recent proliferation of international congresses on CAM and integrative medicine as well as international consortia since the early 2000s.

Acknowledgements This research was funded by the French National Cancer Institute (INCa) from January 2015 to January 2018.

Notes

1. We chose the term 'dietary and herbal supplements' from NCCIH to illustrate both the legal wording and use of most D/HS (sold as dietary supplements) and the focus on botanical-based dietary supplements in the following examples, thus questioning different distinctions between conventional and lab-synthesised drugs and plant-derived dietary supplements.

2. Congressional findings related to Dietary Supplements Health and Education Act of 1994, Pub. L. No. 103–417, § 2, 15 (A), 108 *Stat.* 4325; 4326, October 25 1994 (s).

3. For the most recent one, see: Clarke et al. 2015 (s).
4. As defined by the NCCIH: 'a product that is intended to supplement the diet, contains one or more dietary ingredients (including vitamins, minerals, herbs, or other botanicals), a plant or part of a plant used for its flavor, scent, or potential therapeutic properties (includes flowers, leaves, bark, fruit, seeds, stems, and roots, amino acids, and certain other substances) or their constituents, is intended to be taken by mouth, in forms such as tablet, capsule, powder, softgel, gelcap, or liquid, and is labeled as being a dietary supplement' (https://nccih.nih.gov/health/supplements). Federal institutions such as NCCIH and NCI mention different CAM categories related to botanicals: 'natural products', 'complex natural products', 'dietary supplements', 'nutritional therapeutics', 'botanicals', 'herbs', 'special diets'.
5. An inductive socio-anthropological 'networked ethnography' (Atlani-Duault 2009; Olivier de Sardan 2008), or what we might call 'starfish ethnography', departing from the institutions and expanding back and forth from the investigation to their networks of interactions with other agents involved in this mixed social space of medical research on CAM and cancer CAM.
6. We compiled sources from the institutions we studied ('institutional corpus'), archives from newspapers, scientific journals, legal texts, online sources, and so on. *See* the 'Sources' section in bibliography.
7. We conducted about 60 formal and informal ethnographic interviews, many informal discussions, and observations between November 2014 and June 2017.
8. See Bothwell and Podolsky 2016; Meldrum 2000.
9. Manufacturers only bear the responsibility of their safety before their release on the market, they do not need to report it to the FDA.
10. US Department of Health & Human Services Food and Drug Administration, Center for Drug Evaluation and Research (June 2004), 'Botanical Drug Products' (s).
11. For a long-term history of Ephedra, see: Lee 2011.
12. Haller and Benowitz 2000 (s).
13. US Department of Health and Human Services, Office of Inspector General 2001 (s).
14. *New York Times* 1993 (s).
15. Public Citizen 2001 (s).
16. Bodley 2003 (s); Connolly 2008 (s).

17. NCCIH, 'Minutes', March 2003 (s).
18. Fontanarosa et al. 2003 (s).
19. Wolfe 2003 (s).
20. FDA, 6 February 2004 (s).
21. FDA, June 2004 (s).
22. Regulatory science is defined by the FDA as 'the science of developing new tools, standards and approaches to assess the safety, efficacy, quality, and performance of FDA-regulated products' See: FDA, October 2010. (s).
23. NCCAM, 'Minutes', November 2000 (s).
24. NCCAM, 'Minutes', October 2014 (s).
25. Berman and Larson 1995, x (s).
26. Ibid., ix. (s).
27. Burton 2002 (s).
28. NCCAM, 'Press Release', 5 October 2000 (s).
29. NCCAM, 'Director Testimony', November 2001 and 'Congressional Justification', 2002 (s).
30. Dipaola et al. 1998 (s).
31. NCCIH, 'Minutes', 2004 (s).
32. Burton 2000 (s).
33. Chan et al. 1993 (s); Cumberford 2012 (s).
34. NCCAM, 'Congressional Justification', 2003 (s).
35. NCCAM, 'Congressional Justification', 2004 (s).
36. NCCAM, 'Strategic Plan', 2004 (s).
37. NCCAM, 'Strategic Plan', 2004 (s).
38. Interview with a researcher working on D/HS, February 2017.
39. This term was employed by different researchers when the question of research protocols on CAM was raised.
40. FDA, June 2004 (s).
41. Miller et al. 2004 (s).
42. This first wave of CAM research initiated at NCCAM echoes the decision of extending RCT to every research domain in medicine. It also originates in the 1970s from a FDA recommendation to use such a regime of proof in new drug research and development (Bothwell and Podolsky 2016). Oncology has been the major field of expansion for RCTs, *see*: Bourret and Le Moigne 2014; Cambrosio and Keating 2008; and Cambrosio et al. 2014.
43. Hopp 2015 (s).

44. This term was mentioned during a conference on integrative medicine held at a renowned centre for integrative medicine in the USA, in March 2017.
45. Seifried et al. 2004 (s).
46. Cheng 2011 (s).
47. See, for example, the scholarly work of the former director of the Office of Alternative Medicine (previous name of NCCAM until 1998) who works on a reorganisation of proof production when CAM is concerned: Jonas 2005 (s).
48. Eisenberg et al. 1993 (s).
49. From a booklet given to us by a researcher in integrative medicine: Abrams et al. (2015) 'PRIMIER, A National Integrative Medicine Database', The Bravewell Collaborative (s).
50. Hopp 2015 (s); Barnes et al. 2008 (s).
51. Wang and Arnold 2002 (s); Ron et al. 2002 (s); Mansky and Strauss 2002 (s).
52. In 2009, the FDA released a warning letter with ethical concerns about 'antineoplaston' and the Burzinsky Research Institute investigating and providing this alternative therapy: FDA (5 October 2009), 'Warning Letter, "Burzynski Research Institute/IRB"', ref: 10-HFD-45-09-0 (s). This controversy is also present within the NCCAM unprocessed archives at the Office of NIH History (Cheung Series, Box 8, folder 3; Jonas Series, Box 24, folder 7; OAM series, Box 14, folder 8 & box 25, folder 8; etc.) (s).
53. We anonymised the disease to protect agents we met as they could be easily identified if we had mentioned the specific disease and herbs used in their research study.
54. Zia and White 2009 (s).
55. For an example, see: Banerji et al. 2008 (s).

References

Atlani-Duault, L. (2009). *Au Bonheur des autres: anthropologie de l'aide humanitaire*. Paris: Armand Colin.
Baszanger, I. (1986). Les maladies chroniques et leur ordre négocié. *Revue Française de Sociologie, 27*(1), 3–27.

Bothwell, L. E., & Podolsky, S. H. (2016). The history of clinical trials: The emergence of the randomized, controlled trial. *New England Journal of Medicine, 375*, 501–504.

Bourret, P., & Le Moigne, P. (2014). Essais cliniques, production de la preuve et mutation de la biomédecine. *Sciences sociales et santé, 3*(32), 5–11.

Cambrosio, A., & Keating, P. (2008). Cancer clinical trials: The emergence and development of a new style of practice. In D. Cantor (Ed.), *Cancer in the twentieth century* (pp. 197–223). Baltimore: Johns Hopkins University Press.

Cambrosio, A., Keating, P., & Nelson, N. (2014). Régimes thérapeutiques et dispositifs de preuves en oncologie: l'organisation des essais cliniques, des groupes coopérateurs aux consortiums de recherche. *Sciences sociales et santé, 3*(32), 13–42.

Castel, P., & Friedberg, E. (2010). Institutional change as an interactive process: The case of the modernization of the French Cancer Centers. *Organization Science, 21*(2), 311–330.

Chen, N. (2009). *Food, medicine, and the quest for good health.* New York: Columbia University Press.

Dubet, F. (2002). *Le déclin de l'institution.* Paris: Le Seuil.

Foster, S. (2011). A brief history of adulteration of herbs, spices, and botanical drugs. *HerbalGram, 92*, 42–57.

Fuselier, B., & Marquis, N. (2009). Transaction sociale et négociation: deux notions à articuler. *Négociations, 2*(12), 23–33.

Hess, D. J. (1999). *Evaluating alternative cancer therapies: A guide to the science and politics of an emerging medical field.* New Brunswick: Rutgers University Press.

Hess, D. J. (2002). The raw and the organic: Politics of therapeutic cancer diets in the United States. *The Annals of the American Academy of Political and Social Science, 583*(1), 76–96.

Jasanoff, S. (1990). *The fifth branch: Science advisers as policymakers.* Cambridge, MA and London: Harvard University Press.

Jütte, R. (2001). Alternative medicine and medico-historical semantics. In R. Jütte, M. Eklöf, & M. C. Nelson (Eds.), *Historical aspects of unconventional medicine – Approaches, concepts, case studies* (pp. 11–26). Sheffield: European Association for the History of Medicine and Health Publications.

Lee, M. R. (2011). The history of ephedra (Ma-Huang). *Journal of the Royal College of Physicians of Edinburgh, 41*(1), 78–84.

Markle, G. E., & Petersen, J. C. (1980). *Politics, science, and cancer: The laetrile phenomenon.* Boulder, CO: Westview Press.

Marks, H. (1997). *The progress of experiment: Science and therapeutic reform in the United States (1900–1990)*. Cambridge: Cambridge University Press.

Meimon, J. (2011). Sur le fil. La naissance d'une institution. In M. Offerlé & J. Lagroye (Eds.), *Sociologie de l'institution* (pp. 105–129). Paris: Belin.

Meldrum, M. L. (2000). A brief history of the randomized controlled trial. From oranges and lemons to the gold standard. *Hematology/Oncology Clinics of North America, 14*(4), 745–760.

Micollier, E. (2011). Un savoir thérapeutique hybride et mobile. Éclairage sur la recherche médicale en médecine chinoise en Chine aujourd'hui. *Revue d'anthropologie des connaissances, 1*(5), 41–70.

Offerlé, M., & Lagroye, J. (Eds.). (2011). *Sociologie de l'institution*. Paris: Belin.

Olivier de Sardan, J. P. (2008). *La rigueur du qualitatif: les contraintes empiriques de l'interprétation socio-anthropologique*. Lauvain-la-Neuve: Academia-Bruylant.

Petryna, A. (2009). *When experiments travel: Clinical trials and the global search for human subjects*. Princeton: Princeton University Press.

Smith, M. E. (1992). The Burzynski controversy in the United States and in Canada: A comparative case study in the sociology of alternative medicine. *The Canadian Journal of Sociology/Cahiers Canadiens De Sociologie, 17*(2), 133–160.

Strauss, A. (1978). *Negotiations: Varieties, contexts, processes, and social order*. San Francisco: Jossey-Bass.

Sources

Institutional Archives

NCCAM unprocessed archives at the Office of NIH History and National Library of Medicine

Institutional Corpus

NCCIH-NCCAM:
Congressional Justifications
Minutes of the National Advisory Council for Complementary and Integrative Health Press Releases
Strategic Plans

Other Sources

Abrams, D. et al. (2015). *PRIMIER: A National Integrative Medicine Database.* The Bravewell Collaborative.

Banerji, P., et al. (2008). Cancer patients treated with the Banerji protocols utilising homoeopathic medicine: A best case series program of the National Cancer Institute USA. *Oncology Reports, 20*(1), 69–74.

Barnes, P. M., Blume, B., & Nahin, R. (2008). CDC national health statistics report #12. In *Complementary and alternative medicine use among adults and children: United States, 2007.* Atlanta: Centers for Disease Control.

Berman, B. M., & Larson, D. B. (1995). *Alternative medicine: Expanding medical horizon: A report to the National Institutes of Health on alternative medical systems and Practices in the United States* (pp. 30–34). Washington, DC: US GPO.

Bodley, H. (2003). Medical examiner: Ephedra a factor in Blecher death. *USA Today.*

Burton, T. M. (2000). In trials, potion of herbs slows prostate cancer. *Wall Street Journal,* B1.

Burton, T. M. (2002). Recall of herbal supplement highlights gaps in regulation. *Wall Street Journal.*

Chan, T. Y., Chan, J. C., Tomlinson, B., & Critchley, J. A. (1993). Chinese herbal medicines revisited: A Hong Kong perspective. *Lancet, 342*(8886–8887), 1532–1534.

Cheng, Y. C. (2011). Why and how to globalize traditional Chinese medicine. *Journal of Traditional and Complementary Medicine, 1*(1), 1–4.

Clarke, T. C., Black, L. I., Stussman, B. J., Barnes, P. M., & Nahin, R. L. (2015). Trends in the use of complementary health approaches among adults: United States, 2002–2012. *National Health Statistics Reports, 79*, 1.

Congressional findings related to dietary supplements health and education act of 1994, Pub. L. No. 103–417, § 2, 15 (A), 108 *Stat.* 4325; 4326, Oct. 25, 1994.

Connolly, D. (2008). Steve Blecher's Death Five Years Later. *Baltimore Sun.*

Cumberford, G. (2012). EMI vs EMA: 'Economically motivated integrity' vs. economically motivated adulteration in the natural products supply chain. *HerbalGram, 94*, 40–41.

DiPaola, R. S., Zhang, H., Lambert, G. M., et al. (1998). Clinical and biological activity of an estrogenic herbal combination (PC- SPES) in prostate cancer. *New England Journal of Medicine, 339*, 785–791.

DSHEA, 21 U.S.C. § 321 (ff) (I) (A)–(F), 1994.

Eisenberg, D. M., Kessler, R. C., Foster, C., Norlock, F. E., Calkins, D. R., & Del-Banco, T. L. (1993). Unconventional medicine in the United States: Prevalence, costs, and patterns of use. *New England Journal of Medicine, 328*(4), 246–252.

FDA. (2004). FDA issues regulation prohibiting sale of dietary supplements containing ephedrine alkaloids and reiterates its advice that consumers stop using these products. *FDA Press Release.*

FDA. (2009). Warning Letter, Burzynski Research Institute/IRB. ref: 10-HFD-45-09-0.

FDA. (2010). *Advancing regulatory science for public health.* Washington, DC: U.S. GPO.

FDA, Center for Drug Evaluation and Research. (2004). *Guidance for industry: Botanical drug products.* Washington, DC: U.S. GPO.

Fontanarosa, P. B., Rennie, D., & DeAngelis, C. D. (2003). The need for regulation of dietary supplements – Lessons from ephedra. *JAMA, 289*(12), 1568–1570.

Haller, C. A., & Benowitz, N. L. (2000). Adverse cardiovascular and central nervous system events associated with dietary supplements containing ephedra alkaloids. *New England Journal of Medicine, 343*(25), 1833–1838.

Hopp, C. (2015). Past and future research at national centre for complementary and integrative health (NCCIH) with respect to botanicals. *HerbalGram, 107*, 44–51.

Jonas, W. (2005). Building an evidence house: Challenges and solutions to research in complementary and alternative medicine. *Forsch Komplementärmed Klass Naturheilkd, 12*(3), 159–167.

Mansky, P. J., & Straus, S. E. (2002). St John's wort: More implications for cancer patients. *Journal of the National Cancer Institute, 94*(16), 1187–1188.

Miller, F. G., Emanuel, E. J., Rosenstein, D. L., & Straus, S. E. (2004). Ethical issues concerning research in complementary and alternative medicine. *JAMA, 291*(5), 599–604.

New York Times. (1993). The 1993 Snake Oil Protection Act. *New York Times*, October 5.

Public Citizens' Health Research Group. (2001). Petition requesting a ban of Ephedra.

Ron, H. J., Verweij, M. J., de Bruijn, P., Loos, W. J., & Sparreboom, A. (2002). Effects of St. John's wort on irinotecan metabolism. *Journal of the National Cancer Institute, 94*(16), 1247–1249.

Seifried, H. E., Sorkin, B. C., & Costello, R. B. (2004). Free radicals: The pros and cons if antioxidants – Summary report of the National Institutes of Health symposium. *The Journal of Nutrition, 134*(11), 3143–3163.

U.S. Department of Health and Human Services, Food and Drug Administration Center for Drug Evaluation and Research. (2004). *Guidance for industry: Botanical drug products*. Washington DC: U.S. GPO.

U.S. Department of Health and Human Services, Office of Inspector General. (2001). *Adverse event reporting for dietary supplements: An inadequate safety valve*. Washington, DC: U.S. GPO.

Wang, L., & Arnold, K. (2002). Press release herbal dietary supplement alters metabolism of chemotherapy drug. *Journal of the National Cancer Institute, 94*(16), 1183.

Wolfe, S. (2003). Ephedra – Scientific evidence versus money/politics. *Science, 300*(5618), 437.

Zia, F., & White, J. (2009). Letter to the Editor. *Integrative Cancer Therapies, 8*(2), 113–114.

Index[1]

---

[1] Note: Page numbers followed by 'n' refer to notes.

© The Author(s) 2018   **327**
C. Brosnan et al. (eds.), *Complementary and Alternative Medicine*, Health,
Technology and Society, https://doi.org/10.1007/978-3-319-73939-7